# Drugs and Pregnancy

## Series in Maternal-Fetal Medicine

### About the Series

Published in association with the *Journal of Maternal Fetal and Neonatal Medicine*, the series in *Maternal Fetal Medicine* keeps readers up to date with the latest clinical therapies to improve the health of pregnant patients and ensure a successful birth. Each volume in the series is prepared separately and typically focuses on a topical theme. Volumes are published on an occasional basis, depending on the emergence of new developments.

For more information about this series please visit: www.crcpress.com/Series-in-Maternal-Fetal-Medicine/book-series/CRCSERMATFET

# Drugs and Pregnancy
## A Handbook

### Second Edition

"Bert" (Bertis Britt) Little, MA, PhD,
FAAAS, FRAI, FRSM, FRSPH
Professor of Public Health
School of Public Health and Information Science
Professor of Anthropology (Adj.)
College of Arts and Sciences
University of Louisville
Louisville, Kentucky, USA

Senior Medical Research Scientist
Medical Service, Division of Cardiology
Dallas VA Medical Center
Dallas, Texas, USA

Fellow, American Association for the Advancement of Science (FAAAS)
Fellow, Royal Anthropological Institute (FRAI)
Fellow, Royal Society of Medicine (FRSM)
Fellow, Royal Society of Public Health (FRSPH)

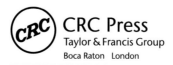

CRC Press
Taylor & Francis Group
Boca Raton   London

CRC Press is an imprint of the
Taylor & Francis Group, an **informa** business

Second edition published 2022
by CRC Press
6000 Broken Sound Parkway NW, Suite 300, Boca Raton, FL 33487–2742

and by CRC Press
2 Park Square, Milton Park, Abingdon, Oxon, OX14 4RN

© 2022 Taylor & Francis Group, LLC

*CRC Press is an imprint of Taylor & Francis Group, LLC*

ISBN: 978-1-032-21678-2 (hbk)
ISBN: 978-1-4987-1451-8 (pbk)
ISBN: 978-0-429-16092-9 (ebk)

DOI: 10.1201/9780429160929

Typeset in Times
by Apex CoVantage, LLC

**Support Materials (References) are available at: https://www.routledge.com/9781498714518**

# Contents

*The woman who taught me everything I know*
*Mildred Denton Little*
*1933–2014*
*"Mother, Author, Poet and Teacher"*

*My dearest friend*
*Kimberly L. Westfall*
*1950–2019*
*"My brother by another mother"*

# Preface

This volume condenses and updates *Drugs and Pregnancy* (Gilstrap and Little, 1992, 1998; Little, 2006). Unfortunately, because of limits on the extent of the typescript, the painful decision was made to have the publisher post and manage the references online to maintain the integrity of referenced material.

My sub-specialty training in human biology was human growth and development. Accordingly, I developed a deep interest in human teratology while developing TERIS, a computerized clinical teratology information system (writing agent summaries, knowledgebase design) from 1985 to 1990 at the University of Texas Southwestern Medical School. I had the unique privilege of working under world class leaders in human clinical teratology (Jan Friedman, Jim Hansen, F. Jose Cordero, Robert Brent, and the late Tom Shepard) who are the expert authorities behind TERIS.

The dedication for this volume includes Kim Westfall for personal reasons, and one that is directly related to this publication. He helped bring the first edition of *Drugs and Pregnancy* (1992) to print by editing, checking sources, and helping prepare the final typescript. Before his premature death following surgery, he intended to help me once again on the present volume.

Dr. Eva Malina contributed greatly to this volume, editing each word in the book. She worked tirelessly, using her incredible eye for detail. Eva is a mathematician and teacher by training, but she spotted infinitesimal details such as an incorrect volume number for the journal *Teratology*. Her assistance and expertise are greatly appreciated.

Giang Vu, DDS, MS, PhD, was my graduate student while I was researching materials for this volume. He researched details in this book and collected over 22,000 pages of publications and book chapters relevant to drug exposure during pregnancy for review.

I would like to express appreciation to my Chairman, Dr. Chris Johnson, for supporting the production of this volume.

My wife, Beverly A. DelHomme, JD, made sacrifices of time and effort to bring this volume to publication.

BL
*Louisville, Kentucky*

# 1 Introduction to Drugs and Pregnancy

Approximately **3.5–5 percent of live-born infants have a birth defect** when examined at birth or neonatally (Polifka and Friedman, 2002), and this is termed the ***background population risk for congenital anomalies***. The prevalence of birth defects may normally be 8 percent, according to a British Columbia universal disease registry (Baird *et al.*, 1989). Estimated teratogenic causes of birth defects (Figure 1.1) show that 1 percent of congenital anomalies are caused by drugs, chemicals, and other exogenous agents (i.e., an estimated one in 400 infants has a birth defect with a teratogenic etiology). Estimates have not changed over several decades, perhaps because genomic research eclipses research in clinical teratology (Polifka and Friedman, 2002). Lack of research funding for research in human birth defects is often attributed to the higher priority given to genomic and other bench science. Little funding goes to birth defects monitoring or epidemiology. Much research remains to be done. The magnitude of the problem of medication use during pregnancy may be underestimated. Approximately 65–70 percent of birth defects have an unknown etiology, some of which may be unrecognized human teratogens not researched because of the lack of resources and funding. Unreported or under-studies of the teratogenic potential of medically prescribed medication contribute to our lack of information on many medications used in pregnancy.

Alcohol use and/or taking drugs of abuse, and other preventable causes of birth defects are likely under-ascertained. **Congenital anomalies** and other pregnancy complications **caused by medication and chemical exposure are unique because these birth defects are potentially preventable**. Key factors in evaluation and prevention of morbidity and mortality due to drug and chemical exposure during pregnancy include knowledge of prenatal exposure effects and the window of opportunity for intervention. Chapters 2–16 summarize information available regarding drug exposure during pregnancy. Drug-specific information obtained from the current medical literature, clinical experience, and science are reviewed for their potential to cause birth defects.

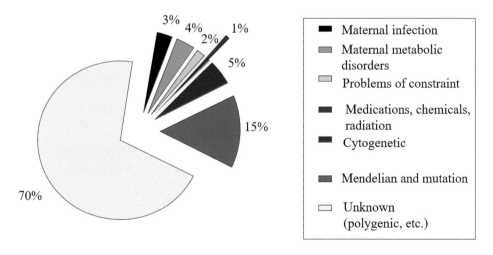

**FIGURE 1.1** Causes of birth defects.

DOI: 10.1201/9780429160929-1

There is a narrow window of opportunity to intervene in medication use during pregnancy because pregnant women do not present for prenatal care until embryogenesis is complete (i.e., after 58 days post-conception). Intervention is further complicated because many women are not aware of the potential adverse effects of drugs and chemicals on pregnancy. For example, more than 60 percent of gravidas had never heard of fetal alcohol syndrome and were not aware of the adverse effects of alcohol on pregnancy in several surveys. The best intervention is patient education prior to conception; however, little to no funding is available for patient education. Social and cultural barriers must be effectively addressed for the patient education process to be successful.

Well-educated obstetrical patients use culturally based "folk etiologies" to explain the occurrence of birth defects and other adverse pregnancy outcomes. Folk etiologies rarely align medically founded causes. Even gravid physicians often incorrectly understand prenatal development and how medications and other environmental exposure can cause birth defects and other untoward pregnancy outcomes. Folk or sociocultural background and education level must be considered when counseling the obstetrical patient regarding specific drug and chemical exposure risks to pregnancy.

The good news is that the rate of birth defects has been reduced over time through avoiding teratogenic medications during pregnancy. The working hypothesis on reduction of congenital anomalies among women with epilepsy could be due to the increased adoption of dose adjustments during pregnancy to maintain an efficacious dose (Tomson *et al.*, 2018). The not-so-good news is that research on drug use during pregnancy has not continued at the pace it could have because of funding and research priority (Adam *et al.*, 2011; Lo and Friedman, 2002; Polifka and Friedman, 2002).

## MAGNITUDE OF THE PROBLEM

The majority of women use a number of drugs during pregnancy, usually before they recognize they are pregnant. Medications are often related to a medical condition being treated before the pregnancy was known. Prevalence of medication use varies widely, <10 percent to more than 95 percent of pregnant women report drug use during gestation. Usually, more than one medication was used during pregnancy. A French study reported 89.9 percent of women used medication during pregnancy (Berard *et al.*, 2019). In the United States, 97.1 percent of women used one medication during pregnancy, and 95.7 percent used medication during the first trimester (Haas *et al.*, 2018). In a Danish study based upon blood samples, 82.6 percent of women used a drug during the first trimester (Aagaard *et al.*, 2018). High prevalence of medication use during pregnancy is clearly a frequent event. Similar prevalences of drug use during pregnancy were reported in Brazil, Australia, New Zealand, and Egypt. Clearly, this is an international pattern and problem. Safety of drugs for use during gestation may be questionable or simply unknown in many instances (Polifka and Friedman, 2002). Paucity of clinical teratology research conducted over the last four decades is the root cause of poor availability of information on drug use in pregnancy (Lo and Friedman, 2002).

Inadvertent drug exposures during pregnancy are due to some medications being: (1) used before pregnancy is recognized, (2) taken without the physician's advice after pregnancy is recognized, and (3) taken with a physician's advice. In practice, the predominant case is that physicians are faced with determining whether or not a medication or drug may be harmful to a pregnant woman, or harm has been induced after the exposure has occurred.

Non-medical exposures to drugs are a concern in 10–20 percent of gravidas. Non-medical exposure to drugs during pregnancy occur in attempted suicide and substance abuse (i.e., recreational use). Suicide gestures in pregnancy occur in an estimated 0.6 percent. Substance abuse during pregnancy (discussed in Chapter 16) is >33-fold more prevalent than suicide gestures. An estimated 10–20 percent of pregnant women use an illicit or social substance of abuse. Cocaine seems to be the most frequently used substance in 2021.

## CLINICAL EVALUATION

Clinical evaluation of drug exposure during pregnancy has five objectives that guide what is entered into the medical record and discussed with the patient (Box 1.1).

---

**BOX 1.1 TERATOGEN EXPOSURE COUNSELING**

1. Estimate date of conception.
2. Obtain the family history medical genetic pedigree.
3. Obtain information on the substances consumed (medications, alcohol, illicit/social substances of abuse), timing in gestation, frequency, and dose.
4. Integrate #1 and #3 to estimate exposure timing. Use the information from the calendar to determine the organ systems being formed during the exposure.
5. Compare the findings in #4 to the published literature and estimate the risk increase if there is one and it is known. If the results are reported in odds ratios, relative risks, or risk ratios, it is possible to estimate percent increases.

---

1. Estimate date of conception. If the ultrasound estimated date of conception is not available, then calculate the date of conception using the pregnancy wheel that every drug company gifts. Determine the estimated date of conception, and use this to evaluate the exposure(s) timing. This is critical to properly evaluating the possible risks because risks vary across different stages of embryonic development (see Figure 1.1). The accuracy of this method assumes accurate maternal recall, assumes regular 28-day cycles, and conception (actually ovulation) occurs on menstrual cycle day 14. Use of LMP day to estimate pregnancy may have an error of >2 weeks.
2. Obtain the family history medical genetic risks through constructing a pedigree and eliciting answers to the standard battery of questions regarding relatives with any abnormality from a missing fingernail to mental retardation. Completed in depth pedigrees often provide the greater risk when compared to teratogens.
3. By interview, obtain information on the substances (medications, alcohol, illicit/social substances of abuse) consumed. Try to determine amount (dose) and frequency (several times a day, daily, every other day, etc.) of each substance used. For medicinal substances, use the amount times daily frequency to calculate dose exposure. For alcohol, determine number of drinks and type of alcohol to obtain an estimated use of alcohol (12 oz. beer (5 percent) = 5 ounces of wine (12 percent) = 1 shot of liquor (40 percent)). For powders (cocaine, methamphetamine), grams or lines is the quantity scale, crack cocaine rocks measure amount, and heroin is sometimes measured in spoons for IV use.
4. Integrate #1 and #3 to estimate exposure timing. Ask the patient for specific dates of the use of the substance(s) in terms of month and day, and note these on a calendar starting as early as the patient can recall, but at least since the estimated date of conception. Write the exposures in the calendar by day/amount. Then write in the estimated date of conception as day 1. Then number each day until you reach 60 days post-conception and you have mapped out the exposure by the stage of embryonic development. Use the information from the calendar to determine the organ systems being formed during the exposure.
5. Compare the findings in #5 to the published literature and estimate the risk increase if there is one and it is known. If the results are reported in odds ratios, relative risks, or risk ratios, it is possible to estimate percent increases (see Box 1.2).

## BOX 1.2   OVERVIEW OF COUNSELING AND KNOWN TERATOGENIC RISK

**Congenital Heart Disease and Cleft Palate: Examples of Risk Estimation**

|  | Background Risk | OR$_{Teratogen}$ | Adjusted Risk | Increased Risk |
|---|---|---|---|---|
| Congenital heart disease[1] | 0.008 | 1.99 | 0.0159 | (3.5%−0.8%) + 1.8% = 0.043 |
|  | 0.8% | 199% | 1.59% | 2.7% + 1.8% = 4.5% |
| Cleft lip w/without palate[2] | 0.0025 | 1.41 | 0.0035 | (3.5%−0.25%) + 0.0035 = 0.036 |
|  | 0.25% | 141% | 0.35% | 3.25% + 0.35% = 3.6% |

[1] Pedersen *et al.*, 2009; Septal heart defects and SSRI antidepressant use.
[2] Hviid and Mølgaard-Nielsen *et al.*, 2011; Cleft lip with/without palate and corticosteroid in pregnancy.
*Abbreviations:* OR: odds ratio; OR$_{Teratogen}$: increased odds due to teratogen exposure.

The evaluation in Box 1.1 brings perspective for the patient who is concerned about possible elevated risk because of a potentially teratogenic or a teratogenic exposure. Stating that the risk of cleft palate is increased 43 percent above baseline because of maternal steroid exposure (Box 1.2) is frightening to exposed gravidas. While it is scientifically correct, perspective must be provided for the patient to understand what the risk assessments mean to their pregnancy. While the risk is increase 43 percent, the net effect of this on the overall risk for birth defects is small, increasing from 3.5 percent to 3.6 percent.

Clinical evaluation of potentially teratogenic and/or toxic exposures during pregnancy has three separate components in normal pregnancy: Maternal, embryonic, and fetal. Marked differences in the physiology of these components exist because of differences in the purposes of the cells, or the end points of cell division (replacement versus morphogenesis versus hyperplastic growth) and the metabolic capabilities of the mother and the developing conceptus. In the embryo, organs are being formed (i.e., organogenesis), and drugs are not metabolized at adult or fetal rates, if at all. The embryo is not a little fetus. The fetus is not a little adult. Most of the fetal period is occupied with growth in size of organs, not usually their formation, and these are growing very rapidly. Exceptions exist (e.g., thyroid, sexual organs, brain cell "arrangement"), but this is generally true for the fetus. Fetal enzyme systems involved in drug metabolism are only beginning to function, and some will not be active until after the neonatal period (e.g., cholinesterase). Pregnant women have the full enzyme complement for metabolizing drugs, but some systems have lower activity during pregnancy, as does cholinesterase (Pritchard, 1955), which metabolizes cocaine and other drugs. In addition, gender differences in the non-pregnant state also exist. For example, alcohol dehydrogenase (ADH) among adult females is approximately 55 percent of adult male activity. Therefore, drug effects on adults, fetuses, embryos, and pregnant women differ markedly in metabolism, pharmacokinetics, pharmacodynamics, and clearance rates (Little, 1999). It is thus important to differentiate the effects of drugs and chemicals based upon these distinctly different components of pregnancy. Drugs and chemicals have different effects on these three components of pregnancy. There is a need for more data and pharmacometric tools to analyze and quantify the impact of pharmacokinetic changes in pregnancy (Dallman *et al.*, 2019).

## HUMAN TERATOLOGY: PRINCIPLES

A teratogen is usually defined as any agent, physical force, or other factor (e.g., maternal disease) that can induce a congenital anomaly through alteration of normal development during any stage of embryogenesis. Agents include drugs and other chemicals. Physical forces include ionizing radiation

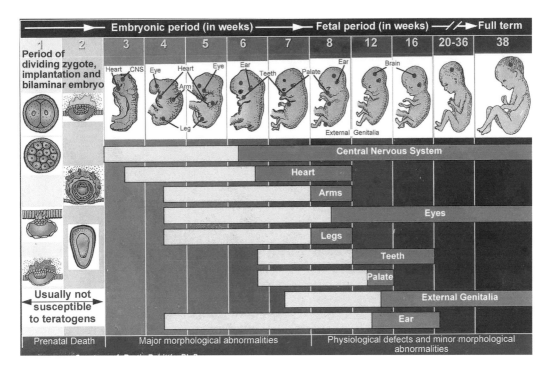

**FIGURE 1.2** Critical times for the development of various organs and structures.

(Redrawn from Moore K., *The Developing Human: Clinically Orientated Embryology*, Third Edition, WB Saunders, Philadelphia, 1982. Used with permission.)

and physical restraint (e.g., amniotic banding). Teratogenic maternal diseases include disorders such as diabetes mellitus and phenylketonuria. Agents that cause defects during the post-embryonic (fetal) period are termed to have the potential for producing adverse "fetal effects," but are not truly teratogens. Not all agents or factors that are teratogens have adverse fetal effects, and vice versa.

A simplified overview of the differences between the embryonic and fetal periods should be presented during consultation to clarify stages for the patient. The embryonic period should be described as the growth of cells that all look alike (i.e., are undifferentiated) into specialized cells that are arranged in special ways (i.e., organs, specialized tissues). Specialized cell lines or lineages grow in number and change in structure and arrangement, giving rise to organs and tissues. Some organs and tissues are formed earlier than are others. For example, the neural tube (brain and spine) forms earlier than do the face and endocrine system. After embryogenesis (58–60 days post-conception) is completed, the conceptus is a fetus (Figure 1.2). With a few exceptions, the morphological architecture for a normal (or abnormal) human is laid down during the embryonic period (embryogenesis or organogenesis), and during the fetal period these structures grow in size and develop normal physiologic function.

Congenital anomalies can be induced during the fetal period through a fetal effect, although they are usually induced during the critical embryonic period. For example, a structure that was formed normally during embryogenesis can be damaged during the fetal period, and the resulting malformation may appear to have arisen during morphogenesis. A classic example of a fetal effect is hemorrhaging due to Coumadin exposure, which may induce brain or eye defects despite the fact that these structures were formed normally during the embryonic period. Alternatively, a limb reduction defect associated with cocaine during the fetal period may be induced through vascular disruption in a normally formed limb.

Thalidomide is the most notorious human teratogen. It is an heuristic example of how such agents might not be identified. Animal models of thalidomide use in pregnancy normally used in drug screening failed to identify this drug as a dangerous substance and it was released to the market and damaged large numbers of children. Thalidomide was one of the most potent human teratogens ever discovered.

Laboratory studies cannot replace large, well-controlled, human epidemiologic studies, but they do play an important role in screening drugs and chemicals for potential to cause human birth defects during pregnancy. Isotretinoin (Accutane) is the only human teratogen discovered through laboratory research. Before isotretinoin was released to the market, its high potential for inducing major congenital anomalies and pregnancy loss was known. This fact was clearly displayed on the manufacturer's package insert. Inadvertent exposures to isotretinoin during early human pregnancy confirmed laboratory findings, with more than 100 pregnancies exposed to isotretinoin have been reported and a pattern of malformations known as isotretinoin embryopathy was observed in >40 percent of exposed offspring. Astute clinicians discovered other human teratogens because they recognized patterns or constellations of anomalies in cases or small clinical series of infants whose mothers used or were exposed to certain drugs or chemicals during early pregnancy. Epidemiological studies of infants whose mothers used certain drugs or chemicals during embryogenesis, as well as research with pregnant animals, served primarily to confirm clinical observations.

Maternal complications and fetal effects due to drug or chemical exposures are not considered under the rubric of classical teratology, but the discovery of drugs and other agents with such potential adverse effects parallels the pattern of the discovery of human teratogens. The untoward fetal effects are called *fetotoxic* or *adverse fetal* effects, and maternal effects are termed *maternal toxic* or *adverse maternal* effects. However, even seasoned human teratologists blur the line between embryonic and fetal effects sometimes.

## ANIMAL STUDIES IN CLINICAL EVALUATION

Rodent animal models are poor predictors of whether or not a drug or chemical is teratogenic in humans. Accuracy and precision (sensitivity and specificity) of animal models in the prediction of human teratogenicity is dependent upon how closely the experimental animal species is phylogenetically to humans. Non-human primates are better predictors of human teratogenicity and fetotoxicity than are rodent models. Animal teratology experiments are further complicated because doses used are often many times greater than therapeutic doses given to humans, approaching maternally toxic doses in experiments. Extremely high doses with toxic effects on the mother confound the interpretation of fetal outcome. Metabolism and absorption of drugs and chemicals are different between species because they differ in placentation, metabolism, pharmacokinetics, pharmacodynamics, embryonic development timing, and innate predisposition to various congenital anomalies. Sensitivity and specificity of rodent studies for prediction of human teratogens are less than 60 percent (Schardein, 2000).

The US Food and Drug Administration (FDA) use rodent animal teratology studies in an accepted drug-approval process to evaluate the safety of medications for use during human pregnancy, despite very poor prediction of human teratogens. Non-human primate teratology studies are considerably better predictors human teratogens, with sensitivity and specificity of 90 percent or greater. Non-human primate studies are orders of magnitude more expensive than rodent teratology studies. The result is few drugs are evaluated in primates. Unfortunately, the ultimate assessment of the safety of medication use in pregnancy must come from human studies (Schardein and Macina, 2006; Shepard and Lemire, 2010). Accordingly, human teratogens are discovered only after numerous children have been damaged. Typically, an astute clinician recognizes a pattern (syndrome) of congenital anomalies, and links the birth defects to exposure during pregnancy. Approximately 2,000 drugs and chemicals were tested in animal models, and 55 percent were teratogenic in animal models (Shepard and Lemire, 2010). The number of known human teratogens is approximately 50 drugs.

## HUMAN STUDIES

Known human teratogens were identified through careful interpretation of data from case reports, clinical series, and epidemiologic studies. A recurrent pattern of anomalies in babies who sustained similar well-defined exposures at similar points during embryogenesis is suggestive that the agent in question may be teratogenic. Case reports are important in raising causal hypotheses. However, most hypotheses from case reports are subsequently proven incorrect. For example, a high incidence of environmental exposure to spermicides by pregnant women and congenital anomalies in offspring is a coincidental occurrence, despite what the legal outcome was. The law and case decisions are not a true reflection of truth, but usually the confluence of political and economic concerns used to beguile a jury. Dr. Robert Brent remarked after a huge failure in judgment found incorrectly found that spermicides caused birth defects that such substances were litogens, substances that cause lawsuits, not birth defects. For the record, **nonoxynols in spermicides are NOT associated with an increased risk of birth defects**.

A teratogen identified through epidemiologic studies, case reports, and animal studies is carbamazepine. For several decades, carbamazepine was assumed safer for the treatment of epilepsy during pregnancy than phenytoin or the other hydantoins. A case report published in 1993 reported a suicide gesture by a non-epileptic gravida during the period of spinal closure. The result was a fetus with a very large meningomyelocele (Little *et al.*, 1993). A case-control study of carbamazepine linked carbamazepine with an increased frequency of birth defects (Jones *et al.*, 1989). Other epidemiologic studies were conducted, and in 2021, the association of neural tubes defects with carbamazepine exposure during early pregnancy is generally accepted. The risk is quantified at about 1 percent, approximately 10 times a 0.1 percent background risk in the general population.

Quantitative estimates of risks for birth defects (strength and statistical significance of associations between agent exposures in pregnant women and abnormalities in their offspring) are obtained only through epidemiological studies. **Investigations in human pregnancy are necessary to demonstrate that an agent is teratogenic because no models of high reliability exist**. Two types of epidemiology studies are used in human teratology: cohort studies and case-control studies. In cohort studies, frequencies of anomalies in offspring of women exposed during embryogenesis (first trimester) are compared to the frequencies in those who are unexposed to the agent in question. A higher frequency of anomalies among exposed pregnancies suggests the drug be scrutinized as a teratogen. In case-control studies, the frequency of prenatal exposure to an agent is compared among children with and without a specific birth defect. If malformed children were more frequently exposed to a drug or agent than unaffected controls, then the drug or agent may be a teratogen. If an agent increases the risk of anomalies in the offspring only slightly, very large studies over a protracted period may be necessary to demonstrate that the increase is causal. The cohort and case-control studies need to incorporate information on potential confounders (e.g., family history, other exposures, maternal disease state(s), poverty). Confounders should be used in a multivariate analysis (e.g., multiple logistic regression) to adjust the odds of a birth defect. Confounders are sometimes the source of risk and not the prenatal drug exposure. Post-marketing surveillance of drugs urgently needs a more rigorous assessment of possible associations with birth defects (Adam *et al.*, 2011).

Epidemiologic studies have several limitations. Spurious associations often occur because many epidemiologists lack medical or biological training, and fail to scrutinize their "statistical associations" for biological plausibility. Other confounders include sample size. Some investigations involve small numbers of exposed or affected subjects because exposures are sometimes rare. Rarity of the maternal disease or situation that led to the exposure may be responsible for an observed association with a congenital anomaly, rather than the agent itself. Of paramount importance is that the observed association be biologically plausible.

1. Exposures that produce malformations in the embryo should do so only during organogenesis or histogenesis.

2. Affected structures should be susceptible to the teratogenic agent only at specific gestational times.
3. Systemic absorption of the agent by the mother and its presence at susceptible sites in the embryo or placenta should be demonstrable.
4. Exposure to higher doses (a greater quantity of the agent) should be associated in a dose-response fashion with an increased frequency of abnormalities.
5. Finally, a causal inference is supported if a reasonable pathogenic mechanism can be established for the observed effect. For example, lower birth weight is associated with maternal antihypertensive therapy, but maternal hypertension is itself strongly associated with decreased birth weight. Is lower birth weight associated with the blood pressure medication, or the disease of hypertension, or some combination?

## KNOWN HUMAN TERATOGENS

The list of known human teratogens is surprisingly small (Box 1.3). The most notorious human teratogen is thalidomide. It is currently available in the United States on a limited basis for treatment of several infectious diseases such as acquired immune deficiency syndrome (AIDS), tuberculosis, and leprosy. In 1996, a new thalidomide embryopathy epidemic was reported in Brazil and other South American countries (Castilla *et al.*, 1996). The astute reader will note that some of the putative teratogens do not fit precisely within the definition of teratogen (i.e., exposure is not strictly confined to the period of organogenesis), sometimes because the agent may also be fetotoxic.

## CRITICAL TIME PERIODS

*In utero* development is divided into three time periods of development, namely, (1) preimplantation, (2) embryogenesis (or organogenesis, or histogenesis), and (3) fetal growth and development. Exposure to drugs during pregnancy must be separated into these periods because the conceptus responds differently in each of the three stages of development.

---

**BOX 1.3   KNOWN HUMAN TERATOGENS**

- ACE inhibitors
- Amiodarone
- Aminopterin
- Antiepileptic drugs
  - Carbamazepine
  - Clonazepam
  - Primidone
  - Phenobarbital
  - Phenytoin/fosphenytoin
  - Valproic acid
- Coumarin derivatives
- Cyclophosphamide
- Danazol
- Diethylstilbestrol
- Lithium

- Methotrexate
- Methylene blue
- Penicillamine
- Quinine
- Radioiodine
- Retinoids (oral)
- Tetracycline and derivatives
- Thalidomide
- Fluconazole
- Methimazole
- Misoprostol
- Trimethadione/paramethadione
- Trimethoprim
- ACE: Angiotensin-converting enzyme

## PREIMPLANTATION

No physiologic interface between the mother and the conceptus exists at conception (ovum penetration by the spermatid to form a single diploid cell). Traditionally, the first two weeks post-conception (until the blastocyst attaches to the wall of the uterus forming chorionic villi) was considered protected from drugs or medications in maternal circulation because the preimplantation embryo does not share maternal circulation. However, evidence (e.g., mitomycin) indicates that the preimplantation embryo may not be as completely protected as previously thought.

## EMBRYONIC DEVELOPMENT

The period of the embryo is the critical stage of development for the induction of birth defects. The embryonic period extends from the time of implantation until 58–60 days post-conception. Organs and tissues are being formed (i.e., organogenesis) during this period. Random biological mistakes that occur during the embryonic period of the embryo may result in malformations (congenital anomalies) or birth defects. Agents that induce abnormal embryonic physical or physiological development by acting during the period of the embryo, or organogenesis are teratogens (Jones, 1988). Lethal embryo malformations present as spontaneous abortion, sometimes before pregnancy is recognized. Similarly, some substances that are directly toxic to the embryo, e.g., methotrexate, also present as spontaneous abortions. The critical times for the development of various organs and structures of the human embryo are given in Figure 1.2.

## FETAL DEVELOPMENT

Normal organogenesis and histogenesis during the embryonic development can be damaged outside the period of the embryo as a fetus. Traditionally, damage to a fetus not considered a teratogenic effect may present as a structural abnormality, but some authorities lump fetal effects into this category. Changes in cellular structures (e.g., brain cell arrangements during neuronal migration) occur during the fetal period. However, the predominant fetal event is hyperplastic growth (increase in cell number) with organs and other tissues becoming larger through cellular proliferation, and only secondarily through hypertrophy (increase in cell size). For example, the thyroid gland appears early in the fetal period, as does fetal endocrine function. Potential adverse effects during fetal development include maldevelopment due to interrupted cell migration and growth retardation (Jones, 1988). If blood flow to an organ or structure is interrupted or obstructed, structures that were normally formed during embryogenesis may become malformed during the fetal period (e.g., vascular disruption and fetal cocaine or warfarin exposure). The structure(s) deprived of blood flow necrose and are resorbed. A defect would result that may mimic an embryonic effect, but the true origin of the defect would be fetotoxicity.

Embryonic and fetal exposure to drugs occurs through the placenta. **The placenta** can (1) **metabolize** some drugs before they reach the conceptus, (2) **allow transfer of most drugs** (~99 percent) by simple diffusion, (3) **not transfer large molecules** (i.e., >1000 molecular weight) unless there is an active transport system (e.g., antibodies), (4) **transfer neutrally charged molecules**, (5) **easily transfer lipid-soluble drugs**, and (6) **not transport charged (+ or –) molecules**. Poor potential for transfer back to the maternal circulation occurs for some drugs (e.g., water-soluble drugs transfer back to the mother's circulation poorly), resulting in accumulation in the embryo-fetal compartment.

## POTENTIAL ADVERSE EFFECTS

### SPONTANEOUS ABORTION

More than 50 percent of early pregnancies (0–58 days) end in spontaneous abortion. *In vitro* fertilization studies suggest that the majority of spontaneous abortions are chromosomally abnormal.

Spontaneous abortion occurs in 15–20 percent of fetuses that survive 59–126 days of gestation. Spontaneous abortion/fetal death risk decreases to 1–2 percent by 18–20 weeks (127–140 days). Weeks 20 to 28 (196 days) post-conception have approximately a 2-percent risk for spontaneous abortion. Excessive spontaneous abortion rates in association with a drug exposure may signal embryo-fetal toxicity. In animal studies, excessive pregnancy losses may predict an increased risk for spontaneous abortion in humans.

## CONGENITAL ANOMALIES

Congenital anomalies or birth defects detected at birth occur in about 3.5–5 percent of live births (Brent and Beckman, 1990). The true frequency of congenital anomalies may increase by up to twofold because some birth defects may not be detected until about 5 years of age. Congenital anomalies are several fold higher among stillbirths and miscarriages than among live births.

## FETAL EFFECTS

Four primary types of fetal effects occur: (1) Damage to structures or organs formed normally during embryogenesis, (2) systems undergoing histogenesis during the fetal period are damaged, (3) growth retardation during gestation, and (4) fetal death or stillbirth.

Fetal effects may be caused by a teratogen, but they may also be caused by agents with no apparent teratogenic potential. Organs, structures, or functions formed normally during embryogenesis can be damaged by environmental (drug, chemical, physical force) exposures during the fetal period.

Fetal growth retardation is the most frequently observed effect of agents given during pregnancy and outside the period of embryogenesis. Frequently it is difficult to distinguish between the effects of agents from those of the disease being treated. Propranolol, for example, is associated with fetal growth retardation, but untreated maternal hypertension is also associated with fetal growth retardation. Some teratogenic agents may be associated with fetal growth retardation. Fetal growth retardation may also occur without embryonic damage. Risks of fetal death, stillbirth, and other adverse effects are increased with exposure to some agents during pregnancy (Table 1.1).

## NEONATAL AND POSTNATAL EFFECTS

Adverse neonatal effects are associated with prenatal exposure to some drugs (e.g., difficulty in adaptation to life outside the womb). Drugs associated with adverse neonatal effects are not always associated with birth defects (i.e., teratogenic effects). Transient metabolic abnormalities, withdrawal, and hypoglycemia are well-documented neonatal effects of certain medications and nonmedical drugs. The floppy infant syndrome and benzodiazepine use near term is an example. Patent ductus arteriosus with the use of NSAIDs (prostaglandin synthetase inhibitors such as aspirin or indomethacin) close to delivery is another well know example. The "gray baby" syndrome with high-dose chloramphenicol near term is another documented example (Table 1.1). Teratogens are frequently associated with developmental delay, but delays are also associated with fetal effects of drugs that are apparently not teratogenic.

## MATERNAL PHYSIOLOGY DURING PREGNANCY

Profound physiological changes occur throughout pregnancy (Table 1.2). Maternal enzymes, particularly cholinesterases (Pritchard, 1955), have lowered activity in pregnancy. Maternal blood volume increases by approximately 40–50 percent during pregnancy to support the developing fetus's requirements (Cunningham *et al.*, 2017). Increased blood volume may lower serum concentrations through increased volume of distribution. Absorption of drugs occurs with kinetics similar to the

**TABLE 1.1**

**Adverse Effects Other Than Birth Defects on the Human Fetus Associated with Drugs**

| Maternal Medication | Fetal/Neonatal Effect |
| --- | --- |
| Acetaminophen | Renal failure |
| Adrenocortical hormones | Adrenocortical suppression; electrolyte imbalance |
| Alcohol | Muscular hypotonia: hypoglycemia (?); withdrawal; intrauterine growth restriction (IUGR); blood changes; affect mental ability |
| Alphaprodine | Platelet dysfunction |
| Amitriptyline | Withdrawal |
| Ammonium chloride | Acidosis |
| Amphetamines | Withdrawal |
| Antihistamines | Infertility (?) |
| Antineoplastics | Transient pancytopenia IUGR |
| Antithyroid drugs | Hypothyroidism |
| Barbiturates/diphenylhydantoin | Coagulation defects; withdrawal (barbiturates only); IUGR |
| Chloral hydrate, excess | Fetal death |
| Chloramphenicol | Death ("gray baby syndrome") |
| Chlordiazepoxide | Withdrawal (?) |
| Chloroquine | Death (?) |
| Chlorpropamide | Prolonged hypoglycemia; fetal death |
| Cocaine | Vascular disruption, withdrawal, IUGR |
| Coumarin anticoagulants | Hemorrhage, death, IUGR |
| Diazepam | Hypothermia; hypotonia; withdrawal |
| Diphenhydramine | Withdrawal |
| Ergot | Fetal death |
| Erythromycin | Liver damage (?) |
| Gold salts | Complications; kernicterus |
| Glutethimide | Withdrawal |
| Heroin/morphine/methadone | Withdrawal; neonatal death |
| Hexamethonium bromide | Neonatal ileus |
| Hykinone | Blood changes; jaundice |
| Immunosuppressants | Transient immune system depression, danger of infection |
| Insulin (shock) | Fetal loss |
| Intravenous fluids, excess | Fluid and electrolyte abnormalities |
| Iophenoxic acid | Evaluation of serum protein-bound iodine (PBI) |
| Lithium | Cyanosis, flaccidity, polyhydramnios, toxicity |
| Magnesium sulfate | Central depression and neuromuscular block |
| Meperidine | Neonatal depression |
| Mepivacaine | Fetal brachycardia and depression |
| Meprobamate | Retarded development (?) |
| Nitrofurantoin | Hemolysis |
| Novobiocin | Hyperbilirubinemia (?) |
| Oral progestogens, androgens, estrogens | Advanced bone age |
| Phenformin | Lactic acidosis (?) |
| Phenobarbital, excess | Neonatal bleeding; death |
| Phenothiazines | Hyperbilirubinemia (?), depression, hypothermia (?), withdrawal |
| Polio vaccine, live | Fetal loss (?) |

## TABLE 1.2
## Physiological Changes during Pregnancy and Medication Disposition

- Changes in total body weight and body fat composition.
- Delayed gastric emptying, prolonged gastrointestinal transit time, and decreased gastric acid secretion, all of which can affect the bioavailability of drugs.[1,2,3]
- Expanded plasma volume and significantly increased extracellular fluid space and total body water content. These vary with the patient's weight and can affect the volume of distribution of drugs.[4]
- Increased cardiac output, stroke volume, heart rate, and blood flow to the uterus, kidneys, skin, and mammary glands. The percentage of cardiac output attributed to hepatic blood flow is lower during pregnancy.[5]
- Decreased concentration of plasma albumin, which can reduce the protein binding of some drugs.[6]
- Increased glomerular filtration rate early in pregnancy, with a continued rise throughout pregnancy.[7]
- Changes in the activity of hepatic enzymes, including the cytochrome P450 enzymes, xanthine oxidase, and *N*-acetyltransferase.[6]

[1] Gryboski and Spiro, 1976.
[2] Frederiksen *et al.*, 1986.
[3] Robson *et al.*, 1990.
[4] Mendenhall, 1970.
[5] Dunlop, 1981.
[6] Tsutsumi *et al.*, 2001; Wadelius *et al.*, 1997.
[7] Lalkin and Koren, 1997.

non-pregnant adult. Renal clearance is increased in pregnancy and enzyme activity is often down-regulated. Increased blood volume exacerbates pregnancy-associated decreased enzyme activity levels, decreasing the overall effective serum concentration of a given dose. Increased renal output causes an increased clearance index for most drugs. Drugs tightly bound to serum proteins have little opportunity to cross the placenta or enter breast milk. Pregnancy changes place increased demands on cardiovascular, hepatic, and renal systems. The gravid uterus is vulnerable to a variety of effects not present in the non-pregnant state, such as hemorrhage, rupture, or preterm contraction.

Pregnancy-imposed demands on these physiological systems are managed without complications under normal maternal conditions. However, disease conditions or other stressors weaken key systems and disrupt normal function. For example, cocaine abuse during pregnancy targets the cardiovascular system that is already stressed. It would, thus, be expected that cocaine use during pregnancy stresses cardiovascular, renal, and hepatic systems more than in the non-pregnant adult. Indeed, these expectations are borne out in the observations of cocaine use during pregnancy.

## PHARMACOKINETICS IN PREGNANCY

Pharmacokinetic data during pregnancy is limited. Results are sometimes conflicting between studies of the same drug, and is related to timing during pregnancy and choice of control/comparison groups. Across pharmacokinetic investigations reviewed, area under the curve was decreased in 41 percent of the studies, volume of distribution was increased in 30 percent, and peak plasma concentration was decreased in 34 percent. Steady-state plasma concentration was decreased in 44 percent of the studies. Half-life ($t^{1/2}$) was decreased in 41 percent. Renal clearance was increased in 55 percent of the studies (Little, 1999).

Pharmacokinetic changes during pregnancy are drug class specific, and stage of pregnancy specific. The individual drug must be considered. Observed changes in pharmacokinetics cause changes, most often decreases, in plasma drug concentrations. Increased doses or schedules are needed to maintain effective systemic drug levels when pharmacokinetic drug behavior is altered in this way. However, information on pharmacokinetics during pregnancy is biased by a lack of information on most therapeutic agents used during pregnancy. Physiologic changes during pregnancy and their effects on the disposition of medications given during gestation found are consistent with previous surveys of the literature (Amon and Hüller, 1984a, 1984b; Cummings, 1983; Kafetzis *et al.*, 1983; Mattison *et al.*, 1992; Philipson, 1978; Reynolds, 1991; Little, 1999; Dawes and Chowienczyk, 2001; Feghali *et al.*, 2015; Pariente *et al.*, 2016; Anger and Piquette-Miller, 2017; Koren and Pariente, 2018).

Multiple confounders, in addition to lack of published literature, make it difficult to interpret available pharmacokinetic data in pregnancy. Very small sample sizes are used in pharmacokinetics in pregnancy studies, frequently fewer than 10 pregnant women. Comparison (control) groups vary in composition. Studies have used non-pregnant women, adult males, the same patients 6–8 weeks postpartum, or published "historical" pharmacokinetic data. Of the options, the optimal comparison is the same woman post-partum because it is a paired comparison that increases statistical power and innately controls for interindividual variation.

Maternal weight-adjusted values are not published for any drug in pharmacokinetic studies in pregnancy. However, maternal weight has a strong influence on area under the curve, volume of distribution, peak plasma concentration, steady-state plasma concentration, half-life, renal clearance, and time to peak plasma concentration. Route of administration also varied, even with the same drug, and is known to be an important influence on time to peak plasma concentration, peak plasma concentration, steady-state plasma concentration, half-life, and area under the curve. Estimated gestational age is an important variable, and is a confounder. Most pharmacokinetic measures differ by the stage of gestation, and the method of determining estimated gestational age was not reported in any of the previously published studies. Quantitative assay of drug levels and inter-laboratory variation are not consistent and further confound studies. Only one group of investigators (Bardy *et al.*, 1982) has reported the empiric effect of pharmacogenetic variation on drug disposition during pregnancy. Polymorphisms in enzymes are known to exist and might result in lower enzyme activity in 10–20 percent of the population, including pregnant women (Vesell, 1997). No data are available to address this variation directly among gravidas, although pharmacogenetic differences must affect drug disposition during pregnancy (Box 1.4). Polymorphisms are infrequently reported, and not systematically used to evaluate pharmacokinetics when they are reported.

## BOX 1.4 PREGNANCY-ASSOCIATED CHANGES IN HEPATIC ENZYME ACTIVITY

| Enzyme | Effect of Pregnancy | Drugs Metabolized by Enzyme |
|---|---|---|
| CYP1A2 | Decreased | Acetaminophen, caffeine, propranolol, theophylline |
| CYP2B6 | Increased | Methadone, efavirenz, sertraline |
| CYP2C8 | Increased | Verapamil, fluvastatin |
| CYP2C9 | Increased | Glyburide, escitalopram, phenytoin, losartan |
| CYP2C19 | Decreased | Proguanil, indomethacin, citalopram |
| CYP2D6 | Increased | Alprenolol, metoprolol, codeine, fluoxetine |
| CYP2E1 | Increased | Disulfiram, theophylline |
| CYP3A4 | Increased | Darunavir, citalopram, nifedipine, lamotrigine, |
| Uridine 5'-diphospho-glucuronosyl-transferases | Increased | Lamotrigine, morphine |

See further Pariente *et al.*, 2016.

Third trimester pregnancy is associated with lower maternal serum concentrations of most medications. Maternal drug concentrations are not routinely measured, and the clinician may not be immediately aware of the lower serum levels. Total drug levels may be lower (i.e., the active component fraction) because of lower protein binding of many drugs in late pregnancy. Higher rates of hepatic metabolism are associated with higher fractions of free drug leading to lower total drug concentrations. Increased volume of distribution in pregnancy leads to lower peak plasma concentrations of drugs and may affect maintenance of therapeutic drug levels. Drug levels may also be lowered by many gravidas attempting to decrease drug exposure during pregnancy because they fear adverse fetal effects. Therefore, general recommendations for dose schedule during pregnancy are very challenging and not practical because of many sources of variation exist that cannot be incorporated into a general guidance. However, it appears the general guidance to assess dose and serum concentration usually finds that some upward adjustment of dose and/or frequency may be necessary in the drugs that were studied (Table 1.3). Drug-specific review of pharmacokinetics in pregnancy shows that the majority of medications require an upward adjustment in dose and/or frequency of dose to maintain therapeutic levels (Table 1.3). Exceptions do exist, and xanthines are an example. Clearance decreases, half-life increases, and concentration increases in pregnancy. For example, theophylline toxicity in pregnancy has been reported (**Carter *et al.*, 1986; Green and Clark, 1989**).

Nonetheless, a general observation is that doses usually need to be adjusted in late pregnancy to maintain therapeutic levels. Some drugs may not require upward adjustment of dose, and in fact may require a lower dose during pregnancy. For example, theophylline toxicity may result in pregnancy if the dose is increased because concentration increases in late pregnancy.

The safest way to approach pharmacokinetics during pregnancy is to titrate doses to achieve a therapeutic level. In 2021, the average cost for blood tests ranges $60 to $200 per test. In a cost-benefit analysis, it is worth an extra several hundred dollars to know what the patient needs in terms of a dose adjustment.

It is important to treat with the proper dose in all cases. The highest risk cases are gravidas with a seizure disorder, infection, or psychological disorders. Dose titration in these cases usually involves a temporary increase of 40–50 percent above the non-pregnant dose. Increased doses of antibiotics, anti-seizure medications, and anti-depressants/anti-psychotics/anti-schizophrenic medications are known to need dose adjustment. The most prudent practice is to adjust doses (titrate) for gravidas with guidance of drug levels to maintain therapeutic levels at different stages of pregnancy.

## PRENATAL DIAGNOSIS

Medication exposure or substance use during pregnancy is not an indication for pregnancy termination. However, this is a common reaction among patients and physicians. Such exposure may be an indication for prenatal diagnosis. Prenatal diagnosis cannot rule out defects that are not related to gross structural abnormalities. Major congenital anomalies, (e.g., spina bifida, structural heart defects, limb reduction) can usually be determined prenatally. The epitome of an overreaction is a patient who was referred to our unit for usual therapeutic acetaminophen (Tylenol) use. Her physician had told the gravida that her child would be born without arms and legs! An ultrasound reassured the patient her child had arms and legs, and she had a normal infant at birth.

Prenatal diagnosis is used to screen for congenital anomalies and other fetal complications following use of drugs during pregnancy. Prenatal diagnosis procedures commonly available include (1) high-resolution ultrasound, (2) maternal serum alpha-fetoprotein (MSAFP), and (3) fetal echocardiography. Ultrasound studies can assess fetal growth and possible detection of specific structural anomalies of major organs. MSAFP is important for screening pregnancies for open neural tube or other open defects (e.g., gastroschisis). Amniocentesis may be performed to assess an abnormal alpha-fetoprotein level, but **a karyotype study is not indicated by drug or alcohol exposure** per se, **except for colchicine**. Fetal echocardiography is used to screen for cardiovascular defects

**TABLE 1.3**
**Possible Changes during Pregnancy to Maintain Therapeutic Levels**

| Drug | Pharmacometric(s) Change in Pregnancy | Dose Change in Pregnancy[*] |
|---|---|---|
| ***Antibiotics*** | | |
| Amoxicillin | Higher Cl | Increase dose/frequency |
| Azithromycin | Higher $V_d$, Lower AUC | Increase dose/frequency |
| Cefatrizine | Lower $C_{max}$, Lower AUC | Increase dose/frequency |
| Cefazolin | Higher free fraction, Lower $t^{1/2}$ | Increase dose/frequency |
| Cefoperazone | Higher free fraction | Increase dose/frequency |
| Cefradine | Lower AUC, Higher Cl, Lower $t^{1/2}$ | Increase dose/frequency |
| Ceftazidime | Higher Cl | Increase dose/frequency |
| Cefuroxime | Lower AUC, Higher Cl, Lower $t^{1/2}$ | Increase dose/frequency |
| Cloxacillin | Higher free fraction | Increase dose/frequency |
| Flucloxacillin | Higher free fraction | Increase dose/frequency |
| Imipenem | Higher $V_d$, Lower $C_{max}$, Lower AUC, Higher Cl | Increase dose/frequency |
| Mecillinam (amdinocillin) | Higher $V_d$, Higher $t^{1/2}$ | Increase dose/frequency |
| Moxifloxacin | Higher $V_d$, Lower $C_{max}$, Lower AUC, Lower $t^{1/2}$ | Increase dose/frequency |
| Penicillin V | Lower AUC, Lower $t^{1/2}$ | Increase dose/frequency |
| Piperacillin | Higher $V_d$, Lower AUC, Lower $C_{max}$, Higher Cl | Increase dose/frequency |
| Trimetoprim/Sulfameth. | Higher $V_d$, Higher Cl | Increase dose/frequency |
| Tazobactam | Higher $V_d$, Lower AUC, Higher Cl | Increase dose/frequency |
| ***Antidepressants*** | | |
| Citalopram | Lower $C_{min}$ | Increase dose/frequency |
| Fluoxetine | Lower $C_{min}$ | Increase dose/frequency |
| Paroxetine | Higher $V_d$ | Increase dose/frequency |
| Venlafaxine | Lower C/D ratio | Increase dose/frequency |
| Clorazepate | Lower $C_{max}$, Higher Cl | Increase dose/frequency |
| Midazolam | Higher free fraction, Lower $C_{max}$, Lower AUC | Increase dose/frequency |
| ***Antiseizure agents*** | | |
| Carbamazepine | Higher Cl, Decreased $C_{ss}$, | Increase dose/frequency |
| Lamotrigine | Higher Cl | Increase dose/frequency |
| Levetiracetam | Higher Cl | Increase dose/frequency |
| Oxcarbazepine | Higher Cl | Increase dose/frequency |
| Phenobarbital | Higher Cl, Decreased $C_{ss}$, Lower $t^{1/2}$ | Increase dose/frequency |
| Phenytoin | Higher Cl, Decreased $C_{ss}$, Lower $t^{1/2}$ | Increase dose/frequency |
| Topiramate | Higher Cl | Increase dose/frequency |
| Valproic acid | Decreased $C_{ss}$ | Increase dose/frequency |
| **EXCEPTIONS: Xanthines** | | |
| [§]Theophylline | Increased AUC, Increased $V_d$, Increased $t^{1/2}$, Decreased Cl | Decreased dose/frequency |
| Caffeine | Increased $C_{max}$ and $C_{ss}$, $t^{1/2}$, Decreased Cl | Decreased dose/frequency |

[*] To maintain therapeutic range serum concentrations.

[§] Aminophylline probably follows the pattern of theophylline.

*Abbreviations:* $V_d$: volume of distribution; $C_{max}$: Maximum concentration; $C_{min}$: Minimum concentration; $C_{ss}$: Steady state concentration; AUC: area under the curve; C/D ratio: concentration/dose ratio; Cl: renal clearance; $t^{1/2}$: half-life

*Sources:* Little, 1999; Koren and Pariente, 2018; Dawes and Chowienczyk, 2001; Feghali *et al.*, 2015; Landmark *et al.*, 2018; Pariente *et al.*, 2016.

that cannot be detected with the basic ultrasound four-chamber heart view (e.g., valvular defects, vascular stenosis).

The patient should be advised of the limitations of prenatal diagnosis not only in the constraints on what can be detected (i.e., gross structural abnormalities), but also in its reliability in detecting defects prenatally (ranging from 40 to 90 percent depending on technology and organ system).

## COUNSELING AND EVALUATION OF THE DRUG-EXPOSED PREGNANT PATIENT

Counseling pregnant patients exposed to drugs or other environmental agents during pregnancy is difficult for several reasons. Patient anxiety from fear that their child will be born with birth defects caused by the exposure. Anxiety is heightened because the mother frequently feels guilt, believing she may have damaged her baby through some action for which she is responsible. Cultural beliefs regarding the causes of congenital anomalies often place blame on the mother, and differ dramatically from scientific explanations. Other factors (educational background, socioeconomic status, ethnic-specific folklore) are barriers to communication during counseling. These influences are important to keep in mind when counseling patients of various backgrounds exposed to potential teratogens.

Rapport with the patient is important, assuring confidentiality and establishing a basis for patience. The counselor must convey to the patient his/her understanding of the patient's concerns. The purpose of the consultation is to deal directly with those concerns by ascertaining the magnitude of the risk for an adverse pregnancy outcome arising from the drug exposure.

### GENERAL PRINCIPLES OF COUNSELING

Patients are often unsatisfied with the counseling they receive for exposure to potential teratogens during pregnancy. Dissatisfaction stems largely from two major issues that cause patient anxiety.

1. The physician is frequently unable to obtain adequate information to make meaningful statements regarding the medical risks of whether the pregnancy was adversely affected by the drug exposure.
2. Most patients do not understand the difference between an embryo and a fetus. Consequently, patients may not be able to grasp the importance of the concept of "critical periods" unless they have been given a proper briefing during the consultation.

It is best practice to explain that there are two distinct phases involved in the growth of a baby, as shown in Figure 1.2, and even provide a copy of that figure. Explain to the patient that the first phase is the **embryonic development**.

During this period, the structure or basic architecture for the baby is established. Embryonic age should be differentiated from menstrual age, which is 2 weeks greater than embryonic age. Explain to patients that organs take shape and the body assumes the form it will have thereafter by day 58 post-conception. All major structures (e.g., heart, brain, liver, kidneys, limbs) have formed by this the 58th day of gestation (or 72 days menstrual).

**Fetal development** during the remainder of pregnancy (second and third trimesters), the second phase of development, is primarily devoted to the growth of these organs and structures, and to augmenting their function.

This heuristic approach to counseling helps the patient understand that most congenital anomalies are caused by early exposures, very frequently before pregnancy was recognized. This ameliorates anxiety and guilt. This counseling component is included early in the consultation because patients will understand why accuracy in answering certain questions on timing and exact exposures are important. This knowledge will empower the patient and increase their cooperation and rapport.

Our policy is to provide in writing all the materials discussed, including research on the specific exposure. The patient should leave the consult with a copy of Figure 1.2, the assessment of patient risk including pedigree, and documentation of any known risks (i.e., publications or a TERIS summary).

## PRECONCEPTIONAL COUNSELING

In an ideal world, all counseling regarding drug or medication use during pregnancy should occur before conception. The opportunity to prevent possible adverse effects is before the exposure occurs. Preconceptional counseling should include all the components of a consultation during the pregnancy, with one exception. Recommendations regarding medication or drug use during pregnancy will be *prospective* for a preventive purpose. Only medically indicated medications known to be safe will be recommended for continued use while attempting to conceive, and during pregnancy.

## COUNSELING THE EXPOSED GRAVIDA

Counseling for drug exposure(s) during pregnancy should follow a protocol as outlined in Figure 1.3. Background risk for major congenital anomalies should be explained in a manner tailored to the patient's level of understanding. This concept is especially important because it must be conveyed to the patient that in the absence of any exposure no guarantee can be given that the fetus she carries will not have a congenital anomaly. The risk for major congenital anomalies is estimated to be 3.5–5 percent. Other identified risks are generally considered additive to background risk.

Determination of exactly what drugs were taken, the dosage, the timing and duration of the exposure(s), the patient's health history, and present state of health is obtained through the consult interview. A thorough physical examination should be used to determine the present state of health. In addition, a medical genetic pedigree, including the patient's parents as well as the baby's father's parents, brothers and sisters, and nieces and nephews, should be constructed. Current state of health of all relatives of the fetus in the pedigree should also be elicited. For deceased individuals in the pedigree, cause of death is important to determine, especially focusing on whether death was related to a birth defect or to a heritable disorder. Ask specifically if the patient's family or the baby's father's family includes a member who was mentally retarded, or has a chromosomal abnormality, Down syndrome, congenital heart disease, spina bifida or another neural tube defect, or any other inherited disease. Discovery of risk factors opens avenues that should be further explored. It is may be desirable to refer the patient for a medical genetic consultation and evaluation when a risk increase above background is greater than zero.

The next step in the consultation is to determine whether or not the agent(s) has known teratogenic potential. This is the most difficult part of the evaluation because there is insufficient information to make such a determination for more than 60 percent of medications. The most reliable source of information regarding drug use during pregnancy is TERIS (Teratogen Information System), a computerized database from which summaries may be purchased (Box 1.2). If it is documented that the agent has no teratogenic risks or adverse fetal effects associated with its use during pregnancy, then no further action is required except to document this in the medical record and counsel the patient accordingly. Emphasize that the background risk of birth defects is 3.5–5 percent.

Some patients may benefit from reassurance offered by high-resolution ultrasound to confirm fetal well-being. This procedure should be offered if the patient's anxiety is not relieved through counseling. The limitations of diagnostic ultrasound and other procedures should also be included in the consultation in writing.

If the drug is known not to be safe for use during pregnancy, or if there are reasons to suspect that a drug with unknown risks is associated with congenital anomalies, then estimated gestational age should be confirmed by ultrasound. It is important to **base the risk assessment and counseling upon embryonic age, not menstrual age**. If the exposure occurred during embryogenesis, then it is necessary to undertake high-resolution ultrasound in an attempt to detect damage to specific organ

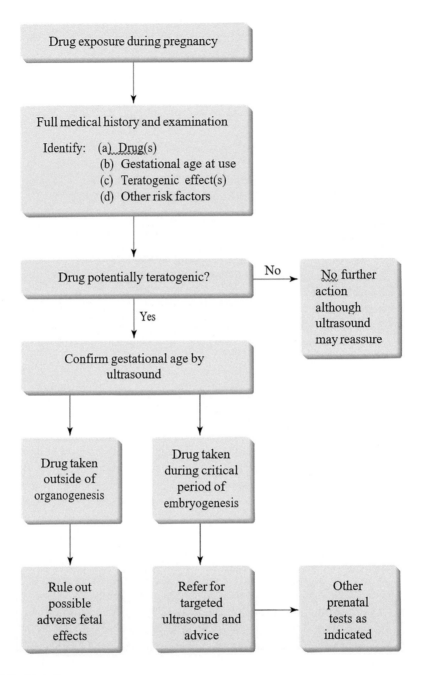

**FIGURE 1.3**   Flow diagram.

systems or structures that were being formed during the time of the exposure. If the ultrasound scan is normal, then it is reasonable to reassure the patient of normal fetal structure within the limits of the sensitivity and specificity of ultrasound, which range from 40 to 90 percent for gross structural abnormalities when the procedure is performed by an experienced sonographer. If the exposure occurred during the fetal period, it is likewise important to evaluate possible fetal effects of the medication (Scwartz *et al.*, 2013; Shroff *et al.*, 2017; Shroukh *et al.*, 2020).

If defects are detected, it is necessary to describe them in detail to the patient and to give a prognosis, as far as available medical knowledge will allow, regarding pregnancy outcome and postnatal development. To assist the patient in making a decision on the disposition of the pregnancy, prognostication should include medically documented risk estimates.

Ethically, pregnancy termination should not be a recommendation made to the patient, her family or significant others. This option may be discussed as one of several possible actions. The ultimate decision of whether to continue the pregnancy should be left to the patient, her family and significant others. The role of teratogen counseling is ultimately to provide the patient with as much information as possible and encourage her to make her own decision regarding whether to continue the pregnancy.

The conversation we have with patients focused on the end goal of having a child. The end goal is to rear a child who will be self-sufficient after parents expire. This context is where parents can think through the long-term consequences of decisions about the pregnancy. Fortunately, these conversations are needed infrequently. Ultimately, this context allows the importance of any theoretical birth defects to be considered. For example, the low empiric risk for a birth defect is certainly not an indication for termination.

**Drug- or chemical-related causes** of maternal complications, congenital anomalies, and fetal toxicity **are unique among adverse pregnancy outcomes because they are potentially preventable**, given the window of opportunity to do so. These complications are also exceptional among obstetric complications in that they are often the focus of malpractice litigation. Attorneys recognize that such adverse outcomes could have been prevented, and litigation ensues despite the fact that the window of opportunity to intervene prudently may not have existed for the physician. More importantly, the drug exposure may not be teratogenic at any time during the pregnancy, but litigation goes forward anyway. This was mentioned earlier as a litogen—it does not cause birth defects but does cause lawsuits, per Dr. Brent.

## FOOD AND DRUG ADMINISTRATION CLASSIFICATION OF DRUGS AND INFORMED CONSENT

Until 1979, most medications were accompanied by disclaimers, the most common of which was that the "safe use in pregnancy has not been established" and that such a medication "should not be used in pregnant women unless, in the judgment of the physician, the potential benefits outweigh the possible hazards" (Brent, 1982). Such disclaimers were given when there existed little to no information upon which to "weigh the possible hazards." Such disclaimers make defense of a litigation case involving a medication extremely difficult for the physician because benefits are not easily weighed against **unknown possible hazards**. With no scientific data relating a specific malformation to a given drug, it is nearly impossible to "prove" in the courtroom that a drug is not a teratogen and is safe for use during pregnancy. Therefore, a jury may be asked to consider the important question of why a physician would prescribe a medication that carried the warning "safe use in pregnancy has not been established." The disclaimer itself implies that a medication may indeed be a teratogen, although the warning is actually little more than legally formulated rhetoric designed to protect the pharmaceutical company (Brent, 1982). Many efforts have encouraged the FDA to (1) change the nature of the labeling on the package insert and (2) change the manner in which drugs are classified with regard to their reproductive risks (Brent, 1982).

In 1979, the FDA attempted to improve labeling policies for the use of medications during pregnancy. Five risk categories (**A, B, C, D, X**) that addressed potential adverse fetal effects, including congenital anomalies, were developed. Although an improvement over the previous labeling disclaimers, the classification is less than perfect (Brent, 1982). In 2015, the FDA discontinued the five risk categories, and will revise the categories to be more informative. These categories have not been published or ascribed to specific drugs as of 2021.

The categories devised by the FDA are "based on the degree to which available information has ruled out risk to the fetus, balanced against the drug's potential benefits to the patient" (*Physicians' Desk Reference*, 2015). FDA categories were intended to provide management guidance for potential teratogenic risks. However, we published a study found that FDA categories have little, if any, correlation to teratogenic risk (Friedman *et al.*, 1990). We compared the teratogenic risk of 157 most frequently prescribed drugs according to TERIS (a computerized database of clinical teratology information) risk rating to the FDA pregnancy categories. It was pointed out that "any classification of agents according to teratogenic risk is incomplete because the risk to a given patient is determined by all of the conditions of exposure." Significant concern must also be given to drug dose, route of administration, and timing of exposure, as well as exposure to multiple agents during the pregnancy (Friedman *et al.*, 1990). The information formerly on the package insert was a joint effort of the FDA and pharmaceutical companies, and fails to provide information about risks that are known. The information does not discuss the option of pregnancy interruption, and provides anxiety-provoking irrelevant information, such as "this drug crosses the placental barrier" (Brent, 1982).

## INFORMED CONSENT AND POST-EXPOSURE COUNSELING

Before initiating informed consent regarding medication exposure during pregnancy, dose, route of administration, and timing must be ascertained as accurately as possible. Even if an agent is a potential teratogen with significant risk of a birth defect or even a proven teratogen such as thalidomide, the actual risk to the fetus may be minimal to none if the timing of exposure occurred during late pregnancy, or after the period of organogenesis. In contradistinction, some teratogens, such as radioactive iodine or the angiotensin-converting enzyme inhibitors may be harmful only after early organogenesis (Brent and Beckman, 1990).

Following a detailed exposure history, the patient should be given "full disclosure" regarding the known or suspected risk(s) of the agent, and various therapeutic and diagnostic alternatives available. This information should be factually accurate, yet easily understandable and tailored to the patient's education level. All information discussed with and provided during counseling should be well documented in the patient's medical chart.

A clinician knowledgeable in both teratology and in counseling should perform all counseling regarding a drug or medication exposure. An authoritative resource such as TERIS or other teratogen information services should be used to provide the patient with the most recent and accurate information on the potential teratogenic effects of a specific agent.

The TERIS summaries are available for a nominal fee by fax from the Department of Pediatrics, University of Washington, Seattle, WA, USA. The contact is Dr. Janine Polifka at +1-206-543-2465. The TERIS website is www.depts.washington.edu/~TERISweb/TERIS.

Experienced counselors may also have their own personal reprint collection dealing with teratogens. We include all such information, especially the TERIS summary in exposure cases, in the patient's chart. It is used as an adjunct in counseling of each exposed pregnant patient. Another source is REPROTOX, available at http://ww.reprotox.org. In additional to TERIS and REPROTOX, information is available from the Organization of Teratology Information Specialists (OTIS). Available at: www.otispregnancy.org.

In counseling, one could also make this statement:

> Although this agent may be associated with an increased risk of malformation when used in the first 8–10 (menstrual) weeks of pregnancy, it would not be expected to be associated with significant risk when given in the latter half of pregnancy.

In the case of an agent such as tetracycline, one might state: "It is logical to conclude that tetracycline would not be expected to cause yellow-brown discoloration of the teeth when given during the first 16–20 weeks of pregnancy."

Another suggested statement would be as follows: "Although the actual teratogenic risk of this agent is unknown, given the dose and route of administration, the fetal risk of this preparation is negligible to non-existent because little to none of it reaches the fetus." Other sources of information regarding the teratogenic risk of specific agents that may be useful in counseling patients, in addition to the present text and TERIS, include Shepard's *Catalog of Teratogenic Agents, Drugs in Pregnancy and Lactation: A Reference Guide to Fetal and Neonatal Risk, Chemically Induced Birth Defects*, and other similar texts.

## SUMMARY

Many patients, as well as attorneys, believe that most congenital anomalies must be secondary to a drug or medication taken during gestation. Counseling these patients requires a significant degree of knowledge and skill. Physicians must appreciate that erroneous counseling by inexperienced health professionals is one of the leading stimuli for non-meritorious litigation (Brent, 1977). The clinician must be aware that drugs and medications represent a bountiful field for litigation. A reasonable likelihood exists that once the family and the attorney have concluded that there is merit to their allegation, they can locate experts who will support the non-meritorious allegation(s). Thus, physicians may focus their attention on attorneys as the cause of the baseless litigation. In reality, non-meritorious litigation could not proceed without the assistance of unknowledgeable or unscrupulous experts who have a degree and qualify under Daubert-Robinson as experts. **Lack of integrity of mercenary experts are a root cause of baseless lawsuits in birth defects cases**. Attorneys and physicians alike call these people with flexible facts and morals whores. Without attacking a specific individual, I should note that experts cited in this volume have given depositions that totally contradict their publications because they were paid handsomely by a plaintiff's attorney to do so. Dr. Brent warned me about the plaintiff's attorneys and manipulation of facts 36 years ago, and his advice was on point then and now.

# 2 Antimicrobials during Pregnancy
## *Bacterial, Viral, Fungal, and Parasitic Indications*

Pregnant women should not be denied appropriate treatment for infection because untreated infections can commonly lead to serious maternal and fetal complications.

(ACOG, 2017)

Antimicrobial use during pregnancy is presented in five sections: antibiotics, antifungals, antivirals, antiparasitics, and a final section on special considerations with specific antibiotic use indications (disease entities), including first-line therapies for each indication:

- Antibiotics
- Antifungals
- Antivirals
- Antiparasitics
- Special considerations

Infections occur relatively frequently during pregnancy with approximately 64 percent of women reporting at least one infection during pregnancy (Collier *et al.*, 2009). Treatment of infections during pregnancy must include a number of treatment considerations because the spectrum of infectious agents (viruses, viroids, prions, bacteria, nematodes) ranges widely in effects (innocuous to severely dangerous) as do the agents used to treat infections that can be harmless to quite damaging to the mother and/or developing embryofetus.

**Management of infection in first trimester of pregnancy**

- Is antimicrobial treatment a medical emergency? *Assess Urgency.*
- Is there a safe alternative to first-line therapy during the first trimester? *Assess Alternatives.*
- Could therapy safely be delayed until after the first trimester? *Weight Benefits and Possible Harm(s).*
- How does pregnancy affect the efficacy and safety of a particular antimicrobial agent(s)? *Evaluate Candidate Regimen Pharmacokinetic/Pharmacodynamics Properties.*
- What do the ***available data*** suggest regarding safety of specific agents during the first trimester? The second and third trimesters of pregnancy? *ABSENCE OF EVIDENCE IS NOT EVIDENCE OF ABSENCE*

The nature and severity (subclinical, clinical grades 1–3) of the infection will drive the clinician's decision when to treat and treatment regimen. Infections such as trichomonal vaginitis or other parasitic infections do not usually require urgent treatment, and therapy may safely begin after the first trimester. In contrast, urinary tract infections treatment should begin upon diagnosis because delayed therapy may have untoward consequences for both mother and fetus.

DOI: 10.1201/9780429160929-2

Ultimately, the 2017 ACOG opinion should be followed (ACOG, 2017). All antimicrobial agents that have been studied cross the placenta, but not all have been studied. Therefore, potential adverse effects are not limited to the mother but extend to the fetus as well. Limited scientific data are available regarding the safety of most antimicrobial agents during pregnancy.

Nonetheless, many of these agents have been used in pregnant women out of necessity. Pregnancy causes physiologic changes that may alter the pharmacokinetics and pharmacodynamics of an antimicrobial agent (Little, 1999). Therapeutically, the most significant pregnancy-associated change is the marked increase in blood volume, increasing to 40–50 percent above the non-pregnant state at term. Increased blood volume begins during the first trimester, with pharmacologically significant increases occurring during the second and third trimesters. There is marked variation from patient to patient in the actual increase in blood volume with a median of 40–50 percent. Additionally, endogenous creatinine clearance is increased, serum-binding proteins are lowered in concentration, and gastrointestinal motility is lower compared to the non-pregnant state. These pregnancy-associated physiologic changes may lower the serum level through increased volume of distribution, altered (usually lowered) metabolism, reduced absorption, and increased clearance. The dose of an antimicrobial usually requires dosage adjustment (increase) during pregnancy to maintain therapeutic levels. For example, β-lactam antimicrobials, fluoroquinolones, and, to a lesser extent, clindamycin cross the placenta. Dose adjustments are usually necessary for the β-lactam antimicrobials and the fluoroquinolones to achieve and maintain therapeutic levels in pregnant women. This is an important consideration in the treatment of certain infectious diseases (e.g., anthrax, syphilis) because the antimicrobial treatment may provide fetal benefit (i.e., protection from congenital infection) in the second and third trimesters of pregnancy (Meaney-Delman *et al.*, 2013).

Pregnancy complications (e.g., hypertension, vascular disease, acute pyelonephritis) may alter "normal" pregnancy-associated physiologic changes, thereby altering drug levels during gestation.

Limited information on pharmacokinetics of most antimicrobial agents during pregnancy is available. A comprehensive review of pharmacokinetics during pregnancy is published (Little, 1999), and Table 2.1 is adapted and updated for antimicrobials.

Serum levels of most antimicrobial agents are reduced during pregnancy, often by approximately 10–15 percent (Landers *et al.*, 1983). For example, serum levels of ampicillin and gentamicin are lower during pregnancy compared to non-pregnant women given the same dose (Duff *et al.*, 1983; Philipson, 1977, 1982; Zaske *et al.*, 1980). Increased blood volume (i.e., increased volume of distribution) is usually the cause of lowered serum drug concentrations, but other pregnancy-associated physiologic changes (e.g., metabolism) also play important roles. For example, lower serum ampicillin concentrations are probably not caused by strong dissociation of ampicillin at physiological pH, which should theoretically interfere with placental transfer. Although ampicillin and methicillin are dissociated, maternal:fetal concentration ratios are 1:1, indicating free transfer across the placenta (Pacifici and Nottoli, 1995).

## ANTIBIOTICS

Antibiotics are commonly prescribed during pregnancy and the postpartum period to treat bacterial infections (e.g., urinary tract infections, chorioamnionitis, endometritis).

### PENICILLINS

The penicillins are bactericidal by virtue of interference with cell wall synthesis. Virtually all the agents in this class cross the placenta, resulting in significant fetal serum levels (Gilstrap *et al.*, 1988a; Landers *et al.*, 1983; Maberry *et al.*, 1990). The ratios of cord blood to maternal blood concentration of several penicillins are shown in Table 2.2.

All penicillins (Box 2.1) cross the placenta. Several recent studies suggested that penicillin and some other antibiotics may be associated with birth defects (Box 2.1).

**TABLE 2.1**
**Pharmacokinetic Study of Antibiotic Agents during Pregnancy: Pregnant Compared with Non-Pregnant**

| | Cl | AUC | Trimester Third T ½ | $V_d$ | Concen. | Pregnancy Dose Adjustment |
|---|---|---|---|---|---|---|
| Amikacin | | | | | = | Monitor levels |
| Amoxicillin | ↑ | | | | | Increase dose |
| Ampicillin | ↑ | | ↓ | ↑ | ↓ | |
| Azithromycin | | ↓ | | ↑ | | Increase dose |
| Azlocillin | | = | = | | | Monitor levels |
| Cefetrizine | | ↓ | | | ↓ | Increase dose |
| Cefazolin | ↑ | = | ↓ | = | ↓ | Increase dose |
| Cefradine (Cephadrine) | ↑ | ↓ | ↓ | ↑ | ↑ | Increase dose |
| Cefoperazone | | | | ↑ | | Increase dose |
| Ceftazidime | ↑ | | | | | Increase dose |
| Cefuroxime | ↑ | ↓ | | | | Increase dose |
| Cloxacillin | | | | ↑ | | Increase dose |
| Flucloxacillin | | | | ↑ | | Increase dose |
| Imipenem | ↑ | ↓ | | ↑ | ↓ | Increase dose |
| Mecillinam (amdinocillin) | | | ↑ | ↑ | | Monitor levels |
| Moxifloxacin | | ↓ | ↓ | ↑ | ↓ | Increase dose |
| Penicillin V | | ↓ | ↓ | | | Increase dose |
| Piperacillin | ↑ | ↓ | | ↑ | ↓ | Increase dose |
| Trimethoprim/Sulfamethoxazole | ↑ | | | ↑ | | Increase dose |
| Tazobactam | ↑ | ↓ | | ↑ | | Increase dose |

Dose adjustment should be made after toxicological assessment of $C_{max}$, and target clinical serum concentrations of the drug. Monitor levels to determine whether or not pharmacokinetic parameters indicate dose adjustment are necessary to maintain therapeutic levels.

**TABLE 2.2**
**Mean Antibiotic Concentration Ratios for Various Penicillins**

| | Antibiotic Cord Blood to Maternal Blood Ratio |
|---|---|
| Ampicillin | 0.71 |
| Ampicillin plus sulbactam | 1.0 |
| Mezlocillin | 0.4 |
| Ticarcillin plus clavulanic acid | 0.8 |

*Sources:* Gilstrap *et al.*, 1988a; Maberry *et al.*, 1990.

**There is no evidence to date that the penicillins are teratogenic,** and they have been used in pregnant women for many years without apparent adverse fetal effects.

Although they are not teratogenic, the penicillins may cause significant adverse effects in the mother, including hypersensitivity reactions, serum sickness, hematologic toxicity, renal toxicity, hypokalemia, gastrointestinal toxicity, and central nervous system toxicity (Box 2.2).

Several investigations recently published analyzed the risks of birth defects after first-trimester exposure to penicillins. However, no pattern of congenital anomalies is apparent (Box 2.2). Given

## BOX 2.1 RECENT STUDIES OF PENICILLIN USE
## IN PREGNANCY AND BIRTH DEFECTS

| Birth Defect Risk | Drug | Trimester Exposure | Cases Exposed | Reference |
|---|---|---|---|---|
| None | Penicillin | First | 9106 | Muanda et al., 2017 |
| None | Amoxicillin | First | 5950 | " |
| Limb deficiency | Penicillin | First | 87 | Crider et al., 2009 |
| Oral clefts | Amoxicillin | First | 144 | Lin et al., 2012 |
| Cleft lip+/-palate | | | | |
| Central nervous sys. | Phenoxymethy Phenoxymethylpenicillin | First | 854 | Muanda et al., 2017 |
| None | Amoxicillin/ Potassium clavulanate | First | 68 | Munda et al., 2017 |

These defects have not been replicated in other studies, including the largest study of penicillin during pregnancy (Heinonen et al., 1977).

## BOX 2.2 POTENTIAL ADVERSE FETAL AND
## MATERNAL EFFECTS OF PENICILLIN

**Fetal effects**

- None known, but fetal penicillin hypersensitivity is a theoretical risk

**Maternal effects**

- Hypersensitivity reactions
- Hematologic toxicity
- Renal toxicity
- Central nervous system toxicity
- Gastrointestinal toxicity

no other complicating factors (e.g., allergy), penicillins should continue to be the mainstay first-line treatment for infections during pregnancy. Until a replicable pattern of anomalies is discovered, the penicillins remain the safest class of antibiotics for use during pregnancy.

The Swedish Registry reported an increased frequency of hypospadias (n = 33) and limb reduction defects (n = 9) among 345 infants exposed to penicillins during the first trimester (Kallen, 2019). Notably, these birth defects were associated with pivmecillinam exposure.

In summary, penicillin antibiotics are not considered an important risk for birth defects (Kallen, 2019).

## MACROLIDE ANTIBIOTICS

Macrolide antibiotics are effective in treatment of a range of aerobic organisms, but have poor activity against most Gram-negative organisms. The major antibiotics in this group are erythromycin, azithromycin, clarithromycin, spiramycin, and telithromycin.

## ERYTHROMYCIN

Erythromycin is bacteriostatic by interfering with bacterial protein synthesis. Unlike most anti-biotics, erythromycin does not cross the placenta well, achieving very low levels in the fetus. For example, erythromycin provides inadequate fetal treatment when given to the mother as prophylaxis for congenital syphilis (see section "Special Considerations" for details). The major preparations are listed in Box 2.3A.

---

### BOX 2.3A   THE ERYTHROMYCINS

- Erythromycin
- Erythromycin estolate
- Erythromycin ethylsuccinate
- Erythromycin gluceptate
- Erythromycin lactobionate
- Erythromycin stearate

---

### BOX 2.3B   BIRTH DEFECTS AND ERYTHROMYCIN ARE LIKELY NOT ASSOCIATED

| Drug | 1st Trimester | 2nd/3rd Trimester | Defects | Source |
|------|---------------|-------------------|---------|--------|
| Erythromycin | 113 | | Club foot | Czeizel *et al.*, 1999 |
| *Erythromycin | 1588 | | Heart defects | Kallen and Olausson, 2003 |
| *Erythromycin | Re-analysis | | Heart defects | Källen *et al.*, 2005 |
| *Erythromycin | Re-analysis | | Heart defects | Kallen and Danielson, 2014 |
| Erythromycin | 1785 | | None | Romoren *et al.*, 2012 |
| Erythromycin | 23 | | None | Cooper *et al.*, 2009 |
| Erythromycin | 46 | | None | Lin *et al.*, 2013 |
| Erythromycin/macrolides | 1789 | | None | Muande *et al.*, 2017 |

*Not replicated in other studies, possible spurious findings (Kallen, 2019).

---

Few reports link erythromycin and congenital anomalies or adverse fetal effects (Box 2.3B). Likewise, few maternal adverse effects (Box 2.4) are reported with the use of this antibiotic during pregnancy, with the exception of gastrointestinal upsets (which may be worse in pregnancy), hyper-sensitivity reactions, and hepatitis (Hautekeete, 1995).

Notably, one study relied on patients' reports of the antibiotic exposure AFTER delivery, and drug exposure was not verified against a prescriber database (Crider *et al.*, 2009). The strength of this study was that it was derived from birth defects registries from 10 states that used a standard-ized protocol and clinical genetic examinations to verify birth defects. In another recent study, drug exposure and timing was validated against a prescriber database, but the birth defect determination was made during the first year of life (Muanda *et al.*, 2017). In a European registry (EUROCAT) analysis, the frequency of atrioventricular septal defects was increased among 119 infants whose

---

**BOX 2.4  POTENTIAL ADVERSE FETAL AND
MATERNAL EFFECTS OF ERYTHROMYCIN**

**Fetal effects**

- None known

**Maternal effects**

- Gastrointestinal intolerance
- Hepatitis
- Hypersensitivity reactions

---

mother used erythromycin during the first trimester (Leke *et al.*, 2021). The association of erythromycin with anencephaly or limb deficiency is unclear because the finding was based upon seven and 14 cases, respectively (Crider *et al.*, 2009).

Importantly, it is possible that associated infection responses (e.g., fever) may be the etiologic agent in the defects observed, and any association with the drug may be spurious.

## AZITHROMYCIN

Azithromycin (Zithromax) is an azalide class antibiotic, similar to the macrolide erythromycin, and is sometimes classed a macrolide. It is an effective for most of the same organisms for which erythromycin is used; Azithromycin is one of the first-line treatments for *Neisseria gonorrhoeae* and *Chlamydia trachomatis* infections.

Azithromycin is well absorbed orally and single-dose therapy is effective for chlamydial infections. This antibiotic was used as single-dose therapy for chlamydial infections during pregnancy without untoward outcomes (Allaire *et al.*, 1995; Bush and Rosa, 1994; Rosenn *et al.*, 1995; Turrentine *et al.*, 1995). It is listed as an FDA category B drug by the manufacturer, and appeared not to cause birth defects (Box 2.4). In a study of 123 first-trimester exposures to azithromycin in the MOTHERISK program the frequency of birth defects was not increased (Sarkar *et al.*, 2006). Among 914 first-trimester exposures to the drug, the frequency of congenital anomalies was not increased (Muanda *et al.*, 2017). Among 914 infants exposed to azithromycin during the first trimester, the frequency of birth defects was not increased (Bérard *et al.*, 2015). The frequency of newborn defects was not increased among 253 infants exposed to azithromycin during the first trimester in the Danish Registry (Andersen *et al.*, 2013). In another study of 234 infants whose mother used azithromycin during the first trimester, the frequency of congenital heart defects was increased (Bar-Oz *et al.*, 2012).

## CLARITHROMYCIN

Clarithromycin (Biaxin) belongs to the macrolide group of antibiotics. Although it is effective against a wide variety of aerobic organisms, it is most commonly used for treatment or prophylaxis against *Mycobacterium avium* complex (MAC) in patients who are human immunodeficiency virus (HIV)-positive. It also has good activity against *Ureaplasma urealyticum* (Reisner, 1996). The manufacturer lists the drug as a category C drug. In one large population-based study, 686 women used clarithromycin during the first trimester, and the frequency of birth defects was not increased (Muanda *et al.*, 2017).

## CEPHALOSPORINS

The drug group "cephalosporins" is probably the most commonly used antibiotics in obstetrics and gynecology. Similar in structure to the penicillins (both contain four-member beta-lactam rings), the cephalosporins also bactericidal and inhibit cell wall synthesis. Cephalosporins are grouped into three sub-classes: First, second, and third generation (Box 2.5).

---

### BOX 2.5   THE CEPHALOSPORINS*

**First generation**

- Cephalothin
- Cephaprin
- Cephradine
- Cefazolin

**Second generation**

- Cefamandole
- Cefoxitin
- Cefotetan
- Cefuroxime
- Cefonicid
- Cefaclor

**Third generation**

- Cefotaxime
- Ceftizoxime (not used with probenecid)
- Cefoperazone
- Ceftriaxone
- Moxalactam
- Cefmenoxime
- Cefmetazole
- Cefuroxime
- Cefixime
- Ceftazidime
- Cefpodoxime proxetil
- Cefprozil
- Cephalexin

* Sometimes given with 1 g probenecid to decrease antibiotic clearance (renal, gut), thus increasing levels.

---

All cephalosporins cross the placenta (Bawdon *et al.*, 1982; Dinsmoor and Gibbs, 1988; Giamarellou *et al.*, 1983; Kafetzis *et al.*, 1983; Martens, 1989). Half-lives ($t_{1/2}$) are shorter and serum levels lower than in non-pregnant women for these antibiotics (Landers *et al.*, 1983). Fetal compartment concentrations for cefotaxime were 35 percent of the mother in one study, and cefotaxime was 100 percent in another study

Among 106 first-trimester exposures to cephalosporin drugs, the frequency of birth defects was not increased (Berkovitch *et al.*, 2000). In a larger study, there was no increased frequency of birth defects of 1,005 infants whose mothers took cephalosporins during the first trimester (Muanda *et al.*, 2017). In a case control study that included 11 infants exposed to cephalosporins during the first trimester, the frequency of anorectal atresia was increased (Ailes *et al.*, 2016).

One study reported cephalosporin use during the first trimester was associated with a statistically significant increased frequency of congenital heart defects (Atrial Septal Defects) among 20 infants exposed during the first trimester (Crider *et al.*, 2009). Animal studies of cephalosporins containing the *N*-methylthiotetrazole (MTT) side chain identified potential adverse fetal effects given to rats at doses 1.5 to 8 times the human dose. Testicular toxicity (failure of seminiferous tubule and spermatozoa development) was observed in male rats exposed during gestation (Martens, 1989). The consequences of this finding for the human fetus is unknown at this time. Most second- and third-generation cephalosporins contain the MTT side chain.

Cephalosporins should be used with caution during pregnancy. Cefoxitin is a second-generation cephalosporin that does not contain the MTT side chain and, at least theoretically, is a better choice when a broad-spectrum cephalosporin is indicated during pregnancy.

Cephalosporins may also have adverse effects in the mother (Box 2.6). In addition, clinically significant bleeding dyscrasias may occur secondary to the MTT side chain, which in turn may cause hypothrombinemia. This complication is reportedly more common with moxalactam, and very uncommon with other MTT-containing cephalosporins, such as cefamandole, cefoperazone, and cefotetan.

---

### BOX 2.6   POTENTIAL FETAL AND MATERNAL ADVERSE EFFECTS WITH CEPHALOSPORINS

**Fetal effects**

- Testicular toxicity[a]

**Maternal effects**

- Gastrointestinal
- Bleeding dyscrasiaa
- Hematologic
- Hepatic
- Hypersensitivity reactions
- Renal

[a] Theoretical risks because these complications have been observed in animal studies only; has not been reported in humans.

---

## TETRACYCLINES

Tetracyclines (Box 2.7) inhibit protein synthesis, are bacteriostatic, and readily cross the placenta. When used in the latter half of pregnancy, yellow-brown discoloration of deciduous teeth are frequent (Kline *et al.*, 1964; Kutscher *et al.*, 1986; Rendle-Short, 1962).

Tetracyclines may also be deposited in the long bones of the developing fetus. However, no scientific evidence is published regarding fetal or neonatal long bone growth effects.

## BOX 2.7   THE TETRACYCLINES

- Demeclocycline (Declomycin)
- Doxycycline (Vibramycin, Vira-Tabs, Dryx, Doxy Caps or tabs, Mondox)
- Minocycline (Minocin, Dynacin)
- Oxytetracycline (Terramycin, Urobiotic, Bio-Tabs)
- Tetracycline (Achromycin)

The frequency of birth defects with exposure to tetracyclines during the first trimester was reported in the Swedish Registry for 2920 infants (Kallen, 2019). This included 1653 infants exposed to doxycycline, 755 to lymecycline, 2 to metacycline, 36 to oxytetracycline, 344 to tetracycline, and 2 to minocycline. The type of tetracycline was not specified in 139 exposures.

The frequencies of heart defects and VSD/ASD were significantly increased in frequency among 2920 infants exposed to tetracyclines during the first trimester (Kallen, 2019).

Tetracyclines may also cause adverse maternal effects (Box 2.8) such as liver toxicity (azotemia, jaundice, acute fatty degeneration, Pancreatitis). As with erythromycin, tetracycline may cause significant gastrointestinal disturbances associated with severe nausea and vomiting.

## BOX 2.8   POTENTIAL ADVERSE FETAL AND MATERNAL EFFECTS OF THE TETRACYCLINES

**Fetal effects**

- Yellow-brown discoloration of the deciduous teeth[a]

**Maternal effects**

- Fatty liver degeneration
- Gastrointestinal intolerance
- Hypersensitivity
- Pancreatitis
- Photosensitivity
- Vestibular disturbances[b]

[a] When given in the latter half of pregnancy.
[b] Minocycline only.

**Tetracyclines are rarely indicated during pregnancy** because of potential adverse fetal effects, **except for penicillin-allergic patients who need treatment for syphilis <u>and</u> for whom desensitization is not available**.

### AMINOGLYCOSIDES

Aminoglycosides interfere with protein synthesis but, unlike erythromycin and tetracycline, they are bactericidal. All aminoglycosides (Box 2.9) cross the placenta.

---

**BOX 2.9   THE AMINOGLYCOSIDES**

- Amikacin (Amikin)
- Gentamicin (Garamycin)
- Netilmicin (Netromycin)
- Streptomycin (Streptomycin)
- Neomycin
- Tobramycin (Nebcin)

---

The Swedish Registry contained only seven infants exposed to aminoglycosides during pregnancy, but none had malformations at birth (Kallen, 2019).

Cord levels of gentamicin concentrations in fetal cord blood were 33, 42, and 62 percent, of maternal levels (Yoshioka *et al.*, 1972; Weinstein *et al.*, 1976; Gilstrap *et al.*, 1988a). Importantly, serum levels aminoglycosides may be sub-therapeutic in the fetus and mother, especially in late pregnancy.

Streptomycin was one of the first aminoglycosides developed and was the primary treatment for tuberculosis for a number of years. Eighth cranial nerve damage of the fetus associated with protracted maternal therapy has been reported (Conway and Birt, 1965; Donald and Sellars, 1981), and is probably a similar risk for streptomycin and other aminoglycosides.

Other than possible congenital deafness linked to eighth cranial nerve damage, no scientific evidence is published to date that the aminoglycosides are associated an increased frequency of birth defects.

Aminoglycosides may cause significant adverse effects in the mother, such as neuromuscular blockade, renal toxicity, and ototoxicity (Box 2.10). Importantly, it may be very difficult to maintain therapeutic levels of aminoglycosides in the mother (or fetus) with usual or standard therapeutic doses, particularly in late pregnancy.

---

**BOX 2.10   POTENTIAL ADVERSE FETAL AND
MATERNAL EFFECTS OF AMINOGLYCOSIDES**

**Fetal effects**

- Eighth cranial nerve damage[a]

**Maternal effects**

- Neuromuscular blockage
- Ototoxicity
- Renal toxicity

[a] Uncommon and not reported for all aminoglycosides.

---

## CLINDAMYCIN

Clindamycin is a derivative of lincomycin, and interferes with protein synthesis. It is a bacteriostatic antibiotic primarily for treatment of serious anaerobic infections, and is used infrequently during pregnancy. Clindamycin crosses the placenta, with the fetus achieving approximately 15 percent of maternal levels in one study (Gilstrap *et al.*, 1988a), and 50 percent of maternal serum levels in two other studies (Philipson *et al.*, 1973; Weinstein *et al.*, 1976).

In one large population-based study in Canada, clindamycin exposure in the first trimester among 380 pregnancies was associated with an increased frequency of major birth defects (musculoskeletal, ventricular/atrial septal defects) (Muanda *et al.*, 2017). In the Swedish registry, 247 infants were born after maternal use of topical clindamycin during pregnancy (Kallen, 2019). In the same registry, systemic use of clindamycin during the first trimester was not associated with an increased frequency of congenital anomalies.

Clindamycin was not teratogenic in laboratory animals (Gray *et al.*, 1972), but as discussed in Chapter 1, animal models are usually poor predictors of human teratogenicity.

In addition, clindamycin is associated with adverse maternal effects, the most serious of which is pseudomembranous colitis (Box 2.11). This latter complication is associated with a toxin produced by *Clostridium difficile* (George *et al.*, 1980).

---

### BOX 2.11   POTENTIAL ADVERSE FETAL AND MATERNAL EFFECTS OF AMINOGLYCOSIDES

**Clindamycin (Cleocin)**

- Gastrointestinal intolerance
- Diarrhea
- Pseudomembranous colitis

**Metronidazole (Flagyl)**

- Antabuse-like effects (disulfiram-like)
- Peripheral neuropathy
- Gastrointestinal intolerance
- Hypersensitivity reaction
- Leukopenia

**Chloramphenicol (Chloromycetin)**

- Aplastic anemia
- Hypersensitivity reaction
- Blood dyscrasias
- Neurotoxicity

---

### LINCOMYCIN

Lincomycin is rarely used in contemporary obstetrics. It is largely replaced by clindamycin in obstetrics and gynecology. The fact that it has been used in the past on large numbers of pregnant women without apparent adverse fetal effects (Mickal and Panzer, 1975) is absence of evidence, which is not evidence of absence. Only one case of exposure to lincomycin was included in the Swedish Registry (Kallen, 2019)

### METRONIDAZOLE

Metronidazole (a nitroimidazole) was first introduced as an antiparasitic and used primarily to treatment trichomoniasis. Later it was discovered to be effective in the treatment of serious anaerobic infections. Use in pregnancy is limited primarily to treatment of trichomonal vaginitis.

Metronidazole interferes with nucleic acid synthesis and causes cell death. It is a small molecule and crosses the placenta, reaching significant concentrations in fetal blood (Heisterberg, 1984).

In one study that included over 1000 women with first-trimester exposure to metronidazole, the frequency of birth defects was not increased (Rosa *et al.*, 1987). The frequency of birth defects in 1387 infants exposed to the drug during the first trimester compared to 1387 control infants (Piper *et al.*, 1993). Among 348 women who used metronidazole during the first trimester, the frequency of birth defects was not increased (Koss *et al.*, 2012). The frequency of congenital anomalies was not increased in a recent study of 412 first-trimester exposures to the drug (Muanda *et al.*, 2017). The findings should be interpreted cautiously because further analyses of the Canadian data associated an increased frequency of spontaneous abortions with first trimester metronidazole use (Muanda *et al.*, 2017). The concern arises because spontaneous abortions are proxies for severe birth defects. Among 228 infants exposed to metronidazole during the first trimester, the frequency of birth defects was not increased (Diav-Citrin *et al.*, 2001). The frequency of birth defects was not increased in the Swedish Registry among 1026 infants exposed during organogenesis (Kallen, 2019).

In animal models, the frequency of congenital anomalies was not increased in in which metronidazole was given at five times the human dose during gestation (Hammill, 1989).

Metronidazole was reported to be carcinogenic in mice and rats (Hammill, 1989) and mutagenic in certain bacteria. Metronidazole has not been shown to be carcinogenic in humans. Because of the tumorigenic effects in animals, however, metronidazole is not recommended for use in the first trimester.

Importantly, this nitroimidazole is the only effective treatment for trichomoniasis. The majority of pregnant women with trichomoniasis infection can be treated with betadine solution or other similar agents until the first trimester is completed. Metronidazole therapy in the second trimester may then begin as necessary.

Metronidazole is excreted in breast milk, reaching concentrations similar to maternal serum (Simms-Cendan, 1996). Adverse maternal effects reported with metronidazole use, include central nervous system manifestation, peripheral neuropathy, gastrointestinal intolerance (nausea, vomiting), and a disulfiram-like reaction associated with alcohol use (nausea, abdominal cramps, headaches). It may also be associated with a metallic after taste (Box 2.11).

## CHLORAMPHENICOL

Chloramphenicol disturbs protein synthesis and is bacteriostatic. It is rarely used today and is not recommended for use in pregnant women, but no scientific evidence suggests that it is teratogenic. The frequency of birth defects was not increased among 100 infants exposed to chloramphenicol in the first trimester (Heinonen *et al.*, 1977). Among 6024 infants whose mothers used chloramphenicol for ophthalmologic indications, no increased frequency of birth defects was found (Thomseth *et al.*, 2015). The 'gray baby syndrome' (cyanosis, vascular collapse, and death) was associated with chloramphenicol in premature neonates given large systemic doses of this drug. Although chloramphenicol does cross the placenta (Scott and Warner, 1950), gray baby syndrome in the fetus or newborn is relatively rare (Landers *et al.*, 1983), and is apparently a dose-related complication. Perhaps the most clinically significant of potential adverse maternal effects (see Box 2.11) is aplastic anemia, which is relatively rare, occurring among approximately one in 100,000 cases.

## SULFONAMIDES

The sulfonamides are analogs of para-aminobenzoic acid, which is necessary for production of folic acid by bacteria, and inhibit folate synthesis (Landers *et al.*, 1983). The sulfonamides (Box 2.12A) are bacteriostatic.

---

### BOX 2.12A    SULFONAMIDES, TRIMETHOPRIM, AND NITROFURANTOIN

**Sulfonamides**

- Sulfisoxazole (Gantrisin)
- Sulfamethoxazole (Gantanol)
- Sulfacytine (Renoquid)
- Sulfamethizole (Thiosulfil)

**Trimethoprim**

- Trimethoprim (Proloprim, Trimpex)
- Trimethoprim plus sulfamethoxazole (Bactrim, Septra, plus many others)[*]

**Nitrofurantoin**

- Nitrofurantoin macrocrystals (Macrodantin)

[*] Folic acid supplementation is recommended.

---

The sulfonamides cross the placenta and reach the fetus, but fetal levels are lower than in the mother (Reid *et al.*, 1975).

Two large studies of sulfonamides during pregnancy have produced different results. In a retrospective case-control study from the US, the frequencies of anencephaly, left side heart defects, coarctation of aorta, transverse limb deficiency, and diaphragmatic hernia were increased among infants born to women who used sulfonamides during the first trimester (Crider *et al.*, 2009). In contrast, no birth defects were increased in frequency among 164 infants born to women who used sulfonamides during the first trimester. An association between sulfonamide exposure during the second trimester and cleft palate was reported (Mølgaard-Nielsen and Hviid, 2012). However, it is unlikely any causal relationship exists, although the authors suggested that an underlying condition may be related to the observed birth defect (cleft palate), but no analysis was done to ascertain whether or not this is the case. Recent analysis of 164 first trimester exposure found no increased risk in birth defects associated with sulfonamide use during organogenesis (Muanda *et al.*, 2017).

Furthermore, ACOG recommends that sulfonamides (and nitrofurantoin) be used during the first trimester only when no other alternative is available. However, second and third trimester use was considered safe (ACOG, 2017). When this class of drugs is necessary for use in pregnancy, folate supplementation should be considered.

Sulfonamides compete for bilirubin-binding sites and, if used near delivery, may cause hyperbilirubinemia, especially in the premature infant, and certain maternal adverse effects (Box 2.12B).

---

### BOX 2.12B    SIDE EFFECTS OF SULFONAMIDES

**Maternal side effects**

- Hypersensitivity
- Photosensitivity
- Blood dyscrasias
- Gastrointestinal intolerance

**Infant side effects**

- Hyperbilirubinemia

## TRIMETHOPRIM

Trimethoprim crosses the placenta.

Older studies reported no increased frequency of birth defects. However, data that are more recent challenge those earlier findings.

In one report of over 100 women treated with a combination of trimethoprim and sulfamethoxazole, there was no increase in the frequency of fetal anomalies (Williams *et al.*, 1969). In another study of 186 pregnant women receiving either a placebo (66 patients) or trimethoprim plus sulfamethoxazole (120 patients), the frequency of congenital malformations was actually lower in the group receiving the antibiotics (3.3 versus 4.5 percent) (Brumfitt and Pursell, 1973). A finding of lower than the control group suggests possible under ascertainment of birth defects.

More recent data from the Denmark health registry on 402 women who took trimethoprim during the 12 weeks prior to conception indicate an approximate doubling in the frequency of specific birth defects (heart, limbs) (Andersen *et al.*, 2013). In contrast, birth defects were not increased in frequency among 6688 infants exposed to trimethoprim during the first trimester (Hansen *et al.*, 2016). Extensive birth defect sub-group analyses were extensively explored possible associations with trimethoprim, but no significant associations were found.

Importantly, trimethoprim is a folate antagonist (at least in bacteria!); it is generally not recommended for use in the first trimester because of the theoretical risk of neural tube defects, although other defects may be associated with folate deficiency. Folate supplementation should be considered if trimethoprim is used.

Like sulfonamides, trimethoprim is associated with several adverse maternal effects (skin rash, gastrointestinal intolerance, and possible hematologic abnormalities).

## NITROFURANTOIN

Nitrofurantoin macrocrystals are used for urinary tract infections during pregnancy. In a case-control study from the US, the frequency of birth defects was increased among 150 infants whose mothers used nitrofurantoin during the first trimester of pregnancy (Box 2.13). Four types of birth defects were increased in frequency: anophthalmia/microphthalmos, heart defects (hypoplastic left heart syndrome, atrial septal defects), cleft lip with cleft palate (Crider *et al.*, 2009). Using the Norwegian health registry, 1,334 women exposed to nitrofurantoin during the first trimester and 979 women in the last 4 weeks of pregnancy, the frequency of birth defects and perinatal complications was not increased compared to controls (Nordeng *et al.*, 2013). In another large study from Canada, no increased frequency of birth defects was found among 874 infants born to women who used nitrofurantoin during the first trimester of pregnancy (Muanda *et al.*, 2017).

### BOX 2.13   STUDIES OF NITROFURANTOIN AND BIRTH DEFECTS

| Birth Defect | First Trimester | Source |
|---|---|---|
| No increase | 1334 | Nordeng *et al.*, 2013 |
| No increase | 874 | Muanda *et al.*, 2017 |
| Increased* | 150 | Crider *et al.*, 2009 |
| Increased** | 2060 | Källén and Otterblad Olausson, 2003 |
| Increased*** | 150 | Ailes *et al.*, 2016 |
| No increase | 76 | Goldberg *et al.*, 2013 |

\* Heart, cleft lip/palate, anophthalmia.
\*\* Heart defects.
\*\*\* Oral clefts.

Meta-analysis was done on 91,115 exposed cases and 1,578,745 controls, and on cohorts of 9,275 exposed and 1,491,933 unexposed infants found that in cohort studies the frequency of birth defects was not increased. However, analysis of nitrofurantoin in case-control studies found an increased frequency of hypoplastic left heart syndrome (Goldberg *et al.*, 2015; Kallen, 2019).

No significant differences in birth weight, head circumference, or body length of the offspring were found among 100 infants born to women who used nitrofurantoin during pregnancy compared to 100 drug-free controls, (Lenke *et al.*, 1983). The frequency of congenital malformations was not reported.

Nitrofurantoin is contraindicated in women with glucose-6-phosphate dehydrogenase deficiency (Powell *et al.*, 1963; ACOG, 2017). This drug crosses the placenta and could theoretically cause hemolytic anemia in fetuses with G6PD enzyme deficiency. However, unpublished experience from a large public hospital of approximately 1,000 pregnant women given nitrofurantoin for urinary tract infections, hemolytic anemia did not occur in either the mother or the fetus. Pneumonitis was reported with this antibiotic, but the association occurs very rarely.

## Vancomycin

Vancomycin is does not belong to any other class of antimicrobial agents with bactericidal and bacteriostatic actions. It is effective for treatment of a wide variety of Gram-positive organisms, including *Enterococci*, *Clostridium-difficile*-associated pseudomembranous colitis, and penicillin-allergic pregnant women for bacterial endocarditis prophylaxis.

No scientific information is available for use of this drug during pregnancy and possible associations with birth defects of other fetal effects. The Swedish Registry included only three infants born after first trimester exposure (Kallen, 2019). However, vancomycin was previously associated with significant maternal side effects, such as nephrotoxicity and ototoxicity. Vancomycin could theoretically result in the same toxicity in the fetus because this drug readily crosses the placenta However, vancomycin use during the second and third trimesters of pregnancy did not produce sensorineural hearing loss or nephrotoxicity in 10 exposed infants (Reyes *et al.*, 1989). The meaning of this small case series is unclear, and does not address possible first trimester effects.

## Aztreonam

Aztreonam belongs to the monobactam class of antibiotics. It is effective in the treatment of aerobic Gram-negative rods or *Enterobacteriaceae*. It is used as an alternative to the aminoglycosides. There are no controlled studies in pregnant humans and aztreonam exposure. Only one exposed infant is included in the Swedish Registry (Kallen, 2019). The manufacturer package insert states that aztreonam was not been teratogenic in several animal models given several times the human dose. Although more based on clinical experience than evidence, a putative advantage of this antibiotic over the aminoglycosides is lack of an association with nephrotoxicity or ototoxicity in the mother or the fetus.

## Imipenem

Imipenem is a carbapenem antibiotic derived from thienamycin. It is usually combined with cilastatin, which inhibits the renal metabolism of imipenem. Cilastatin has no antimicrobial activity. Imipenem is effective against Gram-positive and Gram-negative aerobic and anaerobic organisms. It is often effective as single-agent therapy for polymicrobial pelvic infections in women. No studies of imipenem use in pregnancy and birth defects are published. Imipenem—cilastatin combination was not teratogenic in rats or rabbits, according to the manufacturer package insert. This drug has few indications for use of this very 'potent' antibiotic in pregnant women. Potential maternal side effects include hypersensitivity, central nervous system toxicity, and pseudomembranous colitis.

## QUINOLONES

Ciprofloxacin, norfloxacin, and ofloxacin are fluoroquinolones, and are very effective against the aerobic Gram-negative bacilli. They are thus especially useful for the treatment of urinary tract infections. A range of aerobic Gram-positive organisms is effectively treated with fluoroquinolones, although most anaerobes are resistant. They have also been used to treat *C. trachomatis* and *N. gonorrhoeae*.

Among 549 pregnancies exposed to quinolones during the first trimester, the drugs used were as follows: 318 norfloxacin, 93 ofloxacin, 70 ciprofloxacin, and 57 pefloxacin (Schaefer *et al.*, 1996). Controlling for potential confounding factors, the frequency of congenital anomalies was not increased above background (3.5 percent) for first-trimester exposure to quinolones, except for ofloxacin. However, two of the defects associated with ofloxacin exposure were secondary to prematurity (undescended testicle and inguinal hernia). When the two infants exposed to ofloxacin were excluded from the analysis, the frequency of congenital anomalies was not increased above background.

The frequency of birth defects was not increased in infants born to 42 women who took quinolones during the first trimester (Crider *et al.*, 2009). A recent study (Muanda *et al.*, 2017) found an increased frequency of urinary system defects among 780 first trimester pregnancies exposed to the drug class quinolones.

Analysis of specific agents found an increased frequency of major congenital anomalies in infants exposed to ofloxacin. However, the sample was only six (6) exposed pregnancies of which three (3) had birth defects. This is clarified here because some Internet postings simply state "more birth defects with ofloxacin exposure," and fail to mention that only six total cases were analyzed. In another study of 143 women, 110 of whom were lost to follow-up, who used ofloxacin in early pregnancy, the frequency of birth defects was not increased compared with matched controls (Shin *et al.*, 2018), but it should be noted that no birth defects were reported for any group. Controls should have had ~3.5-percent frequency of birth defects.

Ciprofloxacin exposure during the first trimester in 608 women was not associated with any increased frequency of infants with congenital anomalies. Among 70 pregnancies exposed to levofloxacin during the first trimester, the frequency of infants with birth defects was not increased. First trimester moxifloxacin exposure among 55 mothers was associated with an increased frequency (n=2) of respiratory system defects (Muanda *et al.*, 2017). The study included 37 pregnancies exposed to norfloxacin during the first trimester, and no increased frequency of birth defects. The frequency of birth defects was not increased among 224 infants in the Swedish Registry whose mothers used ciprofloxacin during the first trimester (Kallen, 2019).

Hence, it appears that the drug class "quinolones" does not pose an apparent teratogenic risk given current data on more than 1,300 pregnancy outcomes following first trimester exposure.

The frequency of birth defects was not increased among 948 infants whose mothers took norfloxacin during the first trimester (Kallen, 2019). Norfloxacin was not teratogenic in monkeys dosed during organogenesis (Cukierski *et al.*, 1989). Manufacturer information reports that quinolones may cause lameness or irreversible arthropathy in beagle puppies secondary to lesions in the cartilage (Box 2.13).

### BOX 2.13   POTENTIAL ADVERSE FETAL AND MATERNAL EFFECTS OF QUINOLONES

**Fetal effects**

- None known
- Irreversible arthropathy in immature animals[a]

**Maternal effects**

- Central nervous system toxicity
  - Headache
  - Dizziness
  - Insomnia
  - Gastrointestinal intolerance
  - Nausea
  - Vomiting
  - Anorexia
- Hypersensitivity

This is a theoretical risk for human fetal exposure, but this this class of drugs is not recommended for use during pregnancy. The limited number of serious maternal side effects are summarized in Box 2.13. In addition, approximately 2 percent of pregnant women taking these drugs experienced a reversible skin rash and photosensitivity (Christian, 1996).

Naldixic acid, an early quinolone, was associated with pyloric stenosis (Czeizel *et al.*, 2001), but the relationship is apparently not causal. Data are not adequate to exclude a risk of birth defects following exposure during the first trimester, but it seems unlikely that naldixic acid poses a substantial risk of birth defects. Three quinolones have not been studied during the first trimester of pregnancy: gatifloxacin (Tequin), garebixacin, and gemifloxacin.

### ANTITUBERCULOSIS DRUGS

#### First-Line Therapies

There are several drugs utilized to treat tuberculosis. These are summarized in Box 2.14A. Of 446 pregnancies from 15 studies exposed to rifampin, the frequency of birth defects was 3 to 4 percent, not different from background rate in the general population (Snider *et al.*, 1980). Similarly, the frequency of birth defects was not increased above background over 600 pregnancies exposed to ethambutol and almost 1,500 exposed to isoniazid without evidence of an increase in congenital anomalies (Snider *et al.*, 1980).

---

**BOX 2.14A   POTENTIAL ADVERSE FETAL AND MATERNAL EFFECTS OF RIFAMPIN, ETHAMBUTOL, ISONIAZID, AND PYRAZINAMIDE**

*RIFAMPIN*

**Fetal effects**

- None known

**Maternal effects**

- Discoloration of urine, feces, sweat, sputum, tears
- Gastrointestinal intolerance
- Headache, fatigue, myalgia, fever
- hypersensitivity

### *ETHAMBUTOL*

#### Fetal effects

- None known

#### Maternal effects

- Hypersensitivity
- Hyperuricemia
- Optic and peripheral neuritis

### *ISONIAZID*

#### Fetal effects

- None known

#### Maternal effects

- Gastrointestinal disturbance
- Hepatitis
- Hypersensitivity
- Peripheral neuritis

### *PYRAZINAMIDE*

#### Fetal effects

- Unknown

#### Maternal effects

- Arthralgias
- Elevated liver enzymes
- Gastrointestinal disturbance
- Rash

There is no information regarding the drug pyrazinamide during pregnancy, and CDC guidelines suggest it not be used during pregnancy.

These drugs are excreted into breastmilk, but at low (10–15 percent) levels. Hence, if the infant requires treatment, the baby will need to be treated separately as the mother's breast milk will not provide a therapeutic dose.

It is recommended that pyridoxine supplements be given with isoniazid treatment because this regimen is associated with Vitamin $B_6$ deficiency.

The maternal side effects are also listed in Box 2.14A. *Thalidomide has been used for the treatment of tuberculosis, especially in HIV-infected patients* (Klausner *et al.*, 1996; Peterson *et al.*, 1995; Tramontana *et al.*, 1995; Fourcade *et al.*, 2014). *However, thalidomide is the most potent teratogen should **NEVER** be used in pregnant women or those likely to become pregnant.*

**Second-line therapies:** The second-line therapies are used after first-line therapies fail. Opinions are mixed with respect to information regarding their use in pregnancy. Some are well studied and safe for use during pregnancy, while others are not sufficiently evaluated for their risk of birth defects or untoward perinatal complications (Box 2.14B).

**BOX 2.14B   POTENTIAL ADVERSE EFFECTS OF SECOND-
LINE THERAPIES FOR TUBERCULOSIS**

**Amikacin**

- Electrolyte abnormalities*
- Nephrotoxicity
- Vestibular toxicity/Ototoxicity

**Capreomycin**

- Electrolyte abnormalities*
- Eosinophilia
- Nephrotoxicity
- Vestibular toxicity/Ototoxicity

**Streptomycin**

- Electrolyte abnormalities*
- Giddiness
- Hypersensitivity
- Lichenoid eruptions
- Nephrotoxicity
- Perioral numbness
- Vestibular toxicity/Ototoxicity

* Electrolyte abnormalities include hypocalcemia, hypokalemia, and hypomagnesemia.
*Sources:* Curry International Tuberculosis Center and California Department of Public Health,
2011: Drug-Resistant Tuberculosis: A Survival Guide for Clinicians, Second Edition p. 58–93; Drug
Information Online, 2013: Amikacin. Retrieved August 30, 2013 from www.drugs.com/pro/ amikacin.
html; Lippincott Williams & Wilkins, 2013: Take 5–Z Track Injections. Retrieved August 26, 2013
from www.nursingcenter.com/upload/static/592775/Take5_Ztrack.pdf; Centers for Disease Control and
Prevention, 2003: Treatment of TB.

**Sufficiently studied to be preferred second-line therapies:**
- *Fluoroquinolones*: Not associated with birth defects (see "Quinolones")
- *Amoxicillin/clavulanic acid*: Not associated with birth defects (see "Penicillins")

**Unknown birth defect and side effect risks:**
- Streptomycin and amikacin (limited data suggest an increased risk of congenital deafness
  (streptomycin), but amikacin is not studied during pregnancy
- Capreomycin: Anecdotal association with congenital deafness
- Ethionamide and prothionamide: No studies in human pregnancy
- Cycloserine: No studies in human pregnancy
- Para-aminosalicylic acid: No studies during human pregnancy but animal studies suggest
  embryolethality and ear and limb defects

# ANTIFUNGALS

Commonly prescribed antifungal agents differ by their potential for teratogenicity according to
drug type (-azole versus not) and route of exposure (oral, injection, topical). The most commonly

used antifungals are summarized in Box 2.15. Many of these are for topical application, which is considered a safe route of exposure because minimal systemic absorption occurs. Drugs given in a single large dose seem to pose the greatest risk.

---

**BOX 2.15 ANTIFUNGALS**

- Amphotericin
- Butoconazole
- Ciclopirox
- Clotrimazole
- Fluconazole
- Griseofulvin
- Ketoconazole
- Miconazole
- Nystatin
- Terconazole
- Tolnaftate
- Undecylenic acid

---

One large study of "antifungals" in early pregnancy lumped all such drugs together in analysis of 7,047 infants born to women who has used these drugs during the first trimester (Carter *et al.*, 2008). The frequency of hypoplastic left heart was slightly but significantly increased, but it is not possible to ascribe this finding to any specific drug because of the nature of the authors' analytic methods.

## NYSTATIN, CLOTRIMAZOLE, AND MICONAZOLE

These three agents are utilized primarily for the intravaginal treatment of candidiasis. In at least two recent reports, there were no increases in malformations from their use (Jick *et al.*, 1981; Rosa *et al.*, 1987).

Clotrimazole use during the first trimester by 342 women was apparently not associated with an increased frequency of congenital anomalies (Czeizel *et al.*, 1999).

Oral nystatin use during the first trimester in 106 women resulted in a general finding that the frequency of birth defects was not increased, except for hypospadias (Czeizel *et al.*, 2003).

## BUTOCONAZOLE, TERCONAZOLE, AND KETOCONAZOLE

There are no large studies of the use of these three antifungal agents during pregnancy. Butoconazole is a category B drug, and their manufacturers list the other two as category C. It seems unlikely that these agents would have significant, if any, teratogenic risks.

First trimester use of topical butoconazole among 444 women was associated with no increased frequency of birth defects (Franz Rosa, unpublished). The same unpublished dataset contained 20 first trimester pregnancies that were exposed to ketoconazole, and no birth defects were reported (Franz Rosa, unpublished).

## FLUCONAZOLE

Fluconazole, an azole antifungal similar to ketoconazole, is used for local and systemic fungal infections. It is effective for the treatment of vaginal, oral, and systemic candidiasis, as well as for prophylaxis and treatment of cryptococcal infections in immunocompromised patients (i.e., HIV-infected).

## LOW-DOSE FLUCONAZOLE

Among 60 women who took it during the first trimester of pregnancy, the frequency of birth defects was not increased (Inman *et al.*, 1994).

Four cases of craniosynostosis with radial-humeral bowing and tetralogy of Fallot occurred after repeated high-dose fluconazole for cocci meningitis (Aleck and Bartley, 1997; Lee *et al.*, 1992; Pursley *et al.*, 1996). Importantly, a number of normal healthy children have been born following high-dose fluconazole treatment (Krcmery *et al.*, 1995). First trimester exposure of 226 pregnancies to fluconazole, the frequency of congenital anomalies was not increased (Mastroiacovo *et al.*, 1996). Importantly, fluconazole should not be withheld in HIV-infected pregnant women who require cryptococcal prophylaxis. Maternal side effects may include headache, dizziness, or gastrointestinal upset.

## CICLOPIROX

Ciclopirox is a topical antifungal agent used to treat various dermatophytes such as *Trichophyton* species and *Candida albicans*. No human pregnancy studies of this drug are published. Experimental animal studies (mice, rats, rabbits, monkeys) found no increased frequency of birth defects following oral administration using doses from 13–54 times the recommended human dose. It is a category B drug.

## TOLNAFTATE, UNDECYLENIC ACID, AND TERBINAFINE

Tolnaftate (Tinactin) and undecylenic acid (Desenex) are used for dermatophyte infections such as *tinea pedis* and *tinea corporis*, but are not effective against yeast (Davis, 1995). Terbinafine (Lamisil) is a topical antifungal that is effective against most dermatophytes as well as most *Candida* species (Davis, 1995; PDR, 2018). No reports of these agents being teratogenic are published. These agents are used topically, and it would seem reasonable to classify them as category B agents.

## AMPHOTERICIN B

Amphotericin B, an antifungal agent, is used primarily to treat systemic mycotic infections. No controlled studies of amphotericin B during pregnancy are published. Review of 18 case reports suggested no evidence of teratogenicity of amphotericin B (Briggs *et al.*, 2021).

Potential adverse maternal effects of amphotericin B are summarized in Box 2.16.

---

### BOX 2.16   POTENTIAL ADVERSE FETAL AND MATERNAL EFFECTS OF ANTIFUNGAL AGENTS

*NYSTATIN, CLOTRIMAZOLE, MICONAZOLE,*
*BUTOCONAZOLE, TERCONAZOLE, KETOCONAZOLE*

**Fetal effects**

• None known

**Maternal effects**

• Local irritation

*CICLOPIROX, TOLNAFTATE, UNDECYLENIC ACID, TERBINAFINE*

**Fetal effects**

• None known

**Maternal effects**

- Skin irritation

## *FLUCONAZOLE*

**Fetal effects**

- None known; case reports of skeletal abnormalities

**Maternal effects**

- Headache
- Hypersensitivity
- Liver dysfunction
- Gastrointestinal disturbance

## *AMPHOTERICIN B*

**Fetal effects**

- None known

**Maternal effects**

- Anemia, agranulocytosis
- Hypokalemia
- Hypersensitivity
- Polyneuropathy
- Central nervous system toxicity
- Renal failure

## *GRISEOFULVIN*

**Fetal effects**

- None known (humans)

**Maternal effects**

- Headaches, confusion
- Hepatitis
- Hypersensitivity
- Lcukopenia
- Peripheral neuropathy
- Photosensitivity

*Source:* Adapted in part from the USP DI (United States Pharmacopeial Convention, 2018); PDR, 2018.

## GRISEOFULVIN

Griseofulvin is an antifungal drug effective in treatment of mycotic infections (skin, nails, hair). It is incorporated in the keratin of the epidermis and nails, and is fungistatic (Davis, 1995).

One study included 20 griseofulvin pregnancies exposed in the first trimester, and reported no increased frequency of congenital anomalies. In the same study, the authors sought to test the association of griseofulvin directly by comparing the exposures of 55 conjoined twins, and found no association to the drug (Czeizel *et al.*, 2004). An unpublished cohort of 30 women exposed to griseofulvin during the first trimester reportedly resulted in no increased frequency of congenital anomalies (Briggs *et al.*, 2017).

Rosa and associates (1987) reported two cases of conjoined twins born to mothers who took griseofulvin during early pregnancy. A variety of central nervous system malformations and skeletal anomalies were observed in the offspring of animals treated with several times the human dose of griseofulvin during pregnancy (Klein and Beall, 1972; Scott *et al.*, 1975). Because of these reports, griseofulvin is not recommended for use during pregnancy. The potential maternal adverse effects associated with griseofulvin are summarized in Box 2.16.

## ANTIVIRALS

Commonly used antiviral agents are summarized in Box 2.17. Many of these agents are used to treat life-threatening illnesses.

---

### BOX 2.17   ANTIVIRAL AGENTS

- Amantadine
- Acyclovir
- Cidofovir
- Didanosine (ddI)
- Docosanol
- Famciclovir
- Famvir
- Foscarnet
- Ganciclovir
- Idoxuridine

- Oseltamivir
- Penciclovir
- Ribavirin
- Stavudine (d4T)
- Valacyclovir
- Vidarabine
- Zalcitabine (ddC)
- Zanamivir
- Zidovudine

---

### ACYCLOVIR AND VALACYCLOVIR

Acyclovir, an antiviral drug, is used mainly in the treatment and prophylaxis of herpes simplex infections, and other herpes infections, including varicella. Valacyclovir is the active metabolite of acyclovir, and the use of valacyclovir during pregnancy will have risks similar to those of acyclovir. First trimester exposure to acyclovir was not associated with an increased frequency of birth defects in 1,561 infants (Pasternak and Hviid, 2010). Valacyclovir exposure during the first trimester in 229 pregnancies was not associated with an increased frequency of congenital anomalies. In the same study, 28 first trimester pregnancies exposed to famciclovir resulted in infants with no malformations.

The manufacturer's registry currently contains 712 first trimester acyclovir exposed pregnancies and 14 first trimester valacyclovir pregnancies. They reported no increased risk of congenital anomalies (http://pregnancyregistry.gsk.com/acyclovir.html). In a review of 239 pregnancies in which acyclovir was used in the first trimester (Andrews *et al.*, 1992), there were 47 induced and 24 spontaneous abortions. Of 168 live-born neonates, 159 had no congenital anomalies and of the nine neonates who did, no distinctive pattern of anomalies could be identified (Andrews *et al.*, 1992). The frequency of birth defects was not increased in the Swedish registry, which included 842 infants and 645 infants exposed to acyclovir and valacyclovir, respectively, during the first trimester (Kallen, 2019).

Acyclovir was used during pregnancy to treat varicella pneumonia, disseminated herpes infection, and herpes hepatitis (Johnson and Saldana, 1994; Petrozza *et al.*, 1993; Zambrano *et al.*, 1995). Acyclovir was successfully used during the last 4 weeks of pregnancy to prevent recurrent herpes infections and prevent the need for cesarean delivery (Scott *et al.*, 1996). The potential adverse maternal effects of acyclovir and valacyclovir are summarized in Box 2.18.

---

### BOX 2.18   POTENTIAL ADVERSE FETAL AND MATERNAL EFFECTS OF ANTIVIRAL AGENTS

**ACYCLOVIR AND VALACYCLOVIR**

**Fetal effects**

- None known

**Maternal effects**

- Hypersensitivity
- Acute renal failure
- Hematuria
- Arthralgia
- Gastrointestinal intolerance
- Dizziness
- Insomnia
- Anorexia

**FAMVIR**

**Fetal effects**

- None known

**Maternal effects**

- None known

**RIBAVIRIN**

**Fetal effects**

- Unknown in humans

**Maternal effects**

- Conjunctivitis
- Hypotension

**ZIDOVUDINE**

**Fetal effects**

- None known

**Maternal effects**

- Anemia, granulocytopenia
- Gastrointestinal intolerance
- Headache, dizziness, insomnia
- Agitation, confusion, anxiety
- Hypersensitivity

## *IDOXURIDINE*

**Fetal effects**

- None known (humans)

**Maternal effects**

- Hypersensitivity

## *AMANTADINE*

**Fetal effects**

- None known

**Maternal effects**

- Anticholinergic effects
- Leukopenia
- Orthostatic hypotension
- Gastrointestinal intolerance
- Central nervous system toxicity

## *VIDARABINE*

**Fetal effects**

- None known (humans)

**Maternal effects**

- Hypersensitivity

## ADEFOVIR

This agent is used to treat hepatitis B. It is an FDA category C but no human studies have been published.

## ARBIDOL

Arbidol is an antiviral agent used to treat Zika virus. The viral infection during pregnancy is known to cause multiple congenital anomalies of the central nervous system. In two studies of pregnant rats given the drug at several times the human therapeutic dose, and no birth defects were observed. However, animal models are poor predictors of human teratogenicity.

## PENCICLOVIR (DENAVIR)

Penciclovir is an antiviral cream. The manufacturer states that no systemic absorption occurs following topical application of the drug. However, no studies during pregnancy are reported.

## DOCOSANOL (ABREVA)

Docosanol is a topical cream for the treatment of cold sores. Use by pregnant women has not been reported. The manufacturer states that the drug can be used during pregnancy and breastfeeding.

## EDOXUDINE

Edoxudine is a topical Herpes Simplex treatment that inhibits viral replication.

No human reproduction studies are published, but the manufacturer notes that 49 percent of the topical dose is absorbed systemically.

## ENTECAVIR

Entecavir is an antiviral used to treat hepatitis B. It is classified as category C in the FDA pregnancy risk system. No studies of the use of this drug during pregnancy are published.

## FOSCARNET

Foscarnet is an antiviral used to treat herpes virus infections, including ganciclovir-resistant cytomegalovirus retinitis. It is an FDA category C, and the manufacturer "discourages its use during pregnancy." In rodent and rabbit models given the drug during organogenesis at 1/8 to 1/3 the usual human dose the frequency of birth defects was slightly increased. These results are not usable to evaluate possible teratogenicity because no dose response effect was observed, and the doses were lower than that to which humans are usually exposed.

## FOSFONET

Fosfonet is an antiviral used to treat varicella and herpes simplex virus infections of the eye. It is recommended that the drug be avoided during pregnancy because there are no published data regarding its use in pregnancy.

## IBACITABINE

Ibacitabine is an antiviral drug for topical use. No information is published regarding its use during pregnancy.

## IMIQUIMOD

Imiquimod is an antiviral drug used to treat ano-genital warts and some skin cancers. The topical cream is also used to treat actinic keratosis and superficial cell basal cell carcinoma. No studies are published of imiquimod use during pregnancy. No increased frequency of congenital anomalies was observed after pregnant rats were given up to 8 times the usual human dose during embryogenesis. However, no studies are published of human exposure to the drug during early gestation.

## INDINAVIR

Indinavir is a protease inhibitor antiviral used to treat HIV infection. The Antiviral Registry reported 289 women who used the drug during pregnancy, and the frequency of birth defects was not significantly increased (Antiretroviral Registry, 2018).

## INTERFERONS

The interferons are used to treat a variety of viral infections and immune system modulation. The European Interferon B Registry reported 948 pregnancies that were exposed to interferon B to treat multiple sclerosis, and the frequency of birth defects was not increased above the background rate (Hellwig *et al.*, 2018). However, the timing of drug exposures during the study pregnancies was not reported.

Other interferons have not been studies during human pregnancy.

## GANCICLOVIR

Ganciclovir is a nucleoside analog similar to acyclovir. It has been shown readily to cross the human placenta (Gilstrap *et al.*, 1994; Henderson *et al.*, 1993). Ganciclovir is more toxic than acyclovir, and there is no information regarding its use during pregnancy.

## NEXAVIR

Nexavir is an antiviral used to treat dermatologic conditions. No information about its use during pregnancy in humans or in animals are published, and none have been conducted according to the manufacturer. It has no FDA pregnancy risk category assigned.

## OSELTAMIVIR

Among 44 infants exposed to oseltamivir (Tamiflu) during the first trimester, the frequency of birth defects was not increased (Donner *et al.*, 2010).

## PODOPHYLLOTOXIN

Podophyllotoxin is used to treat genital warts (condylar). It is a topical cytotoxic agent to treatment of genital warts for over 60 years. Review of eight published reports detailed adverse outcomes with podophyllotoxin revealed severe toxicity, resulting in maternal and fetal death (Bargman, 1988). However, the author of the review noted that excessive dosing of the drug may have been associated with large areas being treated (56 cm$^2$ in one case), and increased absorption associated with biopsies or wounds. Nevertheless, safer alternatives exist, and should be first-line treatment.

## RIBAVIRIN

Ribavirin is an antiretroviral drug used to treat hepatitis C. For a number of years animal models that had produced a high frequency of birth defects were the only information regarding this drug during pregnancy. However, a Ribavirin Registry has provided data on 180 live births, but there were only 29 among whom the exposure occurred during the first trimester (Sinclair *et al.*, 2017). There were no defects in the 29 first trimester exposed:

> Based on the patterns of birth defects reported, preliminary findings do not suggest a clear signal of human teratogenicity for ribavirin. However, the current sample size is insufficient for definitive

conclusions, and ribavirin exposure should be avoided during pregnancy and during the 6 months prior to pregnancy, in accordance with prescribing information.

(Sinclair *et al.*, 2017)

### RIMANTADINE (FLUMADINE)

Rimantadine is an antiviral used to treat influenza A. It is an FDA pregnancy category C drug in the old system. No studies of human pregnancies exposed to rimantadine are published.

### SOFOSBUVIR (HARVONI)

Sofosbuvir is an antiviral used WITHOUT ribavirin to treat hepatitis C. It is an FDA pregnancy risk category B drug.

### TENOFOVIR

Tenofovir is an antiviral used to treat hepatitis B infection. The drug was used in 3,715 first-trimester pregnancies, and the frequency of birth defects was not increased (Antiretroviral Registry, 2018). It is reported to account for 15 percent of pregnancies exposed to antivirals.

### TRIFLURIDINE (VIROPTIC)

Trifluridine is used to treat ophthalmic herpes infections. It is an FDA category C drug. The manufacturer reports that it was not teratogenic in rats or rabbits at doses up to 23 times the usual human dose. Systemic absorption of the drug through the eye is reported to be negligible.

## ANTI-HIV DRUGS

### ABACAVIR

Data on the first trimester use of abacavir includes 1131 completed pregnancies from the manufacturer's registry. The frequency of birth defects was not increased compared to population background risk (https://aidsinfo.nih.gov/guidelines/html/3/perinatal/192/abacavir-ziagen-abc-). Fetal drug concentrations are equal to maternal levels, and about 85 percent is excreted into breast milk.

### ATAZANAVIR

This agent (atazanavir) is a protease inhibitor used to treat HIV. 1309 women used Atazanavir during the first trimester, and the frequency of birth defects was not increased (http://pregnancyregistry.gsk.com). The drug was not teratogenic in rabbits and rats given the usual therapeutic dose during pregnancy.

### ATRIPLA

Atripla is an anti-HIV agent that combines efavirenz, emtricitabine, and tenofovir disoproxil fumarate. Please see individual agents for information on use during pregnancy.

### CIDOFOVIR (VISTIDE)

Cidofovir is a nucleoside used to treat cytomegalovirus in HIV patients. It is an FDA category C. This drug was associated with adverse effects in male offspring following exposure to cidofovir during gestation that are associated with infertility. The manufacturer states that the drug is teratogenic and carcinogenic in experimental animals.

## COMBIVIR

This agent is a combination of lamivudine and zidovudine. Please see individual agents for pregnancy risk summary.

## COBICISTAT (TYBOST, COBI)

Cobicistat is used to treat HIV, It does not itself have anti-HIV properties, but when administered with other drugs it can enhance their activity. For example, it increases elvitegravir levels, and has a similar effect on protease inhibitors. It is also co-administered with darunavir for similar purposes.

## DOLUTEGRAVIR

Dolutegravir is an anti-HIV drug. In 116 women who used the drug during pregnancy, there was no significant increase in the frequency of congenital anomalies (Antiretroviral Registry, 2018). Among 426 women in Botswana who took dolutegravir during the first trimester, there were four neural tube defects (Crawford *et al.*, 2020). In another 396 women who used the drug with efavirenz (another anti-HIV agent), there were no neural tubes defects, and no increased frequency of congenital anomalies.

## DARUNAVIR

Darunavir is a protease inhibitor. The frequency of birth defects was not increased among 496 women who took the drug during the first trimester (Antiretroviral Registry, 2018). The registry data is sufficient to rule out a more than twofold increase in the rate of birth defects.

## DELAVIRDINE (RESCRIPTOR)

This drug is a non-nucleoside reverse transcriptase inhibitor that is indicated for the treatment of HIV-1 infection in combination with at least two other active antiretroviral agents. Delavirdine lowers viral titer in an attempt to minimize HIV comorbidities (e.g., Kaposi's sarcoma). It is an FDA pregnancy category C drug in the old system. The registry is actively collecting patients exposed to this drug during pregnancy. Currently, only 10 infants have been born following first trimester exposure, one of whom had a birth defect that was corrected surgically.

The drug was embryotoxic and teratogenic at doses several times that used in humans.

## DIDANOSINE

Didanosine is a nucleoside analog that is used to treat HIV. It was used in the first trimester by 427 women, and there was no increased frequency of birth defects, although it was slightly elevated (4.68 percent) compared to the CDC rate (2.7 percent) (Antiretroviral Registry, 2018). The NIH states that this drug is "not recommended for pregnant women (aidsinfo.nih.gov). The drug was not teratogenic in experimental animals given 12 to 14 times the usual human dose.

## DOLUTEGRAVIR

Dolutegravir is an anti-HIV agent that functions by binding to and blocking sites on the virus necessary for viral replication. The Antiviral Registry reported 258 infants born after first trimester exposure to dolutegravir; no increased frequency of birth defects was observed (Antiretroviral Registry, 2018). Concern for the risk of neural tube defects has been raised because among 426 who took the drug during the first trimester because the rate was approximately nine times the expected rate. Other prior studies of 116 and 396 women who took the drug in the first trimester, and there was no increased frequency of birth defects. There is concern raised by the FDA and WHO that this drug is not safe for use in pregnancy:

> Pending availability of additional data, it would be prudent to avoid the use of dolutegravir (either in ART or PEP) regimens for women who are planning pregnancy or may become pregnant (note that this applies to cis-gender women and also to trans men who may be planning pregnancy). For pregnant women who are taking dolutegravir, there is no need to stop dolutegravir.

(http://hivinsite.ucsf.edu/insite?page=hmq-2018-05-22)

## Efavirenz

Efavirenz is a non-nucleoside reverse transcriptase inhibitor used to treat HIV. Among 1040 infant born after first trimester exposure to Efavirenz there was no increased frequency of birth defects (Antiretroviral Registry, 2018). However, the drug carries a warning that neural tube effects have been observed in human infants and offspring of animals; treat with Efavirenz during organogenesis. Importantly, non-human primates who were given the drug at concentrations similar to the human therapeutic dose had a 15-percent rate of neural tube defects.

## Emtricitabine (Truvada)

Emtricitabine is a nucleoside analog. It is always used with another therapy for the treatment of HIV infection. The Antiretroviral Registry reported 2,785 infants born to women who used the drug during the first trimester of pregnancy, and the frequency of birth defects was not increased (Antiretroviral Registry, 2018). Among 552 women who took Emtricitabine during the first trimester, the frequency of birth defects was not increased above controls (Sibiude *et al.*, 2014).

## Enfuvirtide (Fuzeon)

Enfuvirtide is a member of a new approach to HIV because it blocks the ability of HIV to penetrate cells. No data are published regarding the use of the drug during pregnancy. However, enfuvirtide is an FDA pregnancy risk category B, suggesting it is probably safe for use in pregnancy.

## Elvitegravir (EVG)

An integrase inhibitor, elvitegravir is used to treat HIV infection. 213 women used it during the first trimester (Antiretroviral Registry, 2018). The frequency of congenital anomalies was not increased above background (www.apregistry.com/forms/interim_report.pdf).

## Famciclovir

Famciclovir inhibits viral DNA polymerase by competing with it for a substrate (deoxyguanosine triphosphate). The drug is an FDA pregnancy risk category B. It was tested in experimental animals and no birth defects were observed.

## FOSAMPRENAVIR

Fosamprenavir is a prodrug of amprenavir and protease inhibitor used to treat HIV. It is an FDA pregnancy category C drug, and not recommended for use during pregnancy. The Antiviral Registry reports 109 infants born to women who use the drug during the first trimester of pregnancy, and the frequency of birth defects was not increased (Antiretroviral Registry, 2018).

## LAMIVUDINE

More than 5,300 infants have been born after first-trimester exposure to lamivudine, and the frequency of birth defects was not increased (www.apregistry.com/forms/interim_report.pdf).

## LOPINAVIR

Lopinavir is a protease inhibitor used, in combination with ritonavir, for the treatment of HIV-infected women to prevent vertical transmission of HIV. An aggregate analysis of 10 published studies included 2,800 pregnancies exposed to lopinavir reported no increased frequency of birth defects. One study of 267 women who used the drug during the first trimester, the frequency of birth defects was not increased (Roberts *et al.*, 2009). In another study, 270 women used lopinavir during the first trimester, and the frequency of congenital anomalies was not increased (Shapiro *et al.*, 2010). The Antiretroviral Pregnancy Registry reported 1,418 first trimester exposure to lopinavir and the frequency of birth defects was not increased (Antiretroviral Registry, 2018).

## MARAVIROC

Maraviroc is a biguanide antiretroviral drug that is a CCR5 receptor antagonist. One study reported 18 infants whose mothers took the drug during the first trimester and had no birth defects (Antiretroviral Registry, 2018). It is an FDA pregnancy category B drug.

## MOROXYDINE

Moroxydine is an antiviral drug used for to treat viral infections, including influenza. It is a category C drug according to the FDA pregnancy risk category classification. Among 13 infants exposed to moroxydine during the second and third months of pregnancy, two infants had major congenital anomalies, including one case of anencephaly (Czeizel *et al.*, 2006).

## METHISAZONE (MARBORAN)

Methisazone is a thiosemicarbazone antiviral drug that is effective in the treatment of poxviruses. It is only about 40 percent effective against smallpox. The drug was given at several times the human dose to pregnant rabbits and mice, and no increased frequency of birth defects was shown (Grosenbach *et al.*, 2011).

## NELFINAVIR

Nelfinavir is an antiretroviral drug used to treat HIV infections. 1212 women used it during the first trimester of pregnancy, and the frequency of birth defects was not increased in offspring (Antiretroviral Registry, 2018). It is an FDA pregnancy risk category B drug.

## NEVIRAPINE (VIRAMUNE)

Nevirapine is a non-nucleoside reverse transcriptase inhibitor used to treat HIV. 1148 women used it during the first trimester of pregnancy, and there was no increased frequency of birth defects in babies born (Antiretroviral Registry, 2018). In one study of nevirapine in 1229 pregnant women was associated with a low (<15 percent) rate of liver toxicity, but in an adjusted model the risk was not significantly related to the drug (Ouyang *et al.*, 2009).

## PERAMIVIR

Peramivir is an antiviral used to treat influenza B. It has not been studied during human pregnancy. In pregnant rats, peramivir given by continuous infusion resulted in an increased frequency of renal anomalies (reduced renal papilla and dilated ureters). In rabbits, developmental toxicity (abortion or premature delivery) was increased with exposure during organogenesis at exposures eight times the usual human dose.

## PLECONARIL

Pleconaril is used to treat severe enterovirus, rhinovirus, and other common viral infections. No information has been published regarding the use of this drug during pregnancy.

## RALTEGRAVIR (ISENTRESS)

Raltegravir is an integrase inhibitor used to treat HIV. Among 312 infants whose mothers took raltegravir during the first trimester of pregnancy, the frequency of birth defects was not increased (Antiretroviral Registry, 2018). Notably, the pharmacokinetics of this drug during pregnancy are not sufficiently altered to warrant any dose change, suggesting the regimen dose may remain constant during gestation without loss of efficacy (Blonk *et al.*, 2015).

## REMDESIVIR

Remdesivir is used to treat COVID-19 symptomatic infection, and is sometimes used with other antivirals and/or corticosteroids, usually dexamethasone. In three patients with COVID-19 infection who were treated with remdesivir (two at 25 weeks gestation, one at 34 weeks), the outcome was healthy infants born of mothers in good health (Igbinosa *et al.*, 2020). It is uncertain whether the drug was causally related to the outcome.

## RITONAVIR (NORVIR)

Ritonavir is an antiviral used to treat HIV. A total of 3,155 women used it in the first trimester of pregnancy and the frequency of birth defects was not increased (Antiretroviral Registry, 2018). It appears to have minimal placental transfer at about 5 percent.

## SAQUINAVIR (INVIRASE, SQV)

Saquinavir is a protease inhibitor used to treat HIV infection. It is an FDA pregnancy risk category B drug. The Antiretroviral Registry reported 182 first trimester pregnancies exposed to saquinavir, and the frequency of birth defects was not significantly increased (Antiretroviral Registry, 2018). The Registry states that the sample is not sufficiently large to exclude a possible effect from its use during pregnancy. However, if an effect exists, it must be small.

## SOFOSBUVIR (HARVONI)

Sofosbuvir is an antiviral used WITHOUT ribavirin to treat hepatitis C. It is an FDA pregnancy risk category B drug.

## STAVUDINE

Stavudine is a nucleoside analog reverse transcriptase inhibitor used to treat HIV infection. Among 811 first trimester pregnancies exposed to stavudine, the frequency of birth defects in infants was not increased (Antiretroviral Registry, 2018).

## TIPRANAVIR (APTIVUS, TPV)

Tipranavir is a protease inhibitor used to treat HIV. It is an FDA category C drug. The Antiretroviral Registry included only 13 first trimester pregnancies exposed to tipranavir; none of the infants had congenital anomalies (Antiretroviral Registry, 2018).

## TRIFLURIDINE (VIROPTIC)

Trifluridine is used to treat ophthalmic herpes infections. It is an FDA category C drug. The manufacturer reports that it was not teratogenic in rats or rabbits at doses up to 23 times the usual human dose (Antiretroviral Registry, 2018). Systemic absorption of the drug through the eye is reported to be negligible.

## TROMANTADINE

Tromantadine is an antiviral used to treat herpes infections by interrupting early and late cycle in replication by changing the viral glycoproteins coating. It is used topically. Systemic absorption is unknown.

## VALACYCLOVIR (VALTREX)

Valacyclovir is an active metabolite of acyclovir use to treat herpes infections. It is an FDA category B drug. Among 229 infants born to women who used valacyclovir during pregnancy the frequency of birth defects was not increased (Pasternak and Hviid, 2010). In the Swedish Registry, the frequency of birth defects was not increased among 645 infants whose mothers took valacyclovir during the first trimester (Kallen, 2019).

## VALGANCICLOVIR (VALCYTE)

Valganciclovir is used to prevent CMV infection in those with HIV infection. It is an FDA category C drug. The manufacturer reported that rabbits given this drug during organogenesis at 2 times the usual human dose had offspring with an increased frequency of birth defects. The manufacturer advises against use during pregnancy citing a possible risk of birth defects.

## ZALCITABINE (HIVID)

Zalcitabine is used to treat HIV infection. The Antiretroviral Registry included 41 first trimester exposures to this drug (as a component of a polypharmacy regimen), and the frequency of birth defects was not increased in infants (Antiretroviral Registry, 2018). However, this sample is too small to exclude a possible risk of birth defects.

## Zanamivir (Relenza)

Zanamivir is an antiviral used to treat influenza. Among 180 first trimester pregnancies exposed to zanamivir, the frequency of birth defects in infants was not increased (Dunstan *et al.*, 2014). It is an FDA category C drug.

## Zidovudine (AZT)

Zidovudine (Retrovir) was the first anti-human immunodeficiency virus (HIV) drug, and is a thymidine analog that inhibits viral replication by inhibiting DNA synthesis. The drug is used mainly in treatment of the acquired immunodeficiency syndrome (AIDS). It may also be used as a 'prophylactic agent' to delay the onset of clinical disease or after accidental exposure to the HIV. Zidovudine was not teratogenic in human or animal studies. Some of the maternal side effects secondary to the drug are difficult to distinguish from those caused by the disease process itself. The antepartum (as early as 14 weeks gestation) and intrapartum prophylactic use of this agent is currently recommended to reduce the frequency of perinatal HIV transmission to the fetus (ACOG, 1994). The risk of fetal HIV infection is substantially reduced in women carrying this virus who are treated with zidovudine during pregnancy (Lyall *et al.*, 2001; Minkoff *et al.*, 2001; Mofenson *et al.*, 2002; Mueller and Pizzo, 2001; Watts, 2001). Zidovudine seems unlikely to be associated with an increased risk of congenital anomalies and should be given for the treatment of HIV in pregnancy. First trimester exposure to zidovudine was not associated with an increased frequency of congenital anomalies in 88, 73, 1932 and 1391 infants (Kumar *et al.*, 1994; White *et al.*, 1997; Newschaffer *et al.*, 2000; Watts *et al.*, 2004). In one analysis, hypospadias was increased in frequency (7/382 exposed male infants), but other studies have not replicated this finding (Watts *et al.*, 2007).

## OTHER ANTI-HIV DRUGS

Other anti-HIV drugs include nucleoside/nucleotide reverse transcriptase inhibitors (zalcitabine, tenofovir), protease inhibitors (amprenavir, indinavir, saquinavir, fosamprenavir, ritonavir, darunavir, atazanavir, nelfinavir), and non-nucleoside reverse transcriptase inhibitors (delavirdine, efavirenz, nevirapine). A new type of anti-HIV drug is the "entry inhibitors" that block HIV virus entry into the cell, and there is one currently available: enfuvirtide.

None of these drugs has been adequately studied during human pregnancy, but the life-saving benefit of their use clearly outweighs any theoretical risk.

## Idoxuridine

Idoxuridine is an ophthalmic antiviral agent used primarily for the treatment of herpes simplex eye infections. No adequately controlled scientific studies in humans are published. Idoxuridine was associated with both eye and skeletal malformations in the offspring of pregnant rabbits who received this local antiviral agent in usual human doses (Itoi *et al.*, 1975).

## Amantadine

Amantadine is an antiviral agent used in the treatment and prophylaxis of influenza. No adequately controlled human studies are published. However, this particular agent was not shown to be teratogenic in rats or rabbits. Amantadine is rarely indicated for use during pregnancy. It was reported that one of four fetuses exposed to amantadine had tetralogy of Fallot (Pandit *et al.*, 1994).

### VIDARABINE

Vidarabine is a DNA inhibitor used systemically to treat disseminated herpes simplex infections and locally to treat herpetic ophthalmic infections. There are no adequate human studies available. However, Schardein *et al.* (1977) and Kurtz and associates (1977) reported congenital anomalies in rats given several times the usual human dose. Hillard and colleagues (1982) reported on the use of this drug late in pregnancy for disseminated herpes simplex infections.

### OTHER ANTIVIRALS

Other antivirals (cidofovir, docosanol, famciclovir, penciclovir, foscarnet, valganciclovir, oseltamivir, zanamivir) have not been studied during pregnancy, or assessed for the possible association with birth defects following use during the first trimester.

## ANTIPARASITICS

Parasitic infections are common during pregnancy, but therapy (with a few exceptions) can usually be withheld until after pregnancy since many such infections are mild and asymptomatic. Metronidazole, the only effective antiparasitic agent for trichomoniasis, was discussed earlier. Pediculicides
    Lice (*Pediculosis pubis*) and mite (scabies) infestations during pregnancy require therapy. Several agents are available, summarized in Box 2.19.

---

**BOX 2.19   PEDICULICIDES**

- Lice infestation
- Lindane (Kwell, Scabene)
- Pyrethrins and piperonyl butoxide (RID, A-200)
- Mite infestations
  - Crotamiton (Eurax)
  - Lindane (Kwell, Scabene)
  - Sulfur (6 percent) in petrolatum

---

Lindane (cream, lotion, or shampoo) is the most commonly used agent for both mites and lice. According to its manufacturer, lindane was not teratogenic in a variety of animals, although there are no adequate human reproduction studies. Lindane may be related to an increase in stillbirths in some animal studies (Faber, 1996). However, lindane may be absorbed systemically, which on rare occasions may lead to central nervous system toxicity (Feldman and Maibach, 1974; Orkin and Maibach, 1983). Although this adverse effect could also theoretically occur in the fetus, it would appear to be very unlikely and to date has not been reported. There is no information to suggest that any of the other agents listed in Box 2.19 cause adverse fetal effects, and thus all are apparently safe for use during pregnancy.

### CROTAMITON

Crotamiton is a topical scabicide and antipruritic agent. About 1 percent of topically applied dose is absorbed systemically. No studies of the use of this drug in pregnancy are published. It is an FDA category C drug.

### IVERMECTIN

Ivermectin is an oral medication used to treat a number of parasitic infestations (head lice, scabies, river blindness (onchocerciasis), strongyloidiasis, trichuriasis, lymphatic filariasis). Among

343 infants born after exposure to ivermectin, the frequency of birth defects was not increased (Gyapong *et al.*, 2003). In studies of pregnant rabbits at doses sufficiently high to produce maternal toxicity, an increased frequency of congenital anomalies occurred (cleft palate, exencephaly, clubbed forepaws). Other agents are usually used before turning to an agent such as ivermectin of which little is known. Alternatives such as permethrin are better documented for use during pregnancy. It is an FDA category C drug.

## LINDANE

Lindane is available in the US, but is unavailable in many countries. Among Michigan Medicaid recipients, 1417 infants were born following first trimester maternal use of topical lindane among whom the frequency of birth defects was not increased (Rosa, unpublished data; Briggs *et al.*, 2017). Published warnings include that lindane should be avoided during pregnancy because of potential maternal toxicity associated, and should be avoided during gestation. It is a category C drug. This seems to contradict the information about Lindane cited earlier.

## MALATHION

Animal studies failed to show evidence of teratogenicity or gross fetal abnormalities. A cohort of 22,465 infants born to mothers exposed to aerial malathion spraying in the first trimester did not have an increased risk of congenital malformations (Gerther *et al.*, 1987). It is an FDA pregnancy category B agent.

Malathion should be used only after other safer alternatives have been used (such as mechanical louse extraction treatment or permethrin). Malathion use should be restricted to aqueous solution instead of alcohol solution to minimize absorption.

## PERMETHRIN (LYCLEAR)

Permethrin is a scabicide used topically as a cream (4 percent). Approximately 2 percent of the topical dose is absorbed systemically. According to the manufacturer, animal teratology studies did not indicate teratogenic potential. Of 106 pregnant women exposed to permethrin in the first trimester, and there was no increased frequency of congenital anomalies (Kennedy *et al.*, 2005). Among 185 infants exposed during the first trimester of pregnancy, the frequency of birth defects was not increased (Mytton *et al.*, 2007). Permethrin is considered the first-line agent for topical treatment of parasitic infections. It is an FDA category B drug.

## PRECIPITATED SULFUR POWDER

Sulfur is used to treat initial and recurrent scabies infestations. Less than 2 percent of topical sulfur is systemically absorbed. There is limited information on safe use in human pregnancies. Due to its low systemic absorption and no reported cases of adverse outcomes, topical sulfur is not expected to cause fetal harm. First-line medications such as permethrin should be used before sulfur. It is a category C agent.

## SPINOSAD

Spinosad is a topical mixture of pediculicidal tetracyclic macrolides. Spinosad reached non-detectable systemic concentrations of the agent after topical application because it is poorly absorbed through the skin, and is rapidly metabolized and excreted. No human studies are published of spinosad exposure during pregnancy. Animal studies using oral spinosad were negative for teratogenic effects. It is an FDA category B agent.

## ANTHELMINTICS

Several anthelmintics are available to treated infested women, although it is usually not necessary to treat helminth infections during pregnancy. Both mebendazole (Vermox) and thiabendazole (Mintezol) are effective for a variety of helminths, including pinworms (enterobiasis), whipworm (trichuriasis), roundworm (ascariasis), and hookworm (uncinariasis). According to their manufacturer, none of these drugs was teratogenic in laboratory animals, although there are no adequate human reproduction studies.

Pyrantel pamoate (Antiminth) is used primarily for the treatment of roundworm and pinworm. It may also be of use in treatment of whipworm infestations. Although this agent has not been shown to be teratogenic in animals, there are no adequate studies in humans.

## ANTIMALARIALS

The two major antimalarial drugs are chloroquine and quinine. Chloroquine is the primary drug used for the treatment of malaria, as well as for chemoprophylaxis in pregnant women who must travel to endemic areas (Diro and Beydoun, 1982). Although there have been no studies of infants whose mothers were treated for malaria during pregnancy with chloroquine, one study reported no increased frequency of congenital anomalies among 169 infants whose mothers received weekly low doses of the drug for malaria prophylaxis during pregnancy (Wolfe and Cordero, 1985). Quinine is used primarily for chloroquine-resistant falciparum malaria. Although there are no large studies regarding its use during pregnancy, increased malformations have been reported when large doses were used to attempt abortion (Nishimura and Tanimura, 1976). Quinine sulfate tablets have also been utilized for leg cramps, but their efficacy is unproven. Although not recommended for the treatment of leg cramps during pregnancy, the antimalarial quinines should not be withheld in the seriously ill pregnant woman with chloroquine-resistant malaria.

## PYRIMETHAMINE, SPIRAMYCIN, AND SULFADIAZINE

These agents are used primarily to treat toxoplasmosis. Pyrimethamine, a folic acid antagonist, is also used to treat malaria. There are no adequate scientific studies of its use during pregnancy, but Hengst (1992) reported no increase in the malformation rate in 64 newborns whose mothers had taken this drug during the first half of pregnancy. Spiramycin has been used extensively in Europe during the first trimester with no apparent adverse fetal effects. Sulfadiazine, a sulfonamide, has not been reported to be teratogenic when used in the first trimester. However, as with all sulfonamides, it could potentially be related to hyperbilirubinemia in the newborn, especially in the premature infant.

# SPECIAL CONSIDERATIONS

There is a paucity of information regarding the most efficacious and safe antimicrobial regimens for the treatment of specific infection-related conditions during pregnancy (Table 2.3). The recommendations given in this section are derived from the author's experience or opinion.

## URINARY TRACT INFECTIONS

Urinary tract infections are among the most common infections encountered in pregnant women (Duff, 1993). For example, asymptomatic bacteriuria occurs in 2–10 percent of all pregnant women (Whalley, 1967). The Enterobacteriaceae or enteric group of organisms causes the majority of these infections, with *Escherichia coli* being the single most commonly isolated organism. Although it is often not necessary to treat these infections in non-pregnant women, it is of paramount importance

**TABLE 2.3**

**Summary of Antimicrobial Drugs: Teratogen Information System (TERIS) and Old Food and Drug Administration (FDA)**

| | Risk Estimates | |
|---|---|---|
| **Drug** | **TERIS Risk** | **Old FDA Risk Rating** |
| Acyclovir | Topical: undetermined | B |
| *Systemic: Unlikely* | | |
| Amantadine | Undetermined | C |
| Amoxicillin | Unlikely | B |
| Amphotericin B | Undetermined | B |
| Ampicillin | None | B |
| Azithromycin | Undetermined | B |
| Aztreonam | Undetermined | B |
| Butoconazole | Undetermined | C |
| Cefamandole | Undetermined | B |
| Cefixime | Undetermined | B |
| Chloramphenicol | Unlikely | C |
| Chloroquine | Daily therapeutic dose: minimal | C |
| *Weekly prophylactic dose: None to minimal* | | |
| Ciclopirox | Undetermined | B |
| Ciprofloxacin | Unlikely | C |
| Clarithromycin | Undetermined | C |
| Clindamycin | Undetermined | B |
| Clotrimazole | Unlikely | B |
| Erythromycin | None | B |
| Famvir | | B |
| Fluconazole | Undetermined | C |
| Gentamicin | Undetermined | C |
| Griseofulvin | Undetermined | C |
| Idoxuridine | Undetermined | C |
| Imipenem/cilastatin | Undetermined | C |
| Ketoconazole | Undetermined | C |
| Lindane | Undetermined | B |
| Metronidazole | None | B |
| Nitrofurantoin | Unlikely | B |
| Norfloxacin | Unlikely | C |
| Nystatin | None | C |
| Penicillin | None | B |
| Pyrazinamide | Undetermined | C |
| Pyrimethamine | Minimal | C |
| Quinine | Very large doses: moderate | D[*] |
| Ribavirin | Undetermined | X |
| Spectinomycin | Undetermined | B |
| Spiramycin | Undetermined | C |
| Streptomycin | Deafness: small | D |
| | Malformations: none | |
| Sulfadiazine | Unlikely | NA |
| Sulfamethoxazole | Unlikely | NA |
| Terconazole | Undetermined | C |
| Tetracycline | Unlikely | D |
| Thalidomide | High | X |
| Tolnaftate | Undetermined | NA |
| Trimethoprim | Minimal to small | C |
| Valacyclovir | | B |
| Vancomycin | Undetermined | B |
| Vidarabine | Undetermined | C |
| Zidovudine | Unlikely | C |

[*] Low therapeutic doses: unlikely.

*Abbreviation:* NA, not available.

to screen for and, if possible, eradicate bacteriuria in the pregnant woman, since acute pyelonephritis will develop in as many as 25 percent of untreated pregnant women with bacteriuria (Kass *et al.*, 1976). The majority of pregnant women with asymptomatic bacteriuria can be treated successfully with a short course (3–5 days) of the antimicrobial regimens listed in Box 2.20.

---

**BOX 2.20   OUTPATIENT ANTIMICROBIAL REGIMENS FOR TREATMENT OF ASYMPTOMATIC BACTERIURIA OR CYSTITIS DURING PREGNANCY[a]**

- Ampicillin       250–500 mg qid
- Nitrofurantoin   50–100 mg qid
- Cephalosporins   250–500 mg qid
- Sulfonamides     500 mg to 1 g qid

[a] Oral dose for 3–5 days.

---

An alternative regimen is to use nitrofurantoin macrocrystals, 100 mg given once a day at bedtime, for 7–10 days (Leveno *et al.*, 1981). Single-dose regimens, as listed in Box 2.21, may also prove useful. Regardless of the antimicrobial regimen used, approximately two-thirds of the patients will be cured and remain bacteriuria-free for the remainder of the pregnancy; approximately one-third of the patients will experience a recurrence and require further therapy.

---

**BOX 2.21   SINGLE-DOSE ANTIMICROBIAL REGIMENS FOR THE TREATMENT OF UNCOMPLICATED BACTERIURIA DURING PREGNANCY**

- Amoxicillin      2 g[a]
- Ampicillin       2 g[a]
- Nitrofurantoin   200 mg
- Sulfisoxazole    500 mg

[a] Oral dose, 3–5 days.

---

Symptomatic infection of the lower urinary tract (acute cystitis) can be treated with a variety of antimicrobial regimens similar to that used for asymptomatic bacteriuria, with the exception that there is little information regarding the treatment of pregnant women with single-dose regimens, which are thus not recommended. These women can generally be treated as outpatients with an oral antimicrobial agent for 3–5 days (Box 2.20). As with asymptomatic bacteriuria, recurrence in women with cystitis is common. Therefore, it is important to have frequent surveillance cultures.

Symptomatic infection of the upper urinary tract or acute pyelonephritis is a relatively common complication occurring in approximately 1 percent of all pregnant women. Many of these women experience nausea and vomiting, are dehydrated, and are unable to tolerate oral antimicrobial therapy. These women should be hospitalized for intravenous antibiotic therapy with one of the regimens listed in Box 2.22. As many as 25 percent of women with acute pyelonephritis during pregnancy will experience another such episode during either the antepartum or postpartum periods. Because of the attendant risks associated with acute pyelonephritis during pregnancy, such as septic shock and premature labor, consideration should be given to continuous suppressive antimicrobial therapy following an initial episode of pyelonephritis. One particularly useful regimen is nitrofurantoin macrocrystals, 100 mg orally every night (Hankins and Whalley, 1985).

## BOX 2.22   INPATIENT ANTIMICROBIAL REGIMENS FOR THE TREATMENT OF PREGNANT WOMEN WITH ACUTE PYELONEPHRITIS

- Ampicillin                                    500 mg IV q 6 h
- Cephalosporin (first generation)   500 mg IV q 6 h
- Mezlocillin                                  3–4 g IV q 6 h
- Piperacillin                                 3–4 g IV q 6 h

*Aminoglycoside plus antibiotic listed as follows:*
- Gentamicin 3 mg/kg.day IV in divided doses
- Tobramycin 3 mg/kg.day IV in divided doses
- Cefazolin 1–2 g q 8 h is also useful
- Cefoxitin 1–2 g IV q 6 h

## Acute Chorioamnionitis

Acute chorioamnionitis occurs in approximately 1 percent of all pregnancies (Gibbs *et al.*, 1980; Hauth *et al.*, 1985). The majority of cases occur in the third trimester, although such infections may occur, secondary to invasive procedures such as amniocentesis or chorionic villus sampling, in the late first or early second trimester. There is no unanimity of opinion regarding specific antimicrobial regimens for the treatment of acute chorioamnionitis during pregnancy. Suggested regimens are summarized in Box 2.23. The combination of ampicillin and gentamicin is probably the most often used regimen in the United States (Gibbs *et al.*, 1980; Gilstrap *et al.*, 1988b; Maberry *et al.*, 1991).

## BOX 2.23   ANTIMICROBIAL REGIMENS FOR THE TREATMENT OF ACUTE CHORIOAMNIONITIS

Ampicillin plus                 500 mg to 1 g IV q 6 h
Cefoxitin                         1–2 g IV q 6 h
Gentamicin                      3 mg/kg.day IV in divided doses
Piperacillin/Mezlocillin    3–4 g IV q 6 h
Ampicillin plus gentamicin or plus clindamycin for women with chorioamnionitis requiring cesarean delivery

*Source:* ACOG Committee on Obstetric Practice. Committee Opinion No. 712: Intrapartum Management of Intraamniotic Infection. *Obstet Gynecol.* 2017; 130: e95–e101.

## Protozoal Diarrhea

### Nitazoxanide

Nitazoxanide is an antiprotozoal medication used to treat diarrhea. It has not been studied in human pregnancy. The manufacturer reported no increased frequency of congenital anomalies in pregnant animal models. It is an FDA pregnancy risk category B drug.

## Vaginitis

The two most common forms of vaginitis during pregnancy are fungal and protozoan. Pregnant women with vaginitis secondary to fungi, such as *Candida* species, can be treated with a variety of antifungal agents that are listed in Box 2.24. Women with trichomoniasis present an unusual therapeutic dilemma. Although there is no scientific evidence that metronidazole is either teratogenic or causes adverse effects in the embryo/fetus, the manufacturer has issued a stern warning regarding its use during the first trimester of pregnancy. Fortunately, many of the patients with trichomoniasis can be treated with antiprotozoal agents until they are past the first trimester and then treated with metronidazole—the only effective treatment for this protozoan infection.

---

### BOX 2.24   ANTIFUNGAL AGENTS FOR THE TREATMENT
### OF *Candida vaginitis* DURING PREGNANCY

- Butoconazole
- Clotrimazole
- Miconazole
- Nystatin
- Erconazole

---

## SEXUALLY TRANSMITTED DISEASES

Syphilis is a relatively common sexually transmitted disease in pregnant women, especially in the indigent population. Such women should be treated according to the Centers for Disease Control (CDC) guidelines, as outlined in Box 2.25. Pregnant women with syphilis who are allergic to penicillin present another therapeutic dilemma. For example, erythromycin may eradicate the infection in the pregnant woman, but may not prevent congenital syphilis (Wendel, 1990; Ziaya *et al.*, 1986). Another agent, tetracycline, may be associated with significant yellow-brown discoloration of the fetal deciduous teeth and is currently not recommended for use in the latter half of pregnancy (Genot *et al.*, 1970). The current recommended approach to the pregnant patient with syphilis who is allergic to penicillin is to utilize penicillin desensitization, as outlined in Box 2.26, after skin testing to confirm allergy. Penicillin is the ideal antibiotic choice for the treatment of syphilis during pregnancy (Bofill and Rust, 1996).

---

### BOX 2.25   ANTIMICROBIAL REGIMENS FOR THE
### TREATMENT OF SYPHILIS DURING PREGNANCY

**Early syphilis (less than 1 year)**

Benzathine penicillin G 2.4 million units IM as a single injection

**Syphilis of more than 1 year's duration**

Benzathine penicillin G 2.4 million units IM weekly for 3 doses

**Neurosyphilis**

- Aqueous crystalline penicillin G 2.4 million units IV every 4 h for at least 10 days, followed by benzathine penicillin G 2.4 million units IM weekly for three doses
- Aqueous procaine penicillin G 2.4 million units IM daily, plus probenecid 500 mg orally four times daily, both for 10 days, followed by benzathine penicillin G 2.4 million units IM weekly for three doses
- Benzathine penicillin G 2.4 million units IM weekly for three doses (not recommended for HIV-infected adults)

*Source:* CDC, 2021.

---

**BOX 2.26   PENICILLIN DESENSITIZATION IN PREGNANT
WOMEN ALLERGIC TO PENICILLIN**

- Requires hospitalization for at least 24 h
- Intravenous access, resuscitation medications, and equipment
- Oral protocol—graduated oral doses of phenoxymethyl penicillin (penicillin V suspension)
- Parenteral protocol—graduated intravenous doses of aqueous crystalline penicillin G

---

Gonorrhea is a common sexually transmitted disease encountered during pregnancy, and complicated infections may be treated with amoxicillin, ampicillin, aqueous procaine penicillin G, or ceftriaxone. For women with known strains of *Neisseria gonorrhoeae* that are penicillinase-producing, therapy should consist of either ceftriaxone, 250 mg intramuscular (IM) as a single dose, spectinomycin, 2 g IM as a single dose, or cefixime, 400 mg orally in a single dose. In fact, the CDC (2021) recommends these last three regimens for the treatment of uncomplicated gonococcal infections during pregnancy. *Chlamydia trachomatis* may be isolated in up to 30 percent of women of lower socioeconomic status (unpublished observations, 1990). Erythromycin base or stearate in a dose of 500 mg four times a day for 7–10 days will generally prove satisfactory for the treatment of chlamydial infections during pregnancy. Tetracycline is generally not recommended for use in pregnant women. Other antimicrobial agents such as amoxicillin (with or without clavulanic acid), clindamycin, or azithromycin (1 g single oral dose), may prove satisfactory in eradicating chlamydial infections in pregnant women who are unable to tolerate erythromycin because of its gastrointestinal side effects.

## VIRAL INFECTIONS

Fortunately, the majority of viral infections encountered during pregnancy do not require any specific therapy. Patients with life-threatening disseminated viral infections, such as varicella zoster or herpes infections, should be treated with acyclovir, as the benefits clearly outweigh any potential risk. The same is true for pregnant women with AIDS, who should be treated with zidovudine (Retrovir). Zidovudine is also recommended from 14 weeks gestation onward as prophylaxis for the prevention of perinatal viral transmission in HIV-positive women (Box 2.27). Acyclovir is not recommended for the routine treatment of localized genital tract herpes simplex virus infections (Scott *et al.*, 1996). Valacyclovir and Famvir are also effective and are category B drugs (Table 2.3).

---

**BOX 2.27   RECOMMENDED PROTOCOL FOR PROPHYLACTIC ZIDOVUDINE
TO DECREASE THE RISK OF PERINATAL HIV TRANSMISSION**

- Zidovudine 100 mg five times daily or 200 mg three times daily, beginning at 14–34 weeks and continued throughout pregnancy plus
- Zidovudine intrapartum given as a loading dose of 2 mg/kg IV followed by an infusion of 1 mg/kg and
- Zidovudine syrup orally to the newborn in a dose of 2 mg/kg every 6 h for the first 6 weeks of life

*Sources:* From CDC, 2021; Connor *et al.*, 1994.

## Vaccines

Fortunately, most pregnant women do not require vaccination during pregnancy. However, as with drugs and medications, occasionally a woman will be given an immunization when she does not realize she is newly pregnant. Probably the two most common immunizations given in this instance are rubella and influenza. The four types of immunizing agents are toxoids, killed microbial vaccines, viral vaccines, and immune globulins (ACOG, 2018b).

## Toxoids

The major agent in this class is a combination tetanus–diphtheria that is recommended for pregnant women with no primary immunization or who have not had a booster within 10 years (ACOG, 2018). The mortality to both mother and neonate from tetanus is extremely high, and active immunization to the mother will provide protection to the neonate in the range of 80–95 percent or greater if the mother has received at least two doses 2 weeks before delivery (Faix, 2002; Hayden and Henderson, 1990). This vaccine has no known adverse effects on the fetus. The Hungarian Birth Defects Registry reported no increased frequency of birth defects or untoward outcomes from exposure to tetanus toxoid in the second and third trimesters (Czeizel and Rockenbauer, 1999), but these exposures occurred outside the critical period of organogenesis.

## Inactivated Bacterial Vaccines

The inactivated bacterial vaccines include cholera, meningococcus, plague, pneumococcus, and typhoid, and it is recommended that they not be utilized except for travel requirements or for high-risk close exposure (Committee on Obstetric Practice ACOG, 2012). There are no reports of adverse fetal effects from any of these inactivated bacterial vaccines.

## Immune Globulins

The immune globulins include hepatitis B, rabies, tetanus, and varicella, which are recommended for post-exposure prophylaxis (ACOG, 2018). There are no adverse fetal effects reported with the use of any of these agents.

The dose schedule recommended for hepatitis B immune globulin and for vaccination is summarized in Table 2.4. Although there is general agreement that newborn infants of mothers who develop clinical varicella within 4–5 days before or within 2 days after delivery should receive varicella—zoster immune globulin (VZIG), the efficacy of VZIG in the exposed mother is less than clear. However, several authors have recommended its use in susceptible pregnant women if it can be given within 96 hours (Faix, 1991; MacGregor *et al.*, 1987; Levin *et al.*, 2019) has published the most compelling data to support this recommendation. In this study, in which 25 susceptible pregnant women were given VZIG in a dose of 0.2 mg/kg within 96 hours of exposure, 20 (80 percent) did not develop varicella.

The immune globulins are used primarily for hepatitis A and measles. The recommended dose for hepatitis A exposure is 0.2 ml/kg in one dose for the mother and 0.5 ml to susceptible newborns (ACOG Practice Bulletin, 2007).

The dose of immune globulin for measles is discussed later.

## Viral Vaccines

In general, live attenuated viral vaccines are not recommended for pregnant women, with few exceptions (Table 2.5). Of these vaccines, rubella has probably received the most attention. Although pregnancy is considered contraindicated in women within 3 months of receiving the rubella vaccine,

**TABLE 2.4**
**Hepatitis B Vaccines and Hyperimmune Globulin Prophylaxis**

| | Vaccine | | |
| | Hepatovax-B | Recombivax HB | Engerix-B |
|---|---|---|---|
| Adult | 1.0 mL | 1.0 mL | 1.0 mL |
| Infant of HBV carrier | 0.5 mL | 0.5 mL | 0.5 mL |
| Prophylaxis, hepatitis B immune globulin (HBIG) | | | |
| Adult | 0.6 mL/kg initially and 1 month later | | |

Newborn 0.5 mL initially and at 3 and 6 months.

| | Hepatovax-B | Recombivax HB | Engerix-B |
|---|---|---|---|
| Adult | 1.0 mL | 1.0 mL | 1.0 mL |
| Infant of HBV carrier | 0.5 mL | 0.5 mL | 0.5 mL |
| Prophylaxis, hepatitis B immune globulin (HBIG) | 0.6 mL/kg initially and 1 month later | | |

Newborn 0.5 mL initially and at 3 and 6 months.

*Sources:* From ACOG Practice Advisory, 2018; Pastorek, 1989.

**Table 2.5 The Viral Vaccines Used in Pregnancy: Fetal Risk**

**Live Attenuated Viruses**

| | | |
|---|---|---|
| COVID-19 | Administered as needed | Limited data—low to no risk |
| Measles | Contraindicated | None known |
| Mumps | Contraindicated | None known |
| Poliomyelitis | Only for increased risk of exposure | None known (Fetal death?) |
| Rubella | Contraindicated | None confirmed |
| Yellow fever | Only for high-risk exposure | Unknown |

**Inactivated Viruses**

| | | |
|---|---|---|
| Influenza | Pregnant women with other significant illnesses | None known |
| Rabies | Same as for non-pregnant women | Unknown |

however, the actual risk of congenital rubella syndrome from maternal vaccination would appear to be extremely small, if it exists at all (Preblud and Williams, 1985). However, a number of studies have reported normal infant outcomes following rubella vaccination.

Measles and mumps vaccines are also considered contraindicated during pregnancy, although pooled immune globulin (0.25 mg/kg in a dose up to 15 ml) can be utilized for measles (McLean *et al.*, 2013).

The inactivated viruses include influenza and rabies. Obviously, the benefits of rabies vaccination (considering the high mortality of rabies of nearly 100 percent) far outweigh any theoretical

risk to the fetus, which is actually unknown. Although influenza vaccines are not routinely recommended for all pregnant women, they may be efficacious in certain pregnant women with significant
medical complications.

Recent development of vaccines for COVID-19 (the novel corona-2 virus that caused the pandemic of 2020–2021) has two forms. One contains fragment of the COVID-19 virus, the other is
a new technology that uses mRNA. Guidance from ACOG and Harvard School of Public Health
state:

> There is no virus in the mRNA vaccines. You cannot get COVID, or give your baby COVID, by being
> vaccinated. The components of the vaccine are not known to harm breastfed infants.
> When you receive the vaccine, the small mRNA vaccine particles are used up by your muscle cells at
> the injection site and thus are unlikely to get into breast milk. Any small mRNA particles that reach the
> breast milk would likely be digested.
> When a person is vaccinated while breastfeeding, their immune system develops antibodies that protect
> against COVID-19. These antibodies can be passed through breast milk to the baby. Newborns of vac-
> cinated mothers who breastfeed can benefit from these antibodies against COVID-19.

> (www.health.harvard.edu/blog/wondering-about-covid-19-vaccines-
> if-youre-pregnant-or-breastfeeding-2021010721722)

ACOG COVID-19 Guidance published guidelines for the management of COVID-19 during pregnancy (ACOG COVID-19 Guidance—www.acog.org/-/media/project/acog/acogorg/files/pdfs/clin-
ical-guidance/practice-advisory/covid-19-algorithm.pdf).

Among 63 women who had COVID-19 infection in pregnancy, no evidence of vertical transmission was observed, and infants were born alive with normal birth weight. Preterm birth was 18 percent compared to 8 percent in controls (p = 0.11) (Edlow *et al.*, 2020). The CDC, ACOG and Society
for Maternal; Fetal Medicine support vaccination for pregnant women (Rasmussen *et al.*, 2021). Of
3958, women who were women who were in a COVID-19 pregnancy registry 827 had a completed
pregnancy of those vaccinated in the first trimester. 712 (86.1 percent) of 827 conceptions resulted
in a live birth. 115 (13.9 percent) were a pregnancy loss. Neonatal outcomes were preterm birth
(9.4 percent) and small size for gestational age (3.2 percent), with no neonatal deaths. Proportion
of adverse pregnancy and neonatal outcomes among gravidas vaccinated against COVID-19 was
similar to incidences before the COVID-19 pandemic (Shimabukuro *et al.*, 2021). This included 46
spontaneous abortions (46/712, 5.6 percent).

# 3 Cardiovascular Drugs during Pregnancy

Heart disease occurs among about 1 percent of pregnant women. Pregnant women with heart disease present several medical dilemmas. The physician is concerned with whether a specific medication is safe for the fetus, and maintain awareness that the majority of cardiac medications are used chronically to treat life-threatening conditions. Chronically used cardiac medications cannot be discontinued when pregnancy is diagnosed (Little and Gilstrap, 1989). Hence, embryos/fetuses of women with cardiovascular disease are exposed to these medications during the critical period of organogenesis (i.e., the first eight embryonic weeks of pregnancy) and fetal development. Since heart disease may be inherited in a multifactorial or polygenic fashion, pregnant women with many forms of heart disease may give birth to a newborn with congenital heart disease, and this malformation may in turn be blamed on specific cardiac medications by both the patient and her attorney. Scientific studies regarding the efficacy and safety of most cardiac medications during pregnancy are not conclusive, but the life-threatening nature of cardiovascular disease mandates that treatment be provided, even during pregnancy.

Pharmacokinetic changes during pregnancy affect cardiovascular drug disposition. Based on the limited published data, dose and timing adjustment may be necessary because of (1) decreased drug serum concentrations (C and steady state), (2) decreased half-life, and (3) increased clearance (Table 3.1).

Cardiovascular medications may be classified into six categories: antiarrhythmic, cardiac glycosides, anticoagulants, diuretics, antihypertensives, and antianginals.

## TABLE 3.1
### Pharmacokinetic Studies of Cardiovascular Agents during Pregnancy: Pregnant Compared with Non-Pregnant

| Agent | N | EGA (weeks) | Route | AUC | V | $C_{max}$ | $C_{ss}$ | $T_{1/2}$ | Cl | PPB | Control Group[a] | Authors |
|-------|---|-------------|-------|-----|---|-----------|----------|-----------|----|----|-----------------|---------|
| Labetalol | 8 | 25–34 | PO | = | | = | = | ↓ | | | No | Rogers et al. (1990) |
| Labetalol | 10 | 33–38 | IV | | | = | = | = | = | | Yes (1,2) | Rubin et al. (1983b) |
| Labetalol | 7 | 30–36 | PO | | | = | = | = | = | | No | Saotome et al. (1993) |
| Metoprolol | 5 | 35–38 | IV | ↓ | | ↓ | ↓ | ↓ | = | = | Yes (2) | Hogstedt et al. (1985) |
| Propranolol | 6 | 32–36 | PO, IV | ↓ | = | | = | = | = | | Yes (2) | O'Hare et al. (1984) |
| Sotalol | 6 | 32–36 | PO, IV | | = | | = | = | | | Yes (2) | O'Hare et al. (1983) |
| Digoxin | 15 | 3rd trimester | PO | | | | ↑ | | ↑ | | Yes (2) | Luxford and Kellaway (1983) |
| Digoxin | 7 | Term | PO | | | | ↓ | | | | Yes (2) | Rogers et al. (1972) |

[a] Control groups: 1, non-pregnant women; 2, same individuals studied postpartum; 3, historic adult controls (sex not given); 4, adult male controls; 5, adult male and female controls combined.

*Abbreviations:* EGA, estimated gestational age; AUC, area under the curve; V, volume of distribution; C, peak plasma concentration; $t_{1/2}$, half-life; SS, steady-state concentration; Cl, clearance; PPB, plasma protein binding; PO, by mouth; ↓ denotes a decrease during pregnancy compared to non-pregnant values; ↑ denotes an increase during pregnancy compared with non-pregnant values; = denotes no difference between pregnant and non-pregnant values; IV, intravenous; IM, intramuscular.

*Sources:* Little BB. *Obstet Gynecol*, 1999; 93: 858.

DOI: 10.1201/9780429160929-3

# ANTIARRHYTHMICS

Cardiac arrhythmias are relatively common in women with cardiac disease, and the clinician providing care for such women is faced with a myriad of medications for the treatment of arrhythmias during pregnancy. Arrhythmias may also occur in pregnant women without known heart disease. Antiarrhythmics have been classified into six classes according to their major mode of action or effect (Vaughan-Williams, 1984), as shown in Tables 3.2 and 3.3.

### ADENOSINE

Adenosine is a purine nucleoside approved by the FDA for the treatment of supraventricular tachycardia (Mason *et al.*, 1992). It has also been reported to be effective in the treatment of supraventricular tachycardia in pregnant women (Afridi *et al.*, 1992; Hagley and Cole, 1994; Mason *et al.*, 1992). There are no published studies regarding the teratogenic effects of this adenosine; only three first-trimester exposures occurred in the Swedish Birth Defects Registry (Kallen, 2019).

### AJMALINE

Ajmaline is a potent sodium blocker. Its use in pregnancy has only been published only in case reports for acute treatment of tachyarrhythmias, VT, and SVT. It is recommended that lidocaine or procainamide be used for longer-term treatment because they are better studied for use during pregnancy (Merino and Perez-Silva, 2011).

### AMIODARONE

In pregnancy, amiodarone is used to treat life-threatening ventricular arrhythmias (e.g., ventricular fibrillation, tachycardia) that did not respond to first-line medications (i.e., lidocaine), and should not be used long term except when other regimens fail. Amiodarone is 37 percent iodine by weight. Approximately 10–25 percent of maternal serum levels of amiodarone cross the placenta to reach the fetus (Rotmensch *et al.*, 1987). As predictable from agents with high iodine content, thyroid complications were observed in infants exposed to amiodarone during gestation. Six pregnancies exposed to amiodarone after 10 weeks gestation included 2 cases of hypothyroidism (n = 2), and small size for gestational age (n = 4) was observed (Magee *et al.*, 1995). Among 64 infants born

---

**TABLE 3.2**

**Classification of Antiarrhythmic Agents**

| Class | Action |
|-------|--------|
| I | Interferes directly with depolarization through the sodium (Na+) channel |
| $I_A$ | Prolongation $I_B$ of action-potential duration |
| $I_C$ | Shortening of action-potential duration; No effect |
| II | Anti-sympathetic nervous system effects, mostly beta-blockers |
| III | Markedly prolonged duration of action potential through potassium (K+) efflux |
| IV | Blockade of slow inward (calcium—sodium channel) depolarization current and AV node |
| V | Agents that work through other or unknown mechanisms |

This classification may prove useful in predicting both the efficacy and the toxicity of a specific agent.
*Sources:* Revised from Brown and Wendel, 1989; Vaughan-Williams, 1984.

**TABLE 3.3**

**Classification of Antiarrhythmic Agents**

| Drug | Brand Names | Vaughan Williams Classification |
|---|---|---|
| Adenosine | — | V |
| Ajmaline | Gilurytmal, Ritmo, Aritmia | $I_A$ |
| Amiodarone | Cordarone | III |
| Atenolol | — | II |
| Bisoprolol | Zebeta | II |
| Bretylium | Bretylol | III |
| Carvedilol | Coreg | II |
| Digoxin | Lanoxin | V |
| Diltiazem | Cardizem | IV |
| Disopyramide | Norpace | I |
| Dofetilide | Tikosyn | III |
| Dronedarone | | |
| Encainide | Enkaid | I |
| Esomolol[a] | Brevibloc | II |
| Flecainide | Tambocar | I |
| Ibutilide | — | $III_C$ |
| Lidocaine | Xylocaine, LidoPen | I |
| Magnesium sulfate | — | V |
| Metoprolol | Lopressor | II |
| Mexiletine | Mexitil | I |
| Mibefradil[a] | Posicor | IV |
| Moricizine | Ethmozine | $I_c$ |
| Nebivolol | — | II |
| Phenytoin | Dilantin | $I_B$ |
| Procainamide | Procan, Pronestyl, Promine, Rhthmin | I |
| Propaferone | Rythmol, Rytmonorm | $I_C$ |
| Propranolol | Inderal | II |
| Quinidine | Cardioquin, Quindex, Quinaglute | I |
| Sotalol[a] | Betapace | II, III |
| Tocainide | Tanocard | I |
| Timolol | — | $II_B$ |
| Verapamil | Isoptin, Calan | IV |

[a] No data on use of esomolol, sotalol, or mibefradil during pregnancy have been published.
*Source:* From Vaughan Williams, 1984.

to women who used amiodarone during pregnancy, 11 cases of hypothyroidism (17 percent) were observed (two with goiter, nine without). Learning disabilities were unusually frequent in two small series of children exposed to amiodarone during gestation (Bartalena *et al.*, 2001; Magee *et al.*, 1999). With chronic use of amiodarone during pregnancy, fetal goiter is a major risk after 10 weeks gestation. Fetal death is consistently reported in animal studies of the drug during pregnancy. A possible association between fetal cretinism has also been suggested, especially from direct fetal injection (Pinsky *et al.*, 1991). The frequency of birth defects was not among 30 infants exposed to amiodarone during the first trimester (Bartalena *et al.*, 2001). Under the old FDA system, this drug is a category D for use during pregnancy.

## ATENOLOL

Atenolol is a beta-blocker used to treat arrhythmias. It has been associated with fetal hypoglycemia. Beta-blockers in general have been associated with low birth weight (i.e., IUGR), and limited data on atenolol indicate IUGR is a risk. In one study (Orbach et al., 2013) of 107 women who used atenolol during the third trimester, the frequency of IUGR/LBW was 23.4 percent, significantly higher than expected (3.9 fold). It is an FDA category D drug under the old classification. Among 1,002 infants exposed to atenolol during the first trimester in the Swedish Birth Defects Registry, 47 birth defects occurred (renal mainly), which was an increased frequency with OR = 1.49 (Kallen, 2019)

## BISOPROLOL

Use of bisoprolol during pregnancy was published in only one case report (37 weeks, cleft palate, and unilateral toe abnormalities). Fetal hypoglycemia, bradycardia, and low birth weight are risks associated with this drug because of the third drug class effects on intrauterine development (Kajante et al., 2004). Among 95 infants exposed to bisoprolol during the first trimester, no birth defects were reported in the Swedish Birth Defects Registry (Kallen, 2019).

## BRETYLIUM

Proprietary formulation of bretylium are no longer available but generic forms are. Bretylium is primarily indicated for life-threatening ventricular arrhythmias (e.g., ventricular tachycardia, ventricular fibrillation). No human data are published regarding safety of the drug during pregnancy. Bretylium was reported to be "without effect" in one rat study published by West (1962), but the relevance—if any—of this finding is unknown. It is an FDA category C drug.

## CARVEDILOL

Studies of carvedilol in human pregnancy are not published. The frequency of birth defects was not increased in offspring of experimental animals (rodents). In general, use of beta-blockers during the third trimester of pregnancy probably increases the risk for fetal/neonatal hypotension, bradycardia, hypoglycemia, and respiratory depression in the neonate.

## DIGOXIN

The passage of digoxin to the fetal compartment is reportedly 50 percent to 85 percent of maternal serum. In one uncontrolled series from Michigan Medicaid records, 34 infants were born following first trimester exposure to digoxin. The frequency of birth defects was not increased (Briggs et al., 2021). It is an old FDA category C drug.

The Swedish Birth Defects Registry included only 22 infants whose mothers used digoxin during the first trimester, and no birth defects were reported (Kallen, 2019).

## DILTIAZEM

Maternal hypotension, fetal heart block, depressed cardiac contractility

The frequency of birth defects was apparently increased (14.8 percent) among 27 infants born to mothers who used diltiazem during the first trimester of pregnancy, two of which were congenital heart defects (Briggs et al., 2021). The Swedish Birth Defects Registry included only 6 infants exposed to diltiazem in the first trimester, and no birth defects were reported (Kallen, 2019). However, the number of exposed cases is inadequate to be able to evaluate. It is an old FDA category D drug.

## DISOPYRAMIDE

Disopyramide is similar in action to quinidine, and used to treat supraventricular and ventricular arrhythmias. The drug crosses the placenta with fetal levels reaching approximately half those of the mother (Rotmensch *et al.*, 1983). The drug was embryotoxic in laboratory animals when given at several times the human dose, but no pattern or specific malformations were noted (data from the manufacturer's insert). Disopyramide use during the third trimester has been associated with premature onset of labor (Leonard *et al.*, 1978; Rotmensch *et al.*, 1983). Some authorities have stated this drug is safe for use during the third trimester but no published primary data indicate disopyramide is or is not associated with birth defects. The Swedish Birth Defects Registry included only 3 first trimester exposures (Kallen, 2019).

## DOFETILIDE

Dofetilide is associated with an increased frequency of birth defects in rats (Webster *et al.*, 1996). Most authorities suggest avoidance of dofetilide use during pregnancy, restricting its use to situations in which there are no alternatives. It is an FDA category C drug.

## DRONEDARONE (MULTAQ)

No studies are published of human pregnancies exposed to dronedarone. At doses similar to the usual human dose, the drug was associated with an increased rate of birth defects. In rabbits, doses about 50 percent of the usual human therapeutic dose were associated with an increased frequency of birth defects (Manufacturer's package insert). It is an old FDA pregnancy risk category X drug. The Swedish Birth Defects Registry included only three infants exposed to dronedarone during the first trimester (Kallen, 2019).

## ENCAINIDE (ENKAID)

A lidocaine-related antiarrhythmic medication, encainide, was not teratogenic in rats and rabbits when given at doses up to 9 and 13 times the human dose (Manufacturer's package insert). Encainide is an FDA category B drug. The Swedish Birth Defects Registry contained no infants exposed to encainide during the first trimester.

## ESMOLOL (BREVIBLOC)

Esmolol is a short-acting beta-blocker similar to atenolol. Hypotension has occurred in 50 percent of patients in some trials. The potential for reduced uterine blood flow is a serious risk that should be considered before using this drug in pregnancy. It is an FDA old category C drug. The Swedish Birth Defects Registry contained no infants exposed to esmolol during the first trimester.

## FLECAINIDE

Another lidocaine-related antiarrhythmic medication that is structurally similar to encainide and procainamide, Flecainide has not been studied in human pregnancy. According the manufacturer, Flecainide is associated with an increased incidence of birth defects and embryotoxic effects in certain strains of rabbits given four times the usual human therapeutic dose. However, congenital anomalies were not increased in frequency in rats, mice, and other strains of rabbits given in the usual human dose (Manufacturer insert). A case report suggested an association with birth defects with flecainide. Flecainide has been used to treat fetal arrhythmias, but fetal deaths have occurred with this treatment. Efficacious alternative but related medications available with a better safety profile are available. Thus, flecainide should be avoided, or at least used only as the drug of last resort when others have failed. It is an old FDA category C drug.

## IBUTILIDE (CORVERT)

No human studies of this drug during human pregnancy are published. Animal studies using oral ibutilide revealed evidence of embryocidal and teratogenic effects, but these effects have not been studied in humans. Ibutilide is an FDA pregnancy risk category C drug in the old system; the Swedish Birth Defects Registry contained no infants exposed to ibutilide in the first trimester.

## LIDOCAINE

Lidocaine is commonly used as a local anesthetic. This amide is also effective systemically in the treatment of ventricular and supraventricular tachycardia. Amide-type local anesthetics given for paracervical block are associated with spasm of the uterine arteries, causing decreased uterine blood flow. Lidocaine crosses the placenta quickly with fetal levels attaining approximately 50 percent of maternal levels in less than an hour (Rotmensch et al., 1983). Lidocaine's half-life is two times longer in the fetus/neonate (3 h) than in the mother (1.5–2 h) (Brown et al., 1976). Fetal lidocaine elimination is also prolonged and may persist for up to 48 hours after birth (Garite and Briggs, 1987). IMPORTANT NOTE: most information available regarding pharmacokinetics of lidocaine in pregnant and postpartum women and newborns is from studies of regional or local anesthesia (Rotmensch et al., 1983).

*No published data are available on lidocaine from women who received the drug for cardiac arrhythmias.* However, local anesthetics may be given in toxic doses and may result in central nervous system and cardiac side effects in both the mother and the fetus. Lidocaine is apparently not associated with birth defects at acute therapeutic levels in humans or in chronic doses in animals (Fujinaga and Mazze, 1986; Heinonen et al., 1977; Rotmensch et al., 1983), but timing, duration(s), and dose levels of exposure are not known. Potential for lidocaine toxicity risk is minimized when maternal lidocaine levels are maintained at less than 4 mg/mL (Bhagwat and Engel, 1995). The Swedish Birth Defects Registry contained no infants exposed to lidocaine during the first trimester.

## MEXILETINE

Mexiletine is a local anesthetic similar to lidocaine in action. Also like lidocaine, it is an antiarrhythmic agent (Zipes and Troup, 1978). Primary use of mexiletine is to treat ventricular arrhythmias (ventricular tachycardia, premature ventricular contractions). No studies of congenital anomalies in infants exposed to mexiletine have been published. A few anecdotal case reports suggest no adverse effects on the fetus or on labor, but the importance of such observations is not clear. Mexiletine was not teratogenic in mice, rats, and rabbits (data from the manufacturer's insert). Cord blood concentrations of this drug were similar to maternal levels, and therapeutic levels may be found in breast milk (Timmis et al., 1980). However, breastfeeding is not contraindicated when the mother is using mexiletine (American Academy of Pediatrics, 2001). It is an old FDA category C drug. Only 5 infants were exposed to mexiletine during the first trimester in Swedish Birth Defects Registry (Kallen, 2019).

## MIBEFRADIL

Mibefradil is a calcium channel blocker. No studies of this drug in human pregnancy of this are published. Heart defects were increased in frequency in rodents exposed to three times the usual human dose of mibefradil during organogenesis (Manufacturer package insert). It is an FDA pregnancy category C drug by the old system.

## Moricizine (Ethmozine)

Moricizine is used to treat ventricular tachycardia. According to the manufacturer, the drug is not associated with an increased frequency of birth defects in rodents exposed to the drug during organogenesis. Moricizine is an FDA category B drug.

## Nebivolol

Nebivolol is a beta-blocker. It has not been studied during human pregnancy. In rats and rabbits given up to 10 times the usual human dose during organogenesis, the frequency of birth defects was not increased. Fetal weight and bone ossification were delayed at birth, but was reversible postnatally. Only one infant exposed to nebivolol in the Swedish Birth Defects Registry (Kallen, 2019).

## Procainamide

Procainamide is an amide compound similar to lidocaine used to treat ventricular tachycardia. This drug's pharmacokinetics during pregnancy were reported in a case report; fetal levels were approximately one-fourth maternal levels (Garite and Briggs, 1987). No reports are published of procainamide use during the first trimester of pregnancy and congenital anomalies. The safety profile of a closely related drug, lidocaine, suggests procainamide probably does not pose a great risk when used during pregnancy (Little and Gilstrap, 1989). However, as always, the absence of evidence is not evidence of absence. Breastfeeding is not contraindicated in mothers on procainamide (American Academy of Pediatrics, 2001). A rare complication of chronic use of procainamide is a lupus-like syndrome (serious rash) may occur. Prolonged use should be avoided, unless necessary for life threatening conditions (Rotmensch *et al.*, 1987). It is an old FDA category C drug under the old system. No infants in the Swedish Birth Defects Registry were exposed to procainamide (Kallen, 2019).

## Propaferone

Propaferone is an oral antiarrhythmic used to treat ventricular tachycardia. No epidemiological studies of the use of this drug during the first trimester human pregnancy are published. In rats and rabbits no birth defects were observed at the usual human therapeutic dose, but at 4 and 8 times the usual human therapeutic dose, the frequency of congenital anomalies was increased (manufacturer's package insert). It is an FDA category C drug (old nomenclature).

## Propranolol

The most extensively studied beta-blocker (beta-adrenergic blocker) during pregnancy is propranolol. It is used to treat supraventricular and ventricular tachycardia, hypertension, hyperthyroidism, migraine headaches, and panic attacks. Propranolol is has also been used to treat fetal arrhythmias (Bhagwat and Engel, 1995; McElhinney *et al.*, 2010). Importantly, the information on the use of propranolol is from the treatment of hypertension during pregnancy, a significant confounder because hypertension during pregnancy is associated with IUGR.

No controlled studies of congenital anomalies in infants exposed to propranolol during organogenesis have been published. Among 274 infants exposed to propranolol during the first trimester, the frequency of birth defects (n = 11, 4 percent) was not greater than expected (n = 12, 4.4 percent) in the Michigan Medicaid study (Franz Rosa, unpublished; Briggs *et al.*, 2021). An uncontrolled review of 167 infants from 23 different reports suggested that ~15 percent of chronically exposed fetuses had IUGR, 10 percent had hypoglycemia, and 7 percent had bradycardia (Briggs *et al.*, 2021). However, IUGR and use of propranolol were associated in one study (Pruyn *et al.*, 1979), but not other studies

(Rotmensch *et al.*, 1987). Adverse fetal effects have been reported with the use of propranolol during pregnancy. Importantly, it is also possible that the maternal hypertension, and not propranolol therapy per se, is responsible for decrease in fetal growth. intrauterine growth restriction (IUGR) seemed most frequent with propranolol exposure during the second trimester while reduced placental weight appeared to be the most frequent symptom of restriction in the third trimester (Briggs *et al.*, 2021). The frequency of birth defects was not increased in 1,327 infants exposed to propranolol during the first trimester in the Swedish Birth Defects Registry (Kallen, 2019).

Propranolol was not associated with an increased frequency of congenital anomalies in two animal studies (Fuji and Nishimura, 1974; Speiser *et al.*, 1983).

Decreased fetal growth is one of several other complications associated with beta-blocker use in pregnancy, including, apnea, bradycardia, and hypoglycemia (Bhagwat and Engel, 1995; Habib and McCarthy, 1977; Pruyn *et al.*, 1979; Rubin, 1981; Turnstall, 1969) (Box 3.1).

---

### BOX 3.1  POSSIBLE ADVERSE FETAL EFFECTS OF MATERNAL BETA-BLOCKER THERAPY

- Apnea and respiratory depression:  4 percent
- Bradycardia:                      7 percent
- Hypoglycemia:                     10 percent
- Hyperbilirubinemia:               4 percent
- Intrauterine growth retardation:  14 percent

---

Several other beta-blocker agents are available but are used primarily for the treatment of hypertension. These are discussed later under "Antihypertensives."

## QUINIDINE

Quinidine is used to treat ventricular arrhythmia and supraventricular tachycardia. The drug was successfully used for intrauterine treatment of fetal tachycardia (Spinnato *et al.*, 1984). It was used to treat fetal hydrops (resulting from reciprocating tachycardia) that did not convert with maternal digoxin (Guntheroth *et al.*, 1985). There have been no controlled studies in human pregnancies. Among fewer than 20 pregnancies exposed to quinidine exposure during the first trimester, the frequency of congenital anomalies was not increased above the expected rate (Rosa, personal communication, cited in Briggs *et al.*, 2021). Only two infants exposed to quinidine during the first trimester were included in the Swedish Birth Defects Registry (Kallen, 2019).

## SOTALOL

Sotalol is a beta-blocker that is used to treat hypertension, atrial flutter, supraventricular tachycardia, and ventricular tachycardia. No studies are published of birth defects and first trimester exposure. Studies in pregnant rabbits and rats given up to seven and nine times the usual human dose indicted no increased frequency of birth defects, but at higher doses (up to 16 times the human therapeutic dose) an increased frequency of resorptions and fetal death were observed.

The frequency of birth defects was not increased among 60 infants whose mothers took sotalol during the first trimester in the Swedish Birth Defects Registry (Kallen, 2019).

## TOCAINIDE

Tocainide is a lidocaine-related amide antiarrhythmic agent. The drug was not associated with an increased frequency of congenital anomalies at doses several times the usual adult dose, but the number of pregnancy losses was increased. There are no human studies during pregnancy, but it is closely related to lidocaine and its data may be extrapolated to tocainide. It is an FDA category C drug under the old system.

## TIMOLOL

Timolol is a beta-blocker used to treat hypertension, migraine headaches, and glaucoma (topical). Published reports of timolol in human pregnancy is limited to three case reports. Only 10 infants were exposed to timolol in the first trimester in the Swedish Birth Defects Registry (Kallen, 2019). In animal studies of timolol in pregnant rats, rabbits and mice, the frequency of birth defects was not increased at 40 times the usual human dose; however, the rate of pregnancy loss was increased.

## VERAPAMIL

A calcium channel blocker that is used as an antiarrhythmic, antihypertensive, and antianginal treatment, verapamil is especially efficacious for the treatment of paroxysmal supraventricular tachycardia.

Verapamil is used to treat fetal supraventricular tachycardia transplacentally (Klein and Repke, 1984; Rey *et al.*, 1985; Wolff *et al.*, 1980). Verapamil should be used with caution in pregnant patients because it might reduce uterine blood flow by 25 percent or more (Murad *et al.*, 1985). Importantly, 10–20 percent of neonates who received this drug intravenously for supraventricular tachycardia and congestive heart failure developed cardiac depression and cardiac arrest (Kleinman and Copel, 1991). Therefore, verapamil is not recommended for use in infants of less than 1 year (Garson, 1987). Verapamil might have adverse effects in the fetal heart, especially in the presence of heart failure and hydrops (Shen *et al.*, 1995). Of 78 infants exposed in the first trimester to calcium channel blockers, 33 were exposed to verapamil, and the frequency of congenital anomalies was not increased (Magee *et al.*, 1996). In an uncontrolled series from the Michigan Medicaid surveillance, one of 76 infants born after exposure to verapamil during the first trimester had a birth defect; this was not greater than the expected rate (Franz Rosa in Briggs *et al.*, 2021). The frequency of birth defects was not increased in 94 infants in the Swedish Birth Defects Registry that were exposed verapamil (Kallen, 2019).

Verapamil is not contraindicated in breastfeeding mothers (American Academy of Pediatrics, 2001).

## ANTIARRHYTHMICS

Several other beta-adrenergic blocking agents are available but are used primarily for the treatment of hypertension. These are discussed later under "Antihypertensives."

## CARDIAC GLYCOSIDES

Cardiac glycosides (digitalis, digoxin, Lanatoside C, Deslanoside, Metildigoxin, Gitoformate) are used to treat atrial fibrillation, other supraventricular tachycardia, and for fetal tachycardia.

Cardiac glycosides cause inotropic effects on the heart and antiarrhythmic effects. Various digitalis preparations cross the placenta readily, resulting in fetal levels 50–80 percent of maternal levels (Chan *et al.*, 1978; Rogers *et al.*, 1972).

No scientific studies regarding the safety of cardiac glycosides in pregnant women have been published. Among 34 infants born after exposure to digitalis during the first trimester, the frequency of birth defects (2.9 percent) was not greater than that expected. Fetal digitalis toxicity has been reported but it was secondary to maternal overdose (Sherman and Locke, 1960). In this latter report, it is estimated that the mother ingested 8.9 mg of digitoxin, resulting in significant fetal toxicity and neonatal death. Very limited information supports the view that cardiac glycosides are probably safe for use during pregnancy at therapeutic doses.

## ANTICOAGULANTS AND THROMBOLYTICS

Heparin use in pregnant women is primarily to treat thromboembolic disease and for prophylaxis in women with artificial heart valves. Heparin does not cross the human placenta. Low-molecular-weight heparin is also used to treat thromboembolism in pregnancy, and does not cross the placenta (Feijgin and Lourwood, 1994; Macklon *et al.*, 1995; Schneider *et al.*, 1995).

### WARFARIN DERIVATIVES ARE CONTRAINDICATED FOR USE DURING PREGNANCY

Coumarin derivatives, including warfarin, are ***contraindicated*** for use during pregnancy. The fetal warfarin syndrome is comprised of skeletal and brain defects. Use after the first trimester includes brain and eye defects, and other anomalies associated with vascular disruption. Among 169 infants who received warfarin during the first trimester, six infants had severe birth defects (cleft lip/palate, aortic anomaly, hydrocephaly, VSD, musculoskeletal malformation) (Kallen, 2019). The frequency of 'fetal warfarin syndrome' was increased among 8 of 27 infants whose mothers used coumarin during the first trimester (Iturbe-Alesio *et al.*, 1986). Among 58 infants whose mothers took warfarin during "early pregnancy," three infants had major birth defects, and two were diagnosed with warfarin embryopathy (Vitale *et al.*, 1999). The rate of warfarin embryopathy was estimated to be 7 percent (Hoyer *et al.*, 2010).

No studies are published of human use of thrombolytics (e.g., streptokinase or urokinase) during the first trimester. A review of 172 pregnant women who used thrombolytics compiled from published reports found no increase in congenital anomalies and a pregnancy loss rate of 5.8 percent (Turrentine *et al.*, 1995). However, exposures to the thrombolytics varied from 9 weeks to 40 weeks. Hemorrhagic complications occurred in 8 percent of the women. Among more than 140 infants exposed to heparin during the first trimester, the frequency of congenital anomalies was not increased (Chan *et al.*, 2000). Among 119 infants exposed to heparin in the first trimester in the Swedish birth Defects Registry, the frequency of birth defects was not increased (Kallen, 2019). For low molecular weight heparin findings are similar from a literature review identified more than 440 infants exposed to low molecular weight heparins during pregnancy. The review included nearly 200 infants whose mothers were treated during the first trimester; no congenital anomalies were reported (Sanson *et al.*, 1999). This is a case of ascertainment bias result because seven to 10 infant birth defects were expected in the absence of any drug exposure.

Dalteparin is another heparin that is used to treat ischemic complications. Frequency of birth defects was not increased among 3,390 infants exposed in the first trimester to dalteparin in the Swedish Birth Defects Registry (Kallen, 2019).

Tinzaparin is a heparin that is used to treat DVT and prevent DVT in high risk individuals. The frequency of birth defects was not increased following first trimester exposure to tinzaparin among 699 infants (Kallen, 2019).

Protamine sulfate is used to reverse heparin's anticoagulant effects prior to surgery (e.g., C-section). No studies regarding use of protamine in pregnancy are published. One infant with neonatal depression following maternal protamine sulfate injection was reported (Wittmaack *et al.*, 1994).

## ANTIANGINAL AGENTS

Antianginal agents are potent vasodilators with organic nitrites are the most commonly used agents (Box 3.2). Nitroglycerin is the prototype organic nitrite agent. No human studies of organic nitrites in pregnant women are published. These agents were not associated with an increased frequency of birth defects in rats and rabbit studies when exposure occurred during organogenesis.

---

### BOX 3.2   ANTIANGINAL AGENTS

**Organic nitrites**
- Amyl nitrate Dipyridamole (Persantine)
- Erythrityl tetranitrate (Cardilate)
- Isosorbide dinitrate (Isordil, Sorbitrate)
- Nitroglycerin
- Pentaerythritol tetranitrate (Pentritol, Peritrate)

**Calcium antagonists**
- Aminodipine[a]
- Bepridil[a]

**Calcium channel blockers**
- Mibefradil[a]
- Nicardipine (Cardene)
- Diltiazem (Cardizem) Feldopine[a]

**Beta-blockers**
- Atenolol
- Bisoprolol[a]
- Bucindolol[a]
- Labetalol
- Metoprolol
- Propranolol

**New class**
- Ranolazine[a]

[a] Not studied during pregnancy.
*Source:* Adapted in part from the USP DI (2020).

---

### ANTIHYPERTENSIVES

Intravenous nitroglycerin was used to blunt the hypertensive effect of endotracheal intubation in women with severe preeclampsia undergoing cesarean section (Cheek and Samuels, 1996; Longmire *et al.*, 1991).

Verapamil, the most widely used calcium channel blocker was discussed earlier in this chapter. Other calcium antagonists, such as diltiazem, nicardipine, and nifedipine, are also used to treat angina. Verapamil was not associated with birth defects in rodent studies (Ariyuki, 1975). No studies of the use of *other calcium channel antagonists* use during pregnancy are published.

No information has been published on the use of dipyridamole, a selective coronary vasodilator, in pregnant women. Beta-blockers were discussed earlier, and are again discussed subsequently, under "Antihypertensives."

## ANTIHYPERTENSIVES

### METHYLDOPA

Methyldopa (Aldomet), alpha-adrenergic blocking agent, is used to treat chronic hypertension in pregnant women. No epidemiologic studies are published on methyldopa use during pregnancy. In the Michigan Medicaid study, 242 women used methyldopa in the first trimester, and the frequency of birth defects was not increased compared to the rate expected (Franz Rosa, IN Briggs *et al.*, 2021). The study was not controlled or published. Available data suggest that methyldopa does not pose a significant risk of birth defects, and postnatal growth and development seems unaffected by prenatal exposure. Maternal methyldopa use in the first trimester resulted in 72 infants, and no increased frequency of congenital anomalies in the Swedish Birth Defects Registry (Kallen, 2019).

Methyldopa is not a potent human teratogen and is probably one of the more frequently used antihypertensives during pregnancy.

### HYDRALAZINE

Hydralazine is one of most frequently used antihypertensive drugs, particularly for acutely lowering blood pressure in severe preeclampsia. The mechanism is believed to be action as a peripheral vasodilator (i.e., smooth muscle relaxant). Among 40 infants born after first trimester exposure to hydralazine, there was one newborn with a birth defect; two were expected. This is an uncontrolled, unpublished study. The frequency of birth defects was not increased among 107 infants who were exposed to hydralazine during the first trimester in the Swedish Birth Defects Registry (Kallen, 2019).

No complications were reported from 136 cases exposed anytime during pregnancy (Heinonen *et al.*, 1977), although one case report of three infants associated third trimester use with transient neonatal thrombocytopenia and bleeding,

### BETA-ADRENERGIC BLOCKERS

A number of beta-blockers are available to treat hypertension (Box 3.3) that have been used in pregnant women. Propranolol was discussed previously. Although there are no large human reproduction studies for labetalol, metoprolol, or atenolol use in pregnant women, their use in clinical practice is driven by the perception of lack of apparent adverse fetal effects.

---

**BOX 3.3   ANTIHYPERTENSIVE DRUGS**

- Acebutolol (Sectral)
- Atenolol (Tenormin)
- Betaxolol (Kerlane)
- Captopril (Capoten)
- Carteolol (Cartol)
- Clonidine (Catapres)
- Diazoxide (Hyperstat)
- Enalapril
- Fosinapril
- Hydralazine (Apresoline)
- Labetolol (Normodyne, Trandate)
- Lisinopril
- Methyldopa (Aldomet)
- Metoprolol (Lopressor)
- Nadolol (Corgard)
- Penbutolol (Levatol)
- Propranolol (Inderal)
- Quinapril
- Ramipril
- Sodium nitroprusside (Nipride, Nitropress)
- Timolol (Blocadren)

# LABETOLOL

Investigators who studied drug-free, methyldopa, and labetalol groups reported a higher frequency of fetal growth retardation in the labetalol group with no obvious improvement in neonatal outcome (Sibai *et al.*, 1987, 1990); Labetalol use in the first trimester was not associated with an increased frequency of congenital anomalies in 85 infants (Michael, 1979). The 85 women were being treated for severe hypertension, but no adverse effects were reported in the infants exposed to labetalol during gestation (Michael, 1979). No significant maternal or fetal side effects were observed comparing oral labetalol to intravenous diazoxide for hypertensive crisis during pregnancy (Michael, 1986). Among 104 labetalol- versus methyldopa-treated women with pregnancy-induced hypertension, labetalol caused fewer side effects than methyldopa (el-Qarmalawi *et al.*, 1995). Labetalol is the agent of choice to blunt the hypertensive response to endotracheal intubation because it has fewer maternal, fetal or neonatal side effects than alternatives (Cheek and Samuels, 1996). The frequency of congenital anomalies (n = 41) was increased (OR = 1.6) among 865 infants whose mothers use labetalol during the first trimester (Kallen, 2019). This included infants with severe but unspecified renal/kidney defects.

# ATENOLOL AND METOPROLOL

The beta-blockers metoprolol (Lopressor) and atenolol (Tenormin) are used to treat hypertension during pregnancy. An uncontrolled, unpublished study had 52 infants whose mothers used metoprolol during the first trimester, and there were three newborns with birth defects; two were expected. No increase in adverse maternal or fetal effects, including no significant differences in birth weight, were reported in 120 women treated with atenolol or placebo during pregnancy (Rubin *et al.*, 1983a, 1983b). Similarly, no adverse fetal effects or pregnancy outcomes associated with metoprolol or metoprolol/hydralazine treatment in second and third trimesters of pregnancy were noted (Sundstrom, 1978). Neither drug was associated with birth defects in rodent studies (Manufacturer package insert).

### METOPROLOL

In the Michigan Medicaid study (Franz Rosa, cited in Briggs *et al.*, 2021), the frequency of birth defects among 52 infants born after first trimester exposure was not increased (5.8 percent). Among 57 infants born to women who took metoprolol monotherapy throughout pregnancy, reported mean gestation was 34.1 weeks (13–41 weeks) the rates of IUGR and perinatal mortality was low, not above that which would be expected. β-blockade was not observed in the fetuses or neonates. The frequency of birth defects was not increased among 1565 infants exposed to metoprolol during the first trimester in the Swedish Birth Defects Registry (Kallen, 2019).

Breastfeeding is allowed during maternal therapy with either metoprolol or atenolol (American Academy of Pediatrics, 2001). A case report was published on beta-blocker toxicity in a neonate whose mother was taking atenolol while breastfeeding (Schmimmel *et al.*, 1989).

# ACEBUTOLOL

Acebutolol is a cardioselective beta-adrenergic blocker. No studies of the frequency of congenital anomalies after first trimester exposure to acebutolol. Animal studies (rats, rabbits) of acebutolol during organogenesis at doses 31 times the usual human therapeutic dose resulted in no increased frequency of birth defects (Manufacturer's package insert). Several reports of acebutolol treatment for hypertension during several periods of pregnancy (*n* = 56 infants) have been published that were without adverse maternal or fetal effects (Dubois *et al.*, 1980, 1982; Williams and Morrissey, 1983). Neonatal hemodynamic adaptation failure occurred in five of 11 infants whose mothers were treated with acebutolol during pregnancy (Yassen *et al.*, 1992). It seems unlikely that this drug is associated with an increased risk of congenital anomalies. It is an FDA pregnancy risk category B drug by the old system.

## PINDOLOL

No studies regarding the use of pindolol during the first trimester of pregnancy have been published. Among 51 women with pregnancy-induced hypertension randomized to hydralazine, hydralazine and propranolol, or hydralazine and pindolol, pindolol was associated with fewer maternal and fetal side effects (Paran *et al.*, 1995). However, infants born to mothers who received propranolol had smaller birth weights. In a comparative study of atenolol or pindolol on uterine/fetal hemodynamics and fetal cardiac function, investigators found that pindolol was preferable to atenolol for the treatment of pregnancy-induced hypertension based upon maternal and fetal cardiovascular function (Rasanen and Jouppila, 1995). It is an FDA category B drug under the old classification. The frequency of birth defects was not among 463 infants exposed to pindolol during the first trimester in the Swedish Birth Defects Registry (Kallen, 2019).

## BETAXOLOL, CARTEOLOL, NADOLOL, PENBUTOLOL, AND TIMOLOL

No human teratology or reproduction studies with betaxolol, carteolol, nadolol, penbutolol, or timolol have been published. No increase in congenital malformations was noted in the offspring of pregnant mice who received up to 150 mg/kg/day of carteolol (Tanaka *et al.*, 1979). Only six infants were exposed to betaxolol during the first trimester in the Swedish Birth Defects Registry (Kallen, 2019). Also, no increase in the frequency of malformations was found among the offspring of rats, rabbits, and hamsters that had received nadolol in doses several times higher than the usual human dose (Sibley *et al.*, 1978; Stevens *et al.*, 1984). No increased frequency of adverse fetal effects was found in the offspring of mice treated with penbutolol (Sugisaki *et al.*, 1981).

## CLONIDINE

Clonidine (Catapres) is a centrally acting antihypertensive that blocks alpha-adrenergic receptors. No epidemiologic studies of the frequency of congenital anomalies and clonidine use during early pregnancy have been published. Anecdotal case reports of clonidine use during pregnancy suggest no adverse fetal effects (Horvath *et al.*, 1985). Head size and neurologic examination of 22 children whose mothers received clonidine during pregnancy were normal (Huisjes *et al.*, 1986; Raftos *et al.*, 1973). One rat teratology study found no increased frequency of birth defects (Angelova *et al.*, 1975), but one study found an increase in growth retardation and cleft palates in offspring of mice treated with large doses of this antihypertensive (Chahoud *et al.*, 1985). Clonidine is probably not associated with an increased risk of congenital anomalies when used therapeutically. Among 22 infants exposed to clonidine during the first trimester, the frequency of congenital anomalies was not increased (Kallen, 2019).

## DIAZOXIDE

Diazoxide is a thiazide (Hyperstat) that is used parenterally as an antihypertensive. An oral form of this drug (Proglycem) is also used to treat hypoglycemia secondary to hyperinsulinism. No epidemiologic studies of diazoxide have been published. An anecdotal case report of abnormalities of body and scalp hair, including alopecia, in four neonates of women who received oral diazoxide during the last trimester of pregnancy has been published (Milner and Chonskey, 1972). Maternal diazoxide therapy was also reportedly associated with hyperglycemia in the neonate (Milsap and Auld, 1980). No animal teratology studies are available. Pancreatic islet cell damage was found in the offspring of sheep and goats treated with intravenous diazoxide (Boulos *et al.*, 1971). Diazoxide may inhibit uterine contractions (Landesman *et al.*, 1969) and has been used in the past by some clinicians as a tocolytic agent. Only two infants were exposed to diazoxide in the first trimester in the Swedish Birth Defects Registry (Kallen, 2019).

## SODIUM NITROPRUSSIDE

A potent vasodilator, sodium nitroprusside (Nipride, Nitropress), is used primarily for hypertensive emergencies. It is also used to induce hypotension during certain types of surgical procedures, especially neurosurgical procedures. No epidemiological studies of congenital anomalies in association with nitroprusside use during pregnancy have been published. Nitroprusside was reported to be associated with cyanide toxicity in animals (Lewis *et al.*, 1977), but this is apparently not a significant risk in the human fetus when recommended human doses are used in the mother (Shoemaker and Meyers, 1984). Nonetheless, it is prudent to avoid use of nitroprusside during pregnancy because of the theoretical accumulation of cyanide in the fetal liver. Chronic use of sodium nitroprusside is logically associated with a much higher risk than acute usage.

## DIURETICS

Diuretics are used to treat hypertension, sometimes alone or in conjunction with another drug regimen. Three basic categories of diuretics are: (1) loop diuretics, (2) potassium-sparing diuretics, and (3) thiazide diuretics. Agents in these categories are listed in Boxes 3.4 and 3.5.

### LOOP DIURETICS

Loop diuretics act primarily by inhibiting sodium and water reabsorption by the loop of Henle. Loop diuretics include bumetanide, ethacrynic acid, and furosemide.

## BUMETANIDE

No epidemiological studies of bumetanide (Bumex) during pregnancy have been published. No increase in malformations was found in offspring of animals receiving several times the usual adult human dose of bumetanide (McClain and Dammers, 1981). Five infants were exposed to bumetanide in the first trimester in the Swedish Birth Defects Registry (Kallen, 2019).

## ETHACRYNIC ACID

No animal or human teratology studies of ethacrynic acid (Edecrin) have been reported.

## FUROSEMIDE

Among 350 infants born to women who used furosemide during pregnancy, the frequency of congenital anomalies was not increased (Rosa, personal communication, cited in Briggs *et al.*, 2002). Diuretics given after the first trimester of pregnancy may interfere with normal plasma volume expansion. An adverse effect on plasma volume, no improvement in perinatal outcome (Sibai *et al.*,

1987), and decreased placental perfusion were reported with the use of diuretics during pregnancy (Shoemaker *et al.*, 1973). Furosemide also displaces bilirubin from albumin, increasing the risk for fetal hyperbilirubinemia (Turmen *et al.*, 1982). In animal studies, furosemide exposure in pregnancy was associated with an increase in fetal loss and skeletal anomalies in offspring (Godde and Grote, 1975; Mallie *et al.*, 1985). Furosemide crosses the placenta and assists in assessing fetal urinary tract obstruction and fetal urine production (Barrett *et al.*, 1983; Wladimiroff, 1975). Among 309 infants in the Swedish Birth Defects Registry, the frequency of birth defects was not increased (Kallen, 2019). Furosemide is probably not associated with an increased risk of birth defects.

### POTASSIUM-SPARING DIURETICS

Potassium-sparing diuretics include amiloride, spironolactone, and triamterene, and result in sodium and water loss while sparing potassium. Spironolactone is a competitive inhibitor of aldosterone, while amiloride and triamterene function at the level of the collecting tubules.

## AMILORIDE

No epidemiological studies regarding the use of amiloride in pregnant women are published. No birth defects were noted among 12 infants exposed to amiloride during the first trimester in the Swedish Birth Defects Registry (Kallen, 2019). No increase in malformations in offspring of pregnant hamsters that received small doses of amiloride was found (Storch and Layton, 1973).

## SPIRONOLACTONE

No epidemiological studies of spironolactone (Aldactone) in pregnant women have been published. Spironolactone was not associated with an increased frequency of malformations in offspring of rats (Miyakubo *et al.*, 1977), but feminization of the genitalia in the male offspring of rats that received this diuretic in doses five times that normally used in humans was reported (Hecker *et al.*, 1980). This diuretic is not recommended for use during human pregnancy because of the theoretical risk of feminization of male genitalia. This specific complication has not been reported in humans. Spironolactone for the treatment of pregnant women with Bartter's disease (Groves and Corenblum, 1995; Rigo *et al.*, 1996) has been reported. The frequency of birth defects was not increased among 161 infants whose mothers used spironolactone during the first trimester in the Swedish Birth Defects Registry (Kallen, 2019). None of the three male infants or two female infants had any demonstrable adverse effects, including under-virilization of the male infant.

## TRIAMTERENE

Triamterene (Dyrenium) is another potassium-sparing diuretic. Of 271 pregnant women included in the Collaborative Perinatal Project who were treated with this diuretic (Heinonen *et al.*, 1977), only a few received this diuretic in the first months of pregnancy. The frequency of congenital malformations was not increased in the offspring of these women; neither was the frequency of malformations increased in the offspring of animals who received triamterene (Ellison and Maren, 1972). Triamterene was not included in the Swedish Birth Defects Registry (Kallen, 2019). Notably, triamterene is a folic acid antagonist, and may require supplementation.

### THIAZIDES

Thiazides comprise the largest group of diuretics (Box 3.5). Thiazides function by preventing reabsorption of sodium at the distal renal tubules. No increase in frequency of congenital anomalies in the offspring of over 500 women who took thiazide diuretics in the first trimester of pregnancy was noted (Kraus *et al.*, 1966).

---

**BOX 3.5 THIAZIDE DIURETICS**

| | |
|---|---|
| Bendroflumethiazide (Naturetin) | Hydroflumethiazide (Diucardin, Saluron) |
| Benzthiazide (Exna, Hydrex) | Methyclothiazide (Aquatensen, Enduran) |
| Chlorothiazide (Diuril) | Metolazone (Diulo, Zaroxolyn, Mykrox) |
| Cyclothiazide (Anhydron) | Polythiazide (Renese) |
| | Hydrochlorothiazide (Esidrix, Hydro-Chlor) |
| | Quinethazone (Hydromox) |
| Hydro-D (Hydrodiuril) | Trichlormethiazide (Metahydrin, Naqua, Trichlorex) |

---

## BENDROFLUMETHIAZIDE

Among more than 1000 women included in the Collaborative Perinatal Project who received bendroflumethiazide (Naturetin), only 13 received this diuretic in early pregnancy (Heinonen *et al.*, 1977). In a study of diuretics to prevent preeclampsia, no increase in the frequency of malformations or stillbirths was found in the offspring of over 1,000 women who received this diuretic after the first trimester. Among 154 infants born to women who used bendroflumethiazide during the first trimester in the Swedish Birth Defects Registry (Kallen, 2019).

No increased frequency of congenital anomalies was found among offspring of rats given hundreds of times the usual human dose (Stevens *et al.*, 1984).

## BENZTHIAZIDE

No epidemiological studies are published on the use of this diuretic in pregnant women. No animal teratology studies are available regarding benzthiazide.

## CHLOROTHIAZIDE

Chlorothiazide (Diuril) is the most commonly used thiazide diuretic. The frequency of congenital anomalies was not increased over the expected rate reported among offspring of 63 women who took this diuretic in early pregnancy and of over 5000 women who took this drug after the first trimester of pregnancy (Heinonen *et al.*, 1977).

Neonatal thrombocytopenia was reported in the offspring of several mothers who received chlorothiazide during pregnancy (Rodriguez *et al.*, 1964), but not among infants in another series (Finnerty and Assali, 1964). An increased frequency of hypertension was reported in the offspring of rats treated with chlorothiazide at doses 30 times those employed in humans (Grollman and Grollman, 1962). Another group of investigators (Maren and Ellison, 1972) found no increase in malformations in offspring of rats treated with this agent in doses up to 12 times that used in humans.

## HYDROCHLOROTHIAZIDE

Hydrochlorothiazide is a very commonly used thiazide diuretic. Birth defects were not increased in frequency among offspring of more than 200 women who received this diuretic in early pregnancy (Heinonen *et al.*, 1977; Jick *et al.*, 1981). Neonatal thrombocytopenia was observed with hydrochlorothiazide, as with other thiazide diuretics (Rodriguez *et al.*, 1964). The frequency of congenital anomalies was not increased among 54 infants exposed to hydrochlorothiazide in the first trimester, as reported by the Swedish Birth Defects Registry (Kallen, 2019).

Hydrochlorothiazide was not teratogenic in the offspring of rats who received this agent in doses many times that of the human adult dose (George *et al.*, 1995; Maren and Ellison, 1972).

## HYDROFLUMETHIAZIDE

No human epidemiological studies or animal teratology studies are published for hydroflumethiazide (Diucardin, Saluron). It is reasonable to assume that the potential risks of this diuretic are similar to those of other thiazides.

## METHYCLOTHIAZIDE, POLYTHIAZIDE, AND TRICHLORMETHIAZIDE

No information is available on which to base a risk estimate for these thiazide drugs. For example, the Collaborative Perinatal Project database included only three women treated with methyclothiazide (Aquatensen, Enduran), 10 women treated with polythiazide (Renese), and only two women treated with trichlormethiazide (Metahydrin, Naqua, Trichlorex) in the first 4 months of pregnancy (Heinonen *et al.*, 1977). There are no available animal teratology studies with these three thiazide diuretics. Nonetheless, based upon information for a closely related and better-studied drug, chlorothiazide, it is reasonable to state that the risk of birth defects with these drugs is low, if it exceeds background risk. None of these drugs are included in the Swedish Birth Defects Registry.

### OTHER THIAZIDE-LIKE DIURETICS

Chlorthalidone (Hygroton, Thalitone), metolazone (Diulo, Zaroxolyn), and quinethazone (Hydromox) are not true thiazide diuretics from the standpoint of chemical structure, although their mode of action is very similar to the thiazide group. There is little available information regarding the use of chlorthalidone in women in the first trimester of pregnancy. Over 1300 women who used thiazide diuretics were included in the Collaborative Perinatal Project database, but only 20 used chlorthalidone during the first trimester (Heinonen *et al.*, 1977). Although there was an increased frequency of congenital dislocation of the hip in this latter group, it is difficult if not impossible to draw valid conclusions from such numbers. Only one infant exposed to chlorthalidone in the first trimester was included in the Swedish Birth Defects Registry (Kallen, 2019). There were no reported significant differences in the frequency of birth offspring of mothers exposed to chlorthalidone after 15 weeks gestation, compared to controls (Tervila and Vartianen, 1971). Only eight pregnant women were exposed to quinethazone in the Collaborative Perinatal Project database, and none who received metolazone (Heinonen *et al.*, 1977). No published reports are available on congenital anomalies in the offspring of women who took either of these two diuretics during pregnancy. Metolazone was not found to be teratogenic in one animal study (Nakajima *et al.*, 1978), and no animal teratology studies are available for quinethazone. The Swedish Birth Defects Registry contained 372 infants whose mothers took thiazides during the first trimester (Kallen, 2019), and the frequency of birth defects were not increased in frequency.

## CALCIUM CHANNEL BLOCKERS

Calcium channel blockers are used to treat hypertension and supraventricular tachycardia.

### VERAPAMIL

This calcium channel antagonist was discussed under Antiarrhythmics.

## NIFEDIPINE

Nifedipine has been used as an antihypertensive medication and has been given as an 'off-label' tocolytic agent. Nifedipine was teratogenic in rats given 30 times the usual human dose (data from the manufacturer's insert). There are no studies of nifedipine use during the first trimester of pregnancy. No adverse maternal or fetal effects were reported for the use of nifedipine to treat preeclampsia or hypertension, respectively (Sibai *et al.*, 1992). The frequency of congenital anomalies was not increased among 64 infants born to women treated with nifedipine (or a related calcium channel blocker) (Magee *et al.*, 1996). It is regarded as the "second-line" antihypertensive therapy in pregnant women. Of 102 infants born to women who took nifedipine during the first trimester of pregnancy, the frequency of congenital anomalies was not increased in the Swedish Birth Defects Registry (Kallen, 2019). Nifedipine use during pregnancy is probably safe with "little teratogenic or fetotoxic potential" (Childress and Katz, 1994).

## NICARDIPINE

Treatment of hypertension in pregnancy with nicardipine was more effective than metoprolol in decreasing blood pressure, and neonatal outcomes were not different (Jannet *et al.*, 1994). One study of 40 pregnant women with hypertension reported that intravenous nicardipine "seems to be safe" (Carbonne *et al.*, 1993). Nicardipine was not teratogenic in rats given an oral dose many times the recommended human dose (Sato *et al.*, 1979). The Swedish Birth Defects Registry included only three infants exposed to nicardipine during the first trimester (Kallen, 2019).

## ISRADIPINE

Isradipine, a dihydropyridine calcium channel blocker, is used as an antihypertensive agent. Isradipine was not teratogenic in rats given several times the human dose (data from the manufacturer's insert). The frequency of birth defects was not increased among 80 infants whose mothers took isradipine during the first trimester in the Swedish Birth Defects Registry (Kallen, 2019). Isradipine was evaluated for the treatment of hypertension in pregnancy and was effective for the treatment of non-proteinuric hypertension. No adverse fetal effects were mentioned in this report (Wide-Swensson *et al.*, 1995).

## DILTIAZEM, NIMODIPINE, AND AMLODIPINE

There is limited information regarding the use of these calcium channel blockers during pregnancy. Nimodipine was teratogenic in rabbits (data from the manufacturer's insert).

In the Swedish Birth Defects Registry, the frequency of birth defects was not increased among 133 infants were exposed to amlodipine during the first trimester (Kallen, 2019).

## ANGIOTENSIN-CONVERTING ENZYME INHIBITORS

Angiotensin-converting enzyme (ACE) inhibitors are a class of drugs used to treat hypertension (see Table 3.4). The ACE inhibitor group should be considered contraindicated for use during pregnancy because of the risks discussed later (Shotan *et al.*, 1994). Risks associated with ACE inhibitors are second and third trimester events. First trimester exposures do not seem to present a significant risk for congenital anomalies, but this is an unknown area. The risk of severe birth defects was significantly increased (OR = 1.63) among 30 infants whose mothers used ACE-inhibitors in the Swedish Birth Defects Registry (Kallen, 2019).

**TABLE 3.4**

**Summary of Cardiovascular Drugs: Teratogen Information Service (TERIS) and Food and Drug Administration (FDA) Risk Estimates**

| Drug | Risk | Risk Rating |
|---|---|---|
| Acebutolol | Unlikely | B * |
| Amiloride | Undetermined | B * |
| Amiodarone | Neonatal thyroid dysfunction or goiter: | |
|  | Small to moderate | D |
|  | Congenital anomalies: Undetermined | |
| Atenolol | Undetermined | D |
| Betaxolol | Undetermined | C * |
| Bendroflumethiazide | Undetermined | C * |
| Benzthiazide | Undetermined | C* |
| Bumetanide | Undetermined | C * |
| Captopril | First-trimester use: Undetermined | C * |
|  | Use later in pregnancy: Moderate | |
| Chlorothiazide | Unlikely | C * |
| Chlorthalidone | Unlikely | B * |
| Clonidine | Undetermined | C |
| Diazoxide | Undetermined | C |
| Digoxin | Unlikely | C |
| Diltiazem | Undetermined | C |
| Disopyramide | Undetermined | C |
| Enalapril | First-trimester use: Undetermined | C * |
|  | Use later in pregnancy: Moderate | |
| Encainide | Undetermined | B |
| Flecainide | Undetermined | C |
| Furosemide | Undetermined | C * |
| Heparin | Unlikely | C |
| Hydralazine | Undetermined | C |
| Hydrochlorothiazide | Unlikely | B * |
| Lidocaine | Local administration: None intravenous | B |
|  | Administration: Undetermined | |
| Lisinopril | First-trimester use: None to minimal | C |
|  | *Second or third trimester: Moderate | |
| Methyclothiazide | Unlikely | NA |
| Methyldopa | Undetermined | B |
| Metolazone | Undetermined | B * |
| Nadolol | Undetermined | C * |
| Nifedipine | None to minimal | C |
| Pindolol | Unlikely | B * |
| Polythiazide | Undetermined | C* |
| Procainamide | Undetermined | C |
| Propranolol | Undetermined | C * |
| Quinethazone | Undetermined | D* |
| Quinidine | Undetermined | C |
| Spironolactone | Undetermined | C * |
| Streptokinase | Undetermined | C |
| Timolol | Undetermined | C * |
| Tocainide | Undetermined | C |
| Triamterene | Undetermined | C * |
| Trichlormethiazide | Undetermined | C* |
| Urokinase | Undetermined | B |
| Verapamil | Undetermined | C |

*Abbreviation:* NA, not available.

*Sources:* Compiled from Friedman *et al.*, *Obstet Gynecol*, 1990; 75: 594; Briggs *et al.*, 2021; Friedman and Polifka, 2006.

## CAPTOPRIL

Captopril (Capoten) is an ACE inhibitor used as an oral antihypertensive agent. No epidemiological studies of this antihypertensive agent in pregnant women have been published. No malformations were reported among 22 infants born to mothers who received captopril during the first trimester (Kreft-Jais and Boutroy, 1988), but no controlled studies have addressed whether or not captopril is a potent human teratogen. Case report evidence strongly suggests that captopril and other ACE inhibitors may be associated with anuria, renal failure, and hypocalvaria, possibly contributing to perinatal death (Barr and Cohen, 1991; Boutroy, 1989; Boutroy *et al.*, 1984; Rosa and Bosco, 1991; Rothberg and Lorenz, 1984). Of 29 infants with neonatal renal failure, nine were born to women who had used captopril throughout pregnancy (Rosa and Bosco, 1991). The other 20 infants were born to women who used other ACE inhibitors. **These antihypertensives are, therefore, contraindicated for use during pregnancy**, and should be avoided if possible. Among 14 infants whose mother used captopril during the first trimester, birth defects were not reported in the Swedish Birth Defects Registry (Kallen, 2019). No animal teratology studies have been published for captopril, but an increased frequency of fetal deaths was reported in two animal studies (Pipkin *et al.*, 1980, 1982).

## ENALAPRIL

This drug is an ACE inhibitor. Of 29 cases of perinatal renal failure, 18 occurred following maternal therapy with enalapril during pregnancy (Rosa and Bosco, 1991). This drug is contraindicated in the second and third trimesters. The frequency of birth defects was not increased among 306 infants whose mothers used enalapril during pregnancy in the Swedish Birth Defects Registry (Kallen, 2019).

## LISINOPRIL

Lisinopril is another ACE inhibitor. Among 29 infants with neonatal renal failure, two were born to women who used lisinopril during pregnancy (Rosa and Bosco, 1991). **This drug is contraindicated in the second and third trimesters**. Exposure to Lisinopril during the first trimester was reported among 20 infants, but no birth defects are recorded in the Swedish Birth Defects Registry (Kallen, 2019).

## QUINAPRIL, RAMIPRIL, AND FOSINOPRIL

These ACE inhibitors theoretically carry the same risks of adverse fetal/neonatal effects as the other ACE inhibitors. They are contraindicated in the second and third trimesters. No birth defects were reported among 37 infants exposed to Ramipril during the first trimester in the Swedish Birth Defects Registry (Kallen, 2019).

## ANGIOTENSIN II RECEPTOR BLOCKERS

Angiotensin II receptor blockers (ARBs) are a new class of ACE inhibitors used to treat hypertension. The ARBs include: valsartan, losartan, telmisartan, candesartan, omlesartan, tasosartan, and eprosartan. Based upon case reports, the ARBs have a collection of fetal complications strikingly similar to the ACE inhibitor fetopathy. The risk of congenital anomalies following use during the first trimester is unknown, but use during the second and third trimesters is associated with a significant risk of fetal-neonatal complications. The complications include oligohydramnios, fetal/neonatal renal failure, and decreased calcification of the cranium (Friedman and Polifka, 2006).

## SPECIAL CONSIDERATIONS

Cardiac arrhythmias and hypertension are the two most common cardiovascular diseases that require therapy during pregnancy. A complete review of these disorders is beyond the scope of this book. Only a few of the more common clinical problems are discussed in the following.

## CARDIAC ARRHYTHMIAS

Fortunately, life-threatening cardiac arrhythmias are uncommon during pregnancy. However, certain less serious arrhythmias may be increased in frequency during pregnancy (Brown and Wendel, 1989).

### PAROXYSMAL SUPRAVENTRICULAR TACHYCARDIA

Paroxysmal supraventricular tachycardia occurs among 1–2 per 500 young women, and frequently occurs in those without overt heart disease (Brown and Wendel, 1989). The disease frequently presents with heart rates of over 200 beats per minute. Symptoms include palpitations, light-headedness, and rarely, angina and syncope. Pregnancy may increase risk for this type of arrhythmia (Meller and Goldman, 1982; Szekely and Snaith, 1953). Most cases of paroxysmal supraventricular tachycardia are associated with AV-nodal reentry mechanisms, which can be managed in most patients with maneuvers of vagal stimulation to include carotid massage or Valsalva techniques (Brown and Wendel, 1989; Josephson and Kaster, 1977; Wu *et al.*, 1978). If vagal stimulation is unsuccessful, verapamil at 5–10 mg intravenously will prove successful in most cases in pregnant women. Because of reports of adverse neonatal cardiac effects (including cardiac arrest), ***verapamil should be used with extreme caution during pregnancy***, only after other agents have failed.

Cardioversion appears to be safe for the fetus (Clark *et al.*, 1994). Digoxin and propranolol may also be used (Box 3.6). Recently adenosine, 6-mg dose given as a rapid intravenous bolus, was recommended for treatment of supraventricular tachycardia. As previously noted limited information regarding the safety of this agent during pregnancy. However, there are several reports regarding its efficacy in pregnant women are published (Afridi *et al.*, 1992; Hagley and Cole, 1994; Mason *et al.*, 1992). Electrical cardioversion should be reserved for patients with cardiac decompensation in whom medical therapy has failed.

> ### BOX 3.6    TREATMENT OF ACUTE EPISODES OF PAROXYSMAL SUPRAVENTRICULAR TACHYCARDIA IN THE PREGNANT PATIENT WITHOUT CARDIAC DECOMPENSATION
>
> - Vagal stimulation
> - Carotid sinus massage
> - Valsalva
> - Verapamil, 5–10 mg IV[a]
> - Adenosine, 6 mg as a rapid intravenous bolus
> - Digoxin, 0.5–1.0 mg IV over 15 min (total dose not to exceed 1.5 mg in 24 h)
> - Propranolol, 0.5–1.0 mg/min (total dose not to exceed 3.0 mg)[b]
>
> See manufacturer's recommendations for dosing.
> [a] See text regarding possible fetal effects.
> [b] Caution in patients with heart disease or asthma.

Patients with frequent recurrences of this arrhythmia can usually be treated with digitalis and/or verapamil, quinidine, and propranolol as needed (Zipes, 1988).

### ATRIAL FIBRILLATION

Atrial fibrillation is uncommon in pregnant women, and this event points to underlying cardiac or thyroid disease. Mitral valve disease, secondary to rheumatic heart disease, is the most commonly encountered underlying cause of atrial fibrillation in the pregnant patient. Chronic atrial fibrillation treatment is generally directed at slowing the ventricular rate through medical therapy, with such medications as digitalis, with or without verapamil or propranolol (Brown and Wendel, 1989). Such gravidas may also require heparinization to prevent embolization. β-blocker drug therapy slows ventricular response to physical activity. For new onset atrial fibrillation, intravenous verapamil (5 to 10 mg), or electrocardioversion is given. Chronic fibrillation is treated with digoxin and a β-blocker or a calcium-channel blocker to slow ventricular response. Anticoagulation should be given for persistent fibrillation, left atrial thrombus, and/or an embolism history (Nanna, 2014; Cunningham *et al.*, 2018).

Electrical cardioversion is indicated for significant cardiac decompensation and has been used in pregnant women without apparent adverse effects (Schroeder and Harrison, 1971).

## VENTRICULAR ARRHYTHMIAS

Premature ventricular contractions (PVCs) are relatively common and may actually be increased during pregnancy. They generally do not require therapy, especially in asymptomatic pregnant women. Frequent PVCs should alert the clinician to possible organic heart disease, but medical therapy is rarely necessary for infrequent PVCs. Agents to treat frequent or asymptomatic PVCs include lidocaine, procainamide, quinidine, or disopyramide.

Ventricular tachycardia is a life-threatening arrhythmia. It may lead to ventricular fibrillation, cardiac decompensation, and death. This arrhythmia type is encountered infrequently during pregnancy, and is especially infrequent in the absence of specific cardiac disease (e.g., myocardial infarction). Therapy is primarily electric cardioversion, especially if the patient has hemodynamic instability. Lidocaine (75–100 mg IV bolus followed by 1–4 mg/min infusion) should be given in conjunction with countershock and as initial therapy in the stable patient (Brown and Wendel, 1989). Lidocaine, procainamide, or bretylium may be used to prevent recurrence of tachycardia.

Ventricular fibrillation is a medical emergency of the highest magnitude. Treatment is primarily electrical cardioversion followed by lidocaine or bretylium to prevent further fibrillation.

## HYPERTENSION

Hypertension is one of the most frequent medical complications that occurs during pregnancy. It presents as chronic hypertension, pregnancy-induced hypertension, or preeclampsia. In the case of chronic hypertension, an underlying and potentially correctable etiology should be ruled out.

# CHRONIC HYPERTENSION

Chronic hypertension is hypertension that was present before pregnancy or prior to 20 weeks gestational age, and occurs most frequently among multiparous patients. No unanimity of opinion has been reached regarding the most appropriate antihypertensive for use during pregnancy or the efficacy of such treatment with regard to pregnancy outcome.

Methyldopa (Aldomet) is one of the most commonly used antihypertensives in pregnant women. The initial dose of this agent is 250 mg twice a day with increases up to 2 g per day and a maximum recommended daily dose of 3 g (PDR, 2019).

Beta-adrenergic blockers such as atenolol, propranolol, or labetalol, as well as the calcium channel blockers and the centrally acting agent, clonidine, can also be used during pregnancy to treat hypertension. However, no scientific evidence indicates that they offer any advantage over methyldopa during pregnancy.

A variety of thiazide diuretics may also be employed as an adjunct in the treatment of hypertension. However, they should not be initiated after 20 weeks gestation because they may interfere with the 'normal' pregnancy expansion of blood volume and thus placental perfusion.

In gravidas at high risk for preeclampsia (e.g., prior pregnancy, family history of primary relative), 81mg of aspirin is recommended (ACOG, 2016).

## PREGNANCY-INDUCED HYPERTENSION

Antihypertensives are generally not indicated for the treatment of preeclampsia-associated hypertension, except in severe preeclampsia. In the event of severe, acute hypertension (i.e., diastolic blood pressures greater than 110 mmHg), intravenous hydralazine in 5–10 mg doses will usually be effective. This dose can be increased and repeated every 15–20 min, as necessary. The treatment goal of medical therapy is to achieve a diastolic blood pressure less than 110 mmHg, and in the range of 90–100 mmHg. Caution must be exercised at the lower range to ensure adequate placental perfusion. Labetalol (10 mg IV) may also be given every 10 min. Higher doses (up to a total dose of 300 mg) may be necessary in some women to control hypertension.

Diuretics are generally contraindicated in women with preeclampsia. Diuretics may significantly lower utero-placental blood flow by further decreasing intravascular volume.

### PROPHYLAXIS OF SUBACUTE BACTERIAL ENDOCARDITIS

Pregnant women with significant cardiac lesions should receive antibiotic prophylaxis for invasive procedures, including vaginal and cesarean delivery, as prophylaxis for endocarditis (see Box 3.7).

---

**BOX 3.7    AMERICAN HEART ASSOCIATION PROPHYLAXIS
FOR BACTERIAL ENDOCARDITIS GUIDELINES**

**Non-penicillin allergic**
- Ampicillin 2.0 g IM or IV
- Gentamicin 1.5 mg/kg IM or IV
- To be given 30 min before delivery and repeated once 8 h later

**Penicillin allergic**
- Vancomycin 1.0 g IV given over 60 min
- Gentamicin 1.5 mg/kg IM or IV
- To be given 60 min before delivery and repeated once 8–12 h later

---

### FETAL CARDIAC ARRHYTHMIAS

A variety of fetal arrhythmias may be detected during pregnancy (Box 3.8). It may not be necessary to treat all arrhythmias *in utero*. Factors that influence *in utero* therapy include the type and etiology of the arrhythmia, the potential for fetal compromise (i.e., heart failure or hydrops) and the gestational age of the fetus. Virtually all antiarrhythmic drugs cross the placenta. Frequently, it is difficult to attain sufficient therapeutic blood concentrations in both the mother and fetus with standard therapeutic doses.

---

**BOX 3.8    FETAL ARRYTHMIAS**

- Tachycardia
- Supraventricular tachycardia (sinus or atrial), rate >180 bpm
- Atrial flutter, rate 400–500 bpm
- Atrial fibrillation
- Ventricular tachycardia, rate 180–400

- Bradycardia
- Sinus bradycardia
- Complete heart block
- Irregular rhythms
- Premature atrial contractions
- Premature ventricular contractions

*Source:* From Kleinman and Copel, 1991; Pinsky *et al.*, 1991.

## SUPRAVENTRICULAR TACHYCARDIA

Supraventricular tachycardia is probably the most common fetal arrhythmia associated with fetal congestive heart failure, especially if the condition is long standing (Chitkara *et al.*, 1980; Kleinman *et al.*, 1985a, 1985b; Pinsky *et al.*, 1991). The drug of choice for the initial treatment of supraventricular tachycardia is maternal digitalis therapy (Pinsky *et al.*, 1991). This drug crosses the placenta readily and is safe for the fetus, although it is sometimes difficult to achieve therapeutic levels in the fetus. Recommended maternal doses are summarized in Table 3.5.

Two other drugs that may be given for fetal supraventricular tachycardia: propranolol and procainamide. Verapamil, has been used for this purpose, BUT should be used with extreme caution and usually only after other therapeutic modalities have failed because of potential adverse events. Other efficacious agents include quinidine, disopyramide, flecainide, and amiodarone. The differential treatment decision should be based on the suspected etiology of the tachycardia (Kleinman and Copel, 1991; Copel, 2020).

## ATRIAL FLUTTER

Atrial flutter and fibrillation are uncommon during the fetal period and are often difficult to diagnose. Fetal heart rate may reach 400–500 bpm with atrial flutter. Control of the ventricular rate via atrioventricular nodal blocks with digoxin or verapamil may be inadequate. These agents may worsen fetal hemodynamic status (Kleinman and Copel, 1991; Copel, 2020). Unless the atrial flutter itself is controlled, "there will continue to be actual contractions against a closed or partially closed atrioventricular valve" (Kleinman and Copel, 1991). A type I agent, such as procainamide or quinidine, should be included in the treatment regimen. Atrial fibrillation is even rarer than flutter and is treated similarly (Kleinman and Copel, 1991).

## TABLE 3.5
## Maternal Dose and Serum Level of Medications for Fetal Supraventricular Tachycardia

| | Maternal Dose | Serum Level |
|---|---|---|
| Digoxin | 0.25–0.75 mg (loading dose 1.0–2.5 ng pO) (or 0.5–2.0 ng IV) | 0.5–2 ng/mL |
| Propranolol | 20–160 ng q 6–8 h IV | 20–100 ng/mL |
| Procainamide | 6 mg/kg q 4 h IV | 4–14 ng/mL |
| If above fail: Verapamil | 80–120 mg q 6–8 h IV | 50–100 ng/mL |

*Sources:* From Kleinman *et al.*, 1985a, b; Pinsky *et al.*, 1991.

# 4 Endocrine Disorders, Contraception, and Hormone Therapy during Pregnancy
## *Embryotoxic versus Fetal Effects*

The maternal endocrine system in normal women *is* altered in the gravid patient because of the complex metabolic demands of pregnancy. Endocrine system disorders may be associated with adverse maternal or embryo-fetal effects, including infertility, increased frequencies of spontaneous abortions, fetal malformations, maternal and fetal metabolic dysfunction. Sometimes the complications are sufficiently severe that maternal and/or fetal death occur. Some endocrine disorders, such as gestational diabetes mellitus, emerge precipitously during gestation. Pre-existing endocrine disorders may remain stable, improve, or be exacerbated, during pregnancy.

Abnormal fetal growth and development may occur because of the endocrine disease, from medication(s) used to treat the disease, or from complication of treatment of the disease. Certain drugs have long been considered a potential hazard for the embryo or fetus, particularly if such agents are administered during the first trimester of pregnancy. Endocrine medications may also have untoward effects in the second and third trimesters. Pharmacokinetic disposition of endocrine agents in pregnancy is poorly studied. A specific interest is the metabolism, distribution and excretion of insulin and its homologs, but specific pharmacokinetic parameters are not published.

The limited data available indicate that the volume of distribution ($V_d$) increases for endocrine agents during pregnancy as does clearance for the drugs studied (Table 4.1).

This chapter is designed to address endocrine disorders, hormone therapy during pregnancy, and the possible teratogenic effects of medications. First, it describes briefly the pathogenesis of the major endocrine disorders of pregnancy and second, it enumerates the medications that have been used to treat such disorders and their potential embryotoxic and fetal effects.

## TABLE 4.1
### Pharmacokinetics of Endocrine and Hormone Agents during Pregnancy

| Agent | N | EGA (weeks) | Route | AUC | $V_d$ | $C_{max}$ | $C_{ss}$ | $t_{1/2}$ | Cl | PPB | Control Group[a] | Authors |
|---|---|---|---|---|---|---|---|---|---|---|---|---|
| Dexamethasone | 6 | 33–40 | IV | ↑ | | | = | ↑ | | | Yes (3) | Tsuei *et al.* (1980) |
| Dexamethasone | 10 | 29 | PO, IM | ↑ | | | = | | | | Yes (1) | Elliot *et al.* (1996) |
| Methimazole | 7 | 12–39 | PO | = | | | ↓ | ↑ | | | Yes (3) | Skellern *et al.* (1980) |
| Oxytocin | 9 | 37–40 | BU, IV | = | | | | ↑ | | | Yes (4) | Dawood *et al.* (1980) |
| Propythiouracil | 6 | 37–40 | PO | | | | | | | | No | Gardner *et al.,* 1986 |

[a] Control groups: 1, non-pregnant women; 2, same individuals studied postpartum; 3, historic adult controls (sex not given); 4, adult male controls; 5, adult male and female controls combined $t_{1/2}$-half-life; Cl, renal clearance.

*Abbreviations:* EGA, estimated gestational age; AUC, area under the curve; $V_d$, volume of distribution; $C_{max}$, peak plasma concentration; $C_{ss}$, steady-state concentration; $t_{1/2}$- half life; PPB, plasma protein binding; PO, by mouth; ↓ denotes a decrease during pregnancy compared to nonpregnant values; ↑ denotes an increase during pregnancy compared to nonpregnant values; = denotes no difference between pregnant and nonpregnant values; IV, intravenous; IM, intramuscular.

*Sources:* Little BB. *Obstet Gynecol*, 1999; 93: 858.

DOI: 10.1201/9780429160929-4

## MAJOR ENDOCRINE DISORDERS

### DIABETES MELLITUS

Diabetes mellitus is a chronic disorder caused by a partial or total lack of insulin. It complicates 0.2–0.3 percent of all gestations (Connell *et al.*, 1985a; Cousins, 1991; Gabbe, 1980; Rodman *et al.*, 1976). Clinical manifestations vary with the severity of the disease, and range from an asymptomatic hyperglycemic state to severe diabetic ketoacidosis, coma, and death. Gestational diabetes mellitus is characterized by glucose intolerance presenting in the second to third trimesters, and is found in approximately 2–10 percent of gestations (CDC, 2020). www.cdc.gov/diabetes/basics/gestational.html

In meta-analysis studies, the malformation rate in type 1 diabetic pregnancy did not differ from that of type 2 diabetic pregnancy, estimated at 5–6 percent. Similar malformation rates may be correlated with advanced age and high adiposity in type 2 diabetic women (Eriksson and Wentzel, 2016).

### TYPE 1 DIABETES MELLITUS

The difference between type 1 and type 2 diabetes is that the pancreas produces no insulin and life is entirely dependent on exogenous insulin.

### TYPE 2 DIABETES MELLITUS

In type 2 diabetes, the pancreas may still secrete insulin, although the amount may be insufficient to offer glycemic control. By the time a diagnosis is made with type 2 diabetes, pancreatic insulin secretion is usually 50 percent or less of the normal amount.

Type 1 and type 2 diabetes are chronic disorders. In the 1980s and 1990s gestational diabetes, 0.2–0.3 percent of all gestations (Connell *et al.*, 1985a; Cousins, 1991; Gabbe, 1980; Rodman *et al.*, 1976), but has increased dramaticaly in the past 30 years. In the United States, an estimated 1–2 percent of pregnant women have type 1 or type 2 diabetes, and approximately 6–9 percent of pregnant women develop gestational diabetes. As noted earlier, diabetes during pregnancy has increased since 1990. Recent studies found that from 2000 to 2010, the percentage of pregnant women with gestational diabetes increased 56 percent and the percentage of women with type 1 or type 2 diabetes before pregnancy increased 37 percent.

Diabetes in pregnancy varies by race and ethnicity. Asian and Hispanic women have higher rates of gestational diabetes and black and Hispanic women have higher rates of type 1 or type 2 diabetes during pregnancy.

Clinical manifestations vary with the severity of the disease and range from an asymptomatic hyperglycemic state to severe diabetic ketoacidosis, coma, and death. Gestational diabetes mellitus is characterized by glucose intolerance presenting in the second to third trimesters and is found in approximately 2–3 percent of gestations.

### DIABETIC EMBRYOPATHY

Children of women who have diabetes mellitus prior to pregnancy have a two- to fourfold increase in congenital anomalies compared to the general population (Cousins, 1983, 1987; Mills, 1982). Organ development occurs prior to the eighth week of gestation, the critical window of time during which the teratogenic effect of overt maternal diabetes occurs (Mills *et al.*, 1979). Birth defects seen in infants of diabetic mothers involve cardiovascular, skeletal, and central nervous systems (Box 4.1). It is important to note, however, that infants of women who develop gestational diabetes mellitus are not at an increased risk for such defects because the exposure to the disease is outside the critical period of organogenesis (Mills, 1982).

### BOX 4.1    FEATURES OF DIABETIC EMBRYOPATHY

**Cardiovascular**

- Coarctation of the aorta
- Situs inversus
- Transposition of great vessels
- Ventricular septal defect

**Central nervous system**

- Hydrocephalus
- Microcephaly
- Neural tube defects

**Skeletal**

- Caudal dysplasia syndrome
- Limb defects

**Gastrointestinal**

- Bowel atresia
- Imperforate anus
- Tracheoesophageal fistula

**Genitourinary**

- Absent kidneys
- Double ureters
- Polycystic kidneys

**Miscellaneous**

- Cleft lip or palate
- Polyhydramnios
- Single umbilical artery

*Sources:* Adapted from Becerra *et al.*, 1990; Dignan, 1981; Castori, 2013.

## FETAL COMPLICATIONS

Infants born to women who have diabetes prior to pregnancy and women who acquire gestational diabetes mellitus are at risk for significant neonatal morbidity. These neonates are at increased risk for respiratory distress syndrome, macrosomia, hypoglycemia, hyperbilirubinemia, and hypocalcemia. In addition, the risk of fetal death is two- to threefold greater than in the general population (O'Sullivan, 1980; Rust *et al.*, 1987). It is generally accepted that the frequency of these complications can be reduced with good maternal glucose control. However, national levels investigations found no association between glycemic control and the frequency of congenital anomalies consistent with diabetic embryopathy (Eriksson and Parri Wentzel, 2016).

## MEDICATIONS

The American College of Obstetricians and Gynecologists (ACOG) and the American Diabetes Association (ADA) continue to recommend human insulin as the standard of care in women with gestational diabetes mellitus (GDM) requiring medical therapy. Human insulin does not cross the placenta in the absence of Ig binding.

## INSULIN

Insulin is a hormone secreted by pancreatic beta cells that regulates glucose metabolism and other metabolic processes. Human insulin does not cross the placenta in physiologically significant amounts, but non-human insulin does. Subcutaneous injection is the usual route of administration for insulin, but in an emergency or during a stressful situation where a high degree of control is needed (e.g., labor, surgery), intravenous insulin is used to rapidly lower blood glucose.

Human insulin (semisynthetic or biosynthetic) is preferred over the animal insulins because it is much less antigenic, and animal insulins may cross the placenta. Maternal insulin antibodies can alter insulin pharmacokinetics and cross the placenta, contributing to fetal hypoglycemia, beta-cell hyperplasia, and hyperinsulinemia (Knip *et al.*, 1983). Therefore, most diabetologists agree that immunogenic (animal) insulins should not be used in pregnant women. Maternal glucose freely crosses the placenta, but maternal insulin does not cross the placenta unless bound to IgG antibody. The antibody that transports insulin through the placenta or it is forced through the placenta by high perfusion. Diabetic fetopathy is thought to be the result of fetal hyperinsulinemia. Thus, treatment must be managed to normalize maternal blood glucose concentrations without the use of non-human exogenous insulins that cross the placenta to minimize chances of diabetic fetopathy (Jovanovic and Pettitt, 2007). Insulin lispro, aspart, and detemir are approved for use in pregnancy.

Early studies suggested that the human placenta was impermeable to free insulin as well as insulin antibody complexes, but it appears that considerable amounts of antibody-bound animal insulin can cross the placenta (i.e., 25–59 percent of maternal circulation) (Jovanovic and Pettitt, 2007).

## NON-INSULIN INJECTABLE HYPOGLYCEMIC AGENTS: GLP-1 RECEPTOR AGONISTS

### ALBIGLUTIDE (TANZEUM)

No studies of albiglutide use during human pregnancy are published. The manufacturer states that the drug should not be used in pregnancy because of the potential for harm to the embryofetus, citing studies in mice. Fetal and neonatal loss were increased, but not the frequency of congenital anomalies, in offspring of mice given up to 39 times the usual human dose during gestation. Notably, the manufacture's warnings include discontinuation of albiglutide at least 30 days prior to conception because of the long washout period for the drug.

### EXENATIDE (BYDUREON, BYETTA)

Exenatide is a non-oral drug available to treat diabetes but it has not been studied during pregnancy. No adequate human studies have been published of exenatide use during pregnancy, although a registry was established. The old FDA category was C. Importantly, the manufacturer states the drug should not be used during pregnancy. At doses two to three times the usual human dose of exenatide during gestation in mice, the drug was associated with increased frequency of cleft palate, irregular skeletal ossification, and an increased number of neonatal deaths (Manufacturer's data).

### Liraglutide (Saxenda, Victoza)

Several cases have been reported of normal infants born following exposure to liraglutide, but no epidemiological studies of large numbers of pregnancies exposed to Liraglutide during the first trimester are published. Based on rodent reproductive studies, the manufacturer states that Liraglutide is contraindicated for use during pregnancy. The recommendation is to switch patients to insulin as soon as pregnancy is recognized.

### Pramlintide (Symlin)

No studies of the use of pramlintide during human pregnancy are published. In ex vivo placental experiments, pramlintide had a remarkably low potential for placental transfer (Hiles *et al.*, 2003). The old FDA pregnancy risk category for pramlintide is C, but this is based on rodent studies in which fetal and neonatal survival was markedly reduced.

### Dulaglutide (Trulicity)

Dulaglutide is another GLP-1 inhibitor used to treat T2DM. The drug is not intended for treating type 1 diabetes, and should never be used for this disorder. It has not been studied in human pregnancy. The manufacturer reported increased embryonic loss and skeletal ossification abnormalities in pregnant rats given up to 44 times the usual human dose during organogenesis. Offspring of rabbits given 13 times the usual human dose of dulaglutide during embryogenesis had lung lobe agenesis and vertebral malformations. Under the old FDA category system, dulaglutide is pregnancy risk category C.

### Semaglutide (Ozempic)

Semaglutide is a relatively new GLP-1 inhibitor that has not been studied on human pregnancy. The manufacturer reports that in animal studies birth defects and pregnancy losses occurred in pregnancies exposed to the drug during organogenesis. No pregnancy risk categories are assigned to this agent; however, it is noted in the manufacturer's package literature that the drug should be discontinued two months before conception. No studies of excretion into breast milk are published but the manufacturer states that it is transferred into animal breast milk.

## ORAL HYPOGLYCEMIC AGENTS

Oral hypoglycemic drugs include: **sulfonylureas** (acetohexamide, tolazamide, chlorpropamide, tolbutamide, glyburide, glipizide), biguanides (metformin), **thiazolidinediones or THZs** (rosiglitazone, pioglitazone), and alpha-glucosidase inhibitors (acarbose or Precose).

**Oral hypoglycemics are not recommended for use in pregnancy because they are known to cross the placenta and can stimulate fetal insulin secretion.** These drugs have a very long half-life, and administration near term can result in a severely hypoglycemic neonate (Friend, 1981). **ACOG recommends use of human insulin for management of pregnancy in pregnant patients with diabetes (types 1 and 2).**

## ACETOHEXAMIDE

This drug has been withdrawn from the market and is no longer available in the US. Acetohexamide administration throughout pregnancy was significantly associated with neonatal hypoglycemia (Kemball *et al.*, 1970). Pregnant rats given acetohexamide at many times the usual human dose on days 9 and 10 had approximately 50 percent embryonic death but no abnormalities (Bariljak, 1965).

The frequency of congenital anomalies was increased, other than those expected in diabetes mellitus. Chlorpropamide is a closely related drug.

## CHLORPROPAMIDE

One of 41 children born to women treated with chlorpropamide during the first trimester of pregnancy had a congenital anomaly. However, anomalies were probably the result of diabetic embryopathy, and not the drug exposure (Coetzee and Jackson, 1984).). Rats treated during pregnancy with chlorpropamide in doses 200 to 300 times those usually employed in humans did not produce congenital anomalies in their offspring (Tuchmann-Duplessis and Mercier-Parot, 1959). Unpublished information on 18 infants exposed to chlorpropamide during the first trimester, there were no birth defects (Briggs *et al.*, 2021).

Chlorpropamide is known to cross the placenta (approximately 11 percent of maternal serum concentrations reach the fetus), and therefore use near term is a risk for prolonged neonatal hypoglycemia as a possible risk that requires special management consideration at delivery.

**Importantly,** neonatal hypoglycemia may occur in infants of diabetic mothers treated with chlorpropamide late in pregnancy (Kemball *et al.*, 1970; Zucker and Simon, 1968). Chlorpropamide is excreted into the breast milk, and hypoglycemia is a potential complication with use of the drug postpartum. It is an FDA pregnancy risk category C under the old system.

## TOLBUTAMIDE

The frequency of congenital anomalies was not increased among 42 women who were treated with tolbutamide during pregnancy, but only 12 of these women had been treated during the first trimester. Several clinical series have suggested that the frequency of congenital anomalies among infants born to women who took tolbutamide in pregnancy is no greater than would be expected among infants of diabetic mothers (Coetzee and Jackson, 1984; Dolger *et al.*, 1969; Notelovitz, 1971). Rat and mouse studies show no increase in congenital anomalies with tolbutamide until the doses are maternally toxic. Tolbutamide does not seem likely to cause birth defects in exposed infants, but this is based on fewer than 50 exposed infants.

Given the ratio of maternal serum:breast milk concentrations of the drug, hypoglycemia has potential toxicity for use of tolbutamide post-partum (Committee on Drugs, Am Acad Peds, 2001).

## TOLAZAMIDE

There has been one case report of an ear malformation in an infant exposed to the oral hypoglycemic agent tolazamide during the first 12 weeks of gestation (Piacquadio *et al.*, 1991). It should be avoided in pregnancy since both tolazamide and tolbutamide will not provide good control in pregnant patients who cannot be controlled by di*et al*one (Friend, 1981).

Neonatal hypoglycemia is likely to occur with chronic use near the time of delivery, and is a potential toxicity during breastfeeding because based on molecular properties of the drug placental transfer and excretion into breast milk should be expected.

## GLYBURIDE

The transfer rate of glyburide across the human placenta was reported to be much lower than other oral hypoglycemics using *in vitro* techniques (Elliott *et al.*, 1991). Anencephaly and ventricular septal defect were reported in two infants exposed *in utero* to glyburide during the first 10 and 23 weeks of gestation (Piacquardio *et al.*, 1991). However, as with all of the agents in this class, prolonged neonatal hypoglycemia may be associated with maternal therapy (Coetzee and Jackson,

1984). Among more than 180 infants exposed to glyburide during the first trimester, the frequency of congenital anomalies was not increased (Towner *et al.*, 1995; Rosa, personal communication, cited in Briggs *et al.*, 2021). Given the high background risk for diabetic pregnancies (two- to four-fold higher than the general population), glyburide does not seem to pose a high risk for congenital anomalies. The authors considered glycemic control more important than drug use when they summarized their findings (Kallen, 2019). In contrast, after adjusting for type of diabetes and glycemic control, the insulin-exposed infants had a higher frequency of birth defects in the insulin group (9.6 percent) than in the non-insulin hypoglycemic treated group (1.9 percent) (Rankin *et al.*, 2010).

The risk of neonatal hypoglycemia and macrosomia was significantly increased compared to the insulin group in a comparison of glyburide versus insulin in 1194 patients (including 527 exposed to glyburide) in a meta-analysis (Song *et al.*, 2017). The frequency of congenital anomalies were increased in 883 offspring of mothers who used insulin during the first trimester in the Swedish Birth Defects Registry (Kallen, 2019). CNS malformations, cardiovascular defects, VSD+ASD, hypospadias, and poly/syndactyly were increased in frequency.

## GLIPIZIDE

Glipizide is a sulfonylurea drug used to treat noninsulin-dependent diabetes. In one study of 147 infants born to women who took glipizide during embryogenesis the frequency of congenital anomalies was not increased compared to infants born to women who took another sulfonylurea, used insulin, or controlled their diabetes with diet (Towner *et al.*, 1995).

### GLIMEPIRIDE

Glimepiride is a sulfonylurea agent used to treat type 2 diabetes. No published studies are available that analyzed the frequency of birth defects following exposure to Glimepiride during organogenesis.

### METFORMIN

Metformin is a biguanide that increases insulin sensitivity and reduces hepatic gluconeogenesis. Among 711 infants in the Swedish Birth Defects Registry whose mothers took metformin during the first trimester, 45 were malformed (Kallen, 2019), which was considered significant for severe malformations. However, no individual class of birth defects was increased in frequency. In a case-control analysis of 11 European birth defect registries, the frequency of birth defects was not increased among 168 infants with birth defects who were exposed to metformin during the first trimester (Given *et al.*, 2018).

### GESTATIONAL DIABETES

Gestational diabetes mellitus (GDM) in early pregnancy is associated with poor pregnancy outcomes, similar to pre-gestational diabetes, despite intensive intervention and management. Long term (20-year) analysis of ~4,900 women and pregnancy outcomes with GDM, it was found that GDM treatment for those diagnosed after 24 weeks reduced adverse pregnancy outcomes. Poor pregnancy outcomes associated with GDM (e.g., preeclampsia, preterm delivery, and neonatal jaundice) were significantly higher in frequency in the early GDM group, comparable to gravidas with pre-existing diabetes. Importantly, intensive interventions were made in early GDM patients' group (Sweeting *et al.*, 2016).

> The gradation in risk of poor pregnancy outcomes associated with an early diagnosis of GDM suggests a heterogeneity of the phenotype, with women diagnosed with abnormal glucose tolerance prior to 12 weeks' gestation an especially high-risk cohort. Accordingly, these women require increased

surveillance throughout pregnancy. These findings also indicate the need for further studies to establish the efficacy of earlier diagnostic processes as well as early and/or alternative management approaches to improve outcomes in these high-risk pregnancies.

(Sweeting *et al*., 2017)

## DIPEPTIDYL PEPTIDASE-4 ENZYME (DPP-4) INHIBITORS

This class of medications is poorly studied during pregnancy, with no human experience or only anecdotal case reports. The first-line ACOG recommendation for management of diabetes (types 1 and 2) during pregnancy remains human insulins.

## VILDAGLIPTIN

Vildagliptin is a DPP-4 inhibitor used to treat type 2 diabetes mellitus. The frequency of birth defects was apparently not increased among 69 infants born after first trimester exposure to vildagliptin (Benhalima *et al*., 2018). Renal aplasia and patent ductus arteriosus were the two congenital anomalies observed (2/69).

## ALOGLIPTIN (NESINA)

Studies in women who used alogliptin during first or subsequent trimesters of pregnancy have not been published. The manufacturer reported placental transfer of alogliptin in pregnant rats. Offspring of pregnant rabbits and rats given alogliptin during the period of organogenesis alogliptin at 149 times and 180 times the usual human dose, respectively, did not have an increased frequency of congenital anomalies. Pregnant rats given up to 95 times the usual human dose reportedly did not affect embryo-fetal or postnatal development. The manufacturer also reports that this drug is classified as a pregnancy risk category B drug, but other sources quote a C risk category. The manufacturer reports alogliptin crosses the placenta. One of 18 infants born after exposure to alogliptin during the first trimester had a congenital anomaly (Benhalima *et al*., 2018). Notably, this birth defect was an enlarged kidney.

## SAXAGLIPTIN (ONGLYZA)

No controlled trials in pregnant women are published, and clinical experience with this drug in pregnancy has not been reported. Based solely upon animal studies in rats and rabbits that were negative, the FDA pregnancy risk category assigned is B. Placental transfer of saxagliptin has not been studied, but based upon its molecular weight, lack of protein binding and terminal half-life, it is expected to cross the placenta. First trimester exposure to saxagliptin was reported in 15 pregnancies, but outcomes were available for only two infants (Benhalima *et al*., 2018); one elective termination and one healthy infant, who were normal.

## SITAGLIPTIN (JANUVIA)

Only 16 human pregnancies were reported to the Sitagliptin Registry, and there were no congenital anomalies, but this is purely anecdotal. Animal studies in rabbits and rats given Sitagliptin up to 30 and 20 times the usual human dose during gestation, respectively, had no increased frequency of birth defects. However, the FDA pregnancy risk category is B despite no basis on human experience. The drug crosses the placenta in rodent animal models, but human studies are not published. First trimester exposure to sitagliptin was reported in 30 pregnancies, but only 18 live births resulted (Benhalima *et al*., 2018). Two of these infants had major birth defects (cleft palate, multicystic dysplastic kidney and hypoplastic adenohypophysis and ectopic neurohypophysis).

No human studies of linagliptin during pregnancy are published. The manufacturer provides the only information on linagliptin use during gestation. Placental transfer has not been analyzed for linagliptin, but the long-elimination half-life, molecular weight and charge suggest it will cross the placenta. At doses, nearly 2,000 times the usual human dose given to pregnant rabbits and rats during embryogenesis, no increased frequency of congenital anomalies was reported. The theoretical but probably real risk of hypoglycemia neonatally and during breastfeeding should be monitored. Pregnancy outcome was available for 14 of 33 exposures to linagliptin. Of the 14, two major congenital anomalies were observed (patent ductus and holoprosencephaly) were observed (Benhalima *et al.*, 2018).

## SGLT-2 (SODIUM-GLUCOSE CO-TRANSPORTER-2) INHIBITORS

SGLT-2 inhibitors work by inhibiting reabsorption of glucose back into the blood from the kidneys. The kidneys, thus, lower blood glucose levels with excess glucose being removed through urination. The four drugs in this category are tightly bound to plasma proteins, which may impede in crossing the placenta. Teratogenic concerns are raised regarding the use of these four drugs during pregnancy because of the consistent finding in experimental animals of renal pelvic and tubular dilation in exposed offspring that does not reverse itself.

### CANAGLIFLOZIN (INVOKANA)

#### Canagliflozin/Metformin (Invokamet, Invokamet XR)

The frequency of congenital anomalies in human pregnancies exposed to canagliflozin during the first trimester has not been published.

The frequency of birth defects was not increased in the offspring of rats and rabbits given canagliflozin during organogenesis at doses up to 19 times the usual human dose in pregnant rabbits and rats. However, renal function of fetuses and neonates exposed to canagliflozin during gestation, the equivalent of human second and third trimesters, seem compromised. Concern is raised over human fetal and neonatal renal function after exposure to canagliflozin, and probably other SGLT-2 inhibitors, during mid-to-late gestation. Only 13 of 29 first trimester exposure to canagliflozin had pregnancy outcomes reported. Of those 13, one birth defect occurred (Benhalima *et al.*, 2018).

No data are available regarding excretion of canagliflozin into breast milk, but in rats the transfer of the drug into milk seems equivalent to maternal serum concentrations. It is an FDA category C drug under the old classification system.

### DAPAGLIFLOZIN (FARXIGA)

#### Dapagliflozin/Metformin (Xigduo XR) and Dapagliflozin/Saxagliptin (Qtern)

The manufacturer reported rabbit offspring exposed to dapagliflozin during embryogenesis had no increased frequency of congenital anomalies. The frequency of congenital anomalies was increased among offspring of rats exposed to dapagliflozin at 2344 times the usual human dose during embryogenesis, including blood vessel, rib, and vertebral malformations

Eight first trimester pregnancies were exposed to dapagliflozin. Outcomes included six birth defects: one renal aplasia, one esophageal atresia, one hydrocephaly, two cases of encephalocele, and talipes (Benhalima *et al.*, 2018).

A consistent and particularly worrisome finding of SGLT-2 inhibitors exposure during gestation is renal abnormalities. Among rat offspring whose mothers were exposed to ~1415 times the usual human dose of dapagliflozin during pregnancy, the frequency and severity renal pelvic dilation, as well as at doses ≥19 times the usual human dose of dapagliflozin. Gestational timing equivalent to the human second and third trimester was correlated with the increased frequency and severity of renal pelvic and tubular dilation, which are predictive of renal failure.

It is not known if dapagliflozin crosses the placenta, but its physical properties (molecular weight ~503, long terminal elimination half-life) are consistent with placental transfer. Similarly, dapagliflozin is likely to be excreted into breast milk. Importantly, in animal studies, mammary milk levels 0.49 times the maternal serum levels were associated with renal pelvic and renal tubular dilation.

The FDA has not classified this drug but the Australian pregnancy risk category is D.

## EMPAGLIFLOZIN (JARDIANCE)

### Empagliflozin/Linagliptin (Glyxambi) and Empagliflozin/Metformin (Synjardy, Synjardy XR)

Exposure to empagliflozin during pregnancy was reported for nine conceptuses, none of which had a birth defect (Benhalima *et al.*, 2018).

As with other SGLT-2 inhibitors, empagliflozin may impair renal development and maturation when used in the 2nd and 3rd trimester, as is the case with canagliflozin, dapagliflozin, and ertugliflozin. The frequency of congenital anomalies was not increased in rabbits and rats born following exposure during gestation to doses of empagliflozin 128 and 48 times the usual human dose of empagliflozin, respectively (Manufacturer's information). Long bone defects were found in offspring of pregnant rats given 154 times the usual human dose.

It is not known if empagliflozin crosses the placenta but its chemical characteristics are consistent with other substances that cross the placenta (molecular weight ~451, long elimination half-life) suggest that it is likely to cross the placenta.

## ERTUGLIFLOZIN (STEGLATRO)

### Ertugliflozin/Metformin (Segluromet) and Ertugliflozin/Sitagliptin (Steglujan)

There are no data published regarding use of ertugliflozin in human pregnancy, and the risks remain unknown.

Offspring of pregnant rats given 13 times the usual human dose during organogenesis, including the period for critical renal development, had impaired renal development (renal pelvic/ tubule dilations and renal mineralization) that were not reversible. Higher rates of fetal loss and of visceral malformations (membranous ventricular septal defect) were observed at maternally toxic doses.

The US FDA has not assigned a pregnancy risk category to ertugliflozin, but the Australian equivalent classifies ertugliflozin as a pregnancy risk category D. Placental transfer has not been studied but this drug is a candidate for fetal exposure because molecular weight (~500) and long terminal half-life elimination, but strong binding to maternal proteins may attenuate any potential transfer. Similarly, excretion of ertugliflozin into breast milk may occur, but biding to maternal proteins may minimize transfer to milk.

# THYROID GLAND

Maternal thyroid changes during pregnancy are substantial, and differential diagnosis between normal pregnancy associated changes and true thyroid abnormalities is sometimes unclear.

Volume of the maternal thyroid increases by an estimated 30 percent from the first to the third trimesters. Changes in thyroid function and hormone levels occur throughout pregnancy, and proper assessment depends upon accurate estimation of gestational age at exposure.

Maternal total or bound thyroid hormone levels increase with serum concentrations of thyroxine-binding globulin (or thyroid-binding globulin), Thyrotropin (or thyroid-stimulating hormone

[TSH]) levels decrease in early pregnancy because substantial quantities of human chorionic gonadotropin (hCG) during the first 12 weeks of gestation cause weak stimulation of TSH receptors. This variation is essential in screening for and diagnosis of many thyroid disorders in pregnancy.

This stimulates thyroid hormone secretion, and increases serum free thyroxine ($T_4$) levels and suppresses hypothalamic thyrotropin releasing hormone levels. Successively, this limits pituitary TSH secretion. TSH levels return to baseline levels after the first trimester, progressively increase in the third trimester associated with production of placental deiodinase, and increased placental size (Negro and Mestman, 2011). These physiologic changes must be considered when interpreting thyroid function test results and therapy during pregnancy.

Thyroxine-binding globulin (TBG) concentrations increase to about two times normal values, resulting in significant elevations in serum L-thyroxine (T4) and liothyronine (T3) concentrations, coupled with a decrease in T3 resin uptake (T3RU) to values in the hypothyroid range (Glinoer et al., 1990; Harada et al., 1979; Osathanondh et al., 1976). Shortly after delivery, these values return to normal (Yamamoto et al., 1979). The concentrations of free T4, free T3, and the free thyroid index (FTI) in maternal serum remain normal throughout gestation (Glinoer et al., 1990). Mild diffuse thyromegaly occurs during gestation, probably due to an increased vascularity of the gland, and an increased thyroidal uptake of iodine secondary to elevated renal clearance (Dowling et al., 1961; Pochin, 1952). In addition, the placenta produces two hormones with thyroid-stimulating bioactivity. Human chorionic gonadotropin (hCG) and human chorionic thyrotropin (hCT) are secreted in variable amounts, yet are of questionable physiologic impact (Harada et al., 1979; Kennedy et al., 1992).

Thyrotoxicosis and hypothyroidism are associated with adverse pregnancy outcomes, and should be treated when diagnosed.

## Maternal Hyperthyroidism

The prevalence of hyperthyroidism is approximately two per 1,000 pregnancies (Mestman, 1997; Marx et al., 2008; Cooper and Laurberg, 2013). Graves' disease, Plummer's disease, trophoblastic disease, and Hashimoto's thyroiditis. Hashimoto's disease causes hypothyroidism is believed to cause hyperthyroidism. Hyperthyroidism presents as heat intolerance, tachycardia, tremulousness, palpitations, agitation, hyperreflexia, exophthalmos, lid lag, and weight loss. However, many of these symptoms are observed in a normal pregnancy (Cooper and Laurberg, 2013).

Maternal hyperthyroidism is potentially harmful to the developing fetus and neonate, but this is not due to the direct effect of thyroid hormones because they do not cross the placenta in significant amounts. Thyroid-stimulating immunoglobulins (TSI) readily cross the placenta and may produce fetal and/or neonatal thyrotoxicosis (McKenzie, 1964; Cooper and Laurberg, 2013). Neonatal thyrotoxicosis is typically transient, usually resolving in one to three months in the neonate, until maternal TSI is terminally cleared from the infant's serum. Notably, neonatal syndromes have been described for placental transfer of blocking and stimulating antibodies (Zakarija et al., 1986). Increased incidence of prematurity, preeclampsia, and low birth weight was observed among hyperthyroid gravidas, and maternal weight loss can result in fetal undernutrition (Freedberg et al., 1957; Javert, 1940; Marx et al., 2008; Cooper and Laurberg, 2013).

Treatment of hyperthyroidism during pregnancy is a choice between antithyroid drugs and subtotal thyroidectomy since maternal radioiodine treatment results in fetal thyroid ablation. Ablation should be avoided after 10–12 weeks of gestation, if possible, to avoid fetal thyroid ablation. Antithyroid drugs are commonly employed to control hyperthyroidism in pregnancy to avoid surgical intervention, whereas most instances of exposure to [131]I are inadvertent exposures before pregnancy is recognized. Proper assessment of gestational timing is important during embryo-fetal development because early exposure (before 10–12 weeks) to [131]I exposure pose little to no risk.

### Propylthiouracil

The drug of choice in the therapy of thyrotoxicosis in pregnancy is a thioamide, propylthiouracil (PTU). It is advocated to be monotherapy for thyrotoxicosis after trials with polytherapy. PTU blocks the synthesis but not the secretion of thyroid hormone, and it prevents peripheral conversion of T4 to T3. Early studies suggest that pregnancy does not have a major effect on the pharmacokinetic disposition of PTU (Sitar *et al.*, 1982), but other studies indicate that PTU concentrations during pregnancy are lower in late pregnancy than in non-pregnant women (Gardner *et al.*, 1986). PTU crosses the placenta (Marchant *et al.*, 1977), and the amount in the third trimester was slightly higher in the fetus (Gardner *et al.*, 1986). In 1 to 5 percent of fetuses, PTU-induced hypothyroidism is compensated. PTU is not apparently associated with an increased risk of congenital anomalies (Becks and Burrow, 1991; Davis *et al.*, 1989; Masiukiewicz and Burrow, 1999). Among 99 infants exposed to PTU during pregnancy, the frequency of congenital anomalies was 3 percent (Wing *et al.*, 1994). In 35 infants exposed to PTU in the first trimester the frequency of birth defects was not increased above that expected (2.9 percent) (Briggs *et al.*, 2021). Among 47 infants born following PTU exposure during organogenesis, 10 birth defects were observed (Clementi *et al.*, 2010). The birth defects included three cases of *situs inversus*/dextrocardia, one case of unilateral renal agenesis/dysgenesis, and five cardiac outflow malformations. PTU exposure during the first trimester in 1,399 infants resulted in no increased frequency of birth defects (Yoshihara *et al.*, 2012).

Among 353 infants exposed to PTU during the first trimester in the Swedish Birth Defects Registry, the frequency of birth defects was increased only for hypospadias (Kallen, 2019).

Finally, congenital fetal hyperthyroidism caused by increases in maternal thyroid-stimulating immunoglobulins has been treated by maternal PTU with some success (Check *et al.*, 1982; Serup and Petersen, 1977). Children exposed to PTU *in utero* were not different from unexposed siblings in postnatal intellectual and physical development (Burrow *et al.*, 1968, 1978).

PTU is the drug of choice for treating hyperthyroidism in pregnancy. Fetal goiter is a small risk (< 5 percent), based on a small number of cases.

### Methimazole and Carbimazole

Methimazole (a thioamide) and carbimazole (a thioamide metabolized to methimazole) are not recommended drugs for first-line use during pregnancy. These medications may be considered if other medications (i.e., PTU) do not provide control the condition. The antithyroid action of methimazole and carbimazole block synthesis but not the release of thyroid hormone.

Methimazole crosses the placenta (Marchant *et al.*, 1977). Fourteen cases of aplasia cutis (scalp defect) among infants exposed to methimazole *in utero* are described in the literature (Bachrach and Burrow, 1984; Farine *et al.*, 1988; Kalb and Grossman, 1986; Milham, 1985; Milham and Elledge, 1972; Mujtaba and Burrow, 1975). Scalp, cranium, and cerebral cortex development is complete by the 3rd month of gestation, suggesting that first-trimester exposure to methimazole played a role in induction of scalp defects (Kokich *et al.*, 1982). No relationship between maternal methimazole therapy and scalp malformations in a large case series (n = 243 infants) of methimazole use in pregnancy was reported (Momotani *et al.*, 1984). Apparently, the strength of the association of maternal methimazole or carbimazole use during pregnancy with congenital scalp defects may have been over estimated (Van Dijke *et al.*, 1987). Two cases of fetal goiter development in association with carbimazole use in pregnancy were reported (Sugrue and Drury, 1980). Postnatal follow-up of children exposed to carbimazole *in utero* found no physical growth or development deficits (McCarroll *et al.*, 1976). The Swedish Birth Defects Registry included 155 infants exposed to methimazole during the first trimester. The frequency of birth defects among the 155 exposed infants was increased, but the only significantly increased frequency was for polydactyly (OR=10.3) (Kallen, 2019).

Maternal methimazole therapy for hyperthyroidism is not recommended for use during pregnancy because PTU is better studied. PTU is the recommended therapy for thyrotoxicosis during pregnancy.

Carbimazole has been withdrawn from the market.

### Ethionamide

Maternal ethionamide administration during pregnancy is known to suppress fetal thyroid hormone synthesis and to result in fetal hypothyroidism and goiter. Based on very limited information, ethionamide (thioamide) does appear to pose a high risk of congenital anomalies (Zierski, 1966).

### Propranolol

Propranolol is a beta-adrenergic blocker medication that has been used in pregnancy for a variety of indications. The two most common disorders of pregnancy for which propranolol has been used are hypertension and hyperthyroidism. An extensive review of the use of propranolol in pregnancy is found in in Chapter 3.

### Iodide (Potassium Iodide)

*Iodide compounds are contraindicated for use during pregnancy.*

Iodides cross the placenta, and the fetus is particularly sensitive to the inhibitory effects of excessive iodide (Wolff, 1969). More than 400 cases of neonatal goiter are reported in infants of mothers treated with potassium iodide during pregnancy (Ayromlooi, 1972; Carswell *et al.*, 1970; Galina *et al.*, 1962; Mehta *et al.*, 1983; Miyagawa, 1973; Parmelee *et al.*, 1940). Neonatal goiters are caused by fetal thyroid inhibition with secondary compensatory hypertrophy. Neonatal goiters can be very large. In some cases, goiters developed from iodide exposure can lead to tracheal compression and neonatal death.

A major exception is thyroid storm. One scenario in which potassium iodide is indicated during pregnancy is the case of "thyroid storm." Treatment of "thyroid storm" is acute administration of 1 g of potassium iodide orally with 1 g of propylthiouracil.

### Radioiodine (Iodine 131I)

The fetal thyroid begins to concentrate iodine at approximately 10–12 weeks of gestation. Fetal pituitary thyroid-stimulating hormone (TSH) controls synthesis and secretion of thyroid hormone, and begins at an estimated 18–20 weeks of gestation. Iodine 131I (the iodine isotope) is contraindicated for use during pregnancy. Retrospective analysis of 182 first trimester pregnancies inadvertently exposed to radioiodine therapy for hyperthyroidism showed that six infants (3.3 percent) had hypothyroidism. Four of the six had intellectual deficits (Stoffer and Hamburger, 1976).

Six case reports of congenital or late-onset hypothyroidism after maternal treatment with 131I during various stages of pregnancy are published (Fisher *et al.*, 1963; Goh, 1981; Green *et al.*, 1971; Hamill *et al.*, 1961; Jafek *et al.*, 1974; Russel *et al.*, 1957). While case reports are not usually considered causal evidence, in the case of [131]I the link between exposure is generally accepted as causal.

### Maternal Hypothyroidism

Symptomatic hypothyroidism in women impairs fertility. It increases the frequency of spontaneous abortion, stillbirth, and congenital anomalies (Davis *et al.*, 1988; Mestman, 1980; Montoro *et al.*, 1981; Pekonen *et al.*, 1984). Hypothyroidism is caused by iodine deficiency, iatrogenic (thyroidectomy or 131I therapy) etiologies, or thyroiditis. Hypothyroidism symptoms include cold intolerance, irritability, and difficulty with concentration, dry skin, coarse hair, and constipation. Many of these symptoms are commonly seen in normal pregnancy, making clinical diagnosis difficult.

The mechanism by which maternal hypothyroidism affects the fetus is unknown. Several reports suggest that it is not a major cause of concern (Kennedy and Montgomery, 1978; Montoro *et al.*, 1981), but others have reported a high prevalence of congenital malformations and impaired mental and somatic development among the offspring of hypothyroid women (Pharoah *et al.*, 1971; Potter, 1980).

## MEDICATIONS FOR HYPOTHYROIDISM

### Levothyroxine (L-Thyroxine)

*Thyroxine*

L-Thyroxine (T4) is a hormone normally produced in the thyroid gland. It is used to treat thyroid deficiency and is suitable for use during pregnancy. The frequency of congenital anomalies was not increased among 537 pregnancies exposed to exogenous thyroxine or thyroid hormone during the first trimester, and 1,605 pregnancies exposed at any time during pregnancy (Heinonen *et al.*, 1977a). In another uncontrolled study of 554 infants whose mothers were exposed in the first trimester, the frequency of major anomalies was 4.5 percent, which is not different from background (Briggs *et al.*, 2021).

The Swedish Birth Defects Registry included 1,379 infants whose mothers used thyroxine during the first trimester. It was reported that the frequency of congenital anomalies was increased slightly, but not to a level that reached statistical significance (Kallen, 2019).

Experimental studies agreed with the findings in humans. Thyroxine should be considered safe for use during pregnancy. Importantly, failure to treat maternal hypothyroidism during pregnancy was associated with poorer outcomes compared to controls at 7–12 years of age (Haddow *et al.*, 1999).

*Levothyroxine*

Among 30,067 infants whose mother used levothyroxine during the first trimester the frequency of birth defects was not increased (Kallen, 2019), with one exception.

Choanal atresia was increased in frequency (OR = 2.8), with levothyroxine use during organogenesis. The author states that the analysis was confounded by diabetes, hypothyroidism, and the use of antithyroid drugs. However, this effect was reduced to statistically non-significant when diabetes, hypothyroidism, and the use of antithyroid drugs were controlled. (Kallen, 2019).

Levothyroxine excretion into breast milk is not sufficient to treat a hypothyroid infant disease effects, and does not affect thyroid tests. Levothyroxine has been classified as compatible with breastfeeding.

### Liothyronine

Liothyronine, T3, is normally produced by the thyroid gland. It is used to treat thyroid T3 deficiency. The frequency of birth defects was not increased among 34 infants whose mothers used liothyronine during pregnancy (Heinonen *et al.*, 1977). Excretion of T3 into breast milk does not reach therapeutic levels, and cannot protect an infant from hypothyroidism.

In the Swedish Birth Defects Registry, the frequency of congenital anomalies was not increased among 151 infants whose mothers used liothyronine during the first trimester (Kallen, 2019).

## PARATHYROID GLAND

### MATERNAL PARATHYROID FUNCTION

Parathyroid glands (~4) are located along the posterior border of the thyroid gland. Their function is primarily in the regulation of bone mineral metabolism. Parathyroid hormone (PTH) maintains extracellular fluid calcium concentration. During pregnancy, calcium requirements increase to 3 to 4 times the non-pregnant daily requirement, especially during the latter half of gestation when most of the fetal bone mineral is deposited. Calcium and phosphorus are actively transported across the placenta, resulting in lower maternal serum calcium concentration, an increase in PTH secretion, and decreased calcitonin production (Schedewie and Fisher, 1980). During gestation, 1,25 dihydroxy vitamin D levels and intestinal absorption of calcium increase strikingly (Bouillon and Van Assche, 1982; Heany and Skillman, 1971; Kumar *et al.*, 1979).

## MATERNAL HYPERPARATHYROIDISM

Excess parathyroid hormone secretion during pregnancy causes increased bone resorption, heightened serum calcium, and other clinical manifestations (chronic fatigue, memory loss, poor concentration, sleep disorders, depression, body aches), similar to those in the non-gravid state. Some gravidas may seem asymptomatic, but an estimated 80 percent present have generalized muscle weakness, nausea, vomiting, pain, renal colic, and/or polyuria. Primary hyperparathyroidism is usually caused by an inferior parathyroid gland adenoma. Childhood history of irradiation to the head or neck is associated with an exceptionally high frequency of hyperparathyroidism (Gelister *et al.*, 1989; van der Spuy and Jacobs, 1984). Effects of maternal hyperparathyroidism contain an increased frequency of kidney stone formation caused by hypercalciuria and hyperphosphaturia, bone trabeculae and thinning, secondary to increased bone resorption (Peacock., 1978; Stanbury *et al.*, 1972). Embryo and fetal effects include a high incidence of spontaneous abortion, stillbirth, neonatal death, and low birth weight (Delmonico *et al.*, 1976; Johnstone *et al.*, 1972; Kristofferson *et al.*, 1985; Ludwig, 1962; Mestman, 1980; Wagner *et al.*, 1964). The incidence of severe hypocalcemia and tetany in infants born to mothers with hyperparathyroidism approaches 50 percent (Butler *et al.*, 1973; Mestman, 1980; Pederon and Permin, 1975), and is caused by elevated maternal ionized calcium crossing the placenta (active transport) and blunting, ultimately suppressing the fetal parathyroid. Infants are usually unable to maintain normal serum calcium concentration in the perinatal period. Neonatal calcium supplementation is usually needed, but this effect is transient and usually resolves by 2 weeks of age without sequelae (Pederon and Permin, 1975).

Treatment of choice for primary hyperparathyroidism during the pregnant or non-pregnant state is surgery to avoid maternal, fetal, and perinatal complications.

## MATERNAL HYPOPARATHYROIDISM

Inadequate PTH characterizes hypoparathyroidism, and presents as severe hypocalcemia. Symptoms during pregnancy are similar to the non-pregnant state, including weakness, fatigue, tetany (by Chvostek's sign and Trousseau's sign tests) and seizures. The etiology of hypoparathyroidism is usually idiopathic, autoimmune, or iatrogenic (surgical removal of parathyroid glands or compromised blood supply during thyroid surgery). In contrast, pseudohypoparathyroidism is caused by deficient end-organ response to the endogenous PTH.

Maternal hypoparathyroidism affects the fetus in different ways. Untreated maternal hypoparathyroidism is associated with neonatal hyperparathyroidism, hypercalcemia, and osteomalacia (Aceto *et al.*, 1966; Bronsky *et al.*, 1970; Goloboff and Ezrin, 1969; Landing and Kamoshita, 1970). Neonatal symptoms are transient, usually resolving over time (Landing and Kamoshita, 1970). Neonatal hyperparathyroidism secondary to low maternal calcium (Loughhead *et al.*, 1990) is associated with neonatal skeletal disease and bone demineralization.

## MEDICATIONS FOR HYPOPARATHYROIDISM

### Vitamin D

Calcium and vitamin D are used to treat maternal hypoparathyroidism during pregnancy and the non-gravid state. Vitamin D is available in a variety of commercially available forms that have a similar metabolic fate, and have a very similar effect on the mother and fetus. Pregnant patients treated for hypoparathyroidism with vitamin D apparently do not have an increased incidence of embryotoxic effects or fetal malformations (Goodenday and Gordon, 1971a, 1971b; Sadeghi-Nejad *et al.*, 1980; Wright *et al.*, 1969), even high doses of 1,25 dihydroxy vitamin D were used (Marx *et al.*, 1980). Among 27 infants born to 15 women following high dose vitamin D during pregnancy, all were normal at follow-up at 16 years of age (Goodenday *et al.*, 1971a, 1971b). Birth defects were not increased in frequency among 1221 infants in the Swedish Birth Defects Registry whose mothers took a vitamin D supplement during the first trimester (Kallen, 2019).

## PITUITARY GLAND

### MATERNAL PITUITARY FUNCTION

The anterior lobe of the pituitary gland (adenohypophysis) doubles or triples in size during normal pregnancy due to hypertrophy and hyperplasia of the lactotrophs (Goluboff and Ezrin, 1969). Physiologic changes during pregnancy are outlined in Box 4.2.

---

**BOX 4.2   PITUITARY GLAND FUNCTION CHANGES DURING PREGNANCY**

- Low basal luteinizing hormone (LH) and follicle-stimulating hormone (FSH) levels, blunted gonadotropin response to gonadotrophin-releasing hormone (GnRH) infusion (Jeppsson *et al.*, 1977; Reyes *et al.*, 1976) secondary to a negative feedback inhibition from elevated levels of estrogen and progesterone.
- Low basal growth hormone (GH) levels and blunted response to insulin-induced hypoglycemia and arginine infusion (Spellacy *et al.*, 1970; Tyson *et al.*, 1969).
- Normal to low adrenocorticotropic hormone (ACTH) levels, that rise markedly during labor and delivery (Beck *et al.*, 1968; Carr *et al.*, 1981).
- Normal levels of thyroid-stimulating hormone (TSH) with a similar response to thyroid-releasing hormone (TRH) stimulation, as in the nonpregnant state (Fisher, 1983a).
- Ten- to 20-fold increase in serum prolactin levels (Rigg *et al.*, 1977; Tyson *et al.*, 1972), secondary to marked hypertrophy and hyperplasia of the lactotrophs.
- Neurophysins are intraneuronal protein carriers for oxytocin and vasopressin that are present in the neurohypophysis, and their plasma concentrations may be elevated during pregnancy (Robinson *et al.*, 1973). However, maternal plasma oxytocin and vasopressin levels are low and do not vary throughout gestation (Fisher, 1983b).

---

Abnormal pituitary function is associated with infertility (e.g., hyperprolactinemia, Cushing's disease). However, hormonal therapy restores fertility in most instances. Pituitary disorders that may complicate pregnancy include enlargement of a prolactinoma, acromegaly, Cushing's disease, and diabetes insipidus.

### PROLACTINOMA

The pituitary gland increases in size during pregnancy. A prolactinoma and its enlargement in pregnant women is concerning. A review of 16 investigations and among 246 pregnant patients showed a low incidence of symptomatic microadenoma (less than 10 mm in size), an increase in size of 1.6 percent. The incidence of symptomatic macroadenoma (more than 10 mm in size) showed 15.5 percent enlargement during pregnancy (Gemzell and Wang, 1979).

## MEDICATIONS FOR PROLACTINOMAS

### Bromocriptine (Parlodel)

A dopamine agonist and ergot alkaloid, bromocriptine, has prolactin-lowering activity. Bromocriptine is frequently used to treat hyperprolactinemia associated with infertility. Bromocriptine crosses the placenta and is associated with fetal hypoprolactinemia (del Pozo et al., 1977, 1980). Effects on fetal neuroendocrine development are unknown.

Outcomes of 1,410 pregnancies in 1,135 women who received bromocriptine in the early weeks of pregnancy was associated with a higher frequency of spontaneous abortion (11.1 percent), but birth defect rate (3.5 percent) was similar to that observed in the general population (Turkalj et al., 1982). Children (n = 212) from this study who were followed for up to six years were normal on mental and physical development assessments. Other investigators (Canales et al., 1981; Hammond et al., 1983; Konopka et al., 1983) reported similar findings with fewer patients. Evidence indicates that there is no increased risk to the fetuses of women treated with bromocriptine during pregnancy, and if symptomatic tumor enlargement should occur, bromocriptine therapy is preferred to surgical intervention during pregnancy (MacCagnan et al., 1995).

Among 2,587 infants whose mother used bromocriptine during organogenesis, the frequency of birth defects was not increased (Krupp and Monka, 1987). In a review of published data on 5,213 infants whose mothers used bromocriptine during early pregnancy, the frequency of birth defects was not increased (Molitch, 2015).

A recent review of 5,213 reported cases of bromocriptine exposure in pregnancy found the frequency of birth defects was not increased (1.8 percent) (Nana and Williamson, 2019).

## CABERGOLINE

Cabergoline is another drug used to treat acromegaly. In a review, the frequency of congenital anomalies was not increased (3.6 percent) among 83 newborns exposed to cabergoline during the first trimester (Stalldecker et al., 2010). In a single center study of 250 live births to women who used cabergoline during pregnancy the frequency of birth defects was high at 9 percent (n = 23), but only 8 of these pregnancies were exposed during the first trimester (Colao et al., 2008). Among 629 infants whose mothers took cabergoline during the first trimester, the frequency of birth defects was not increased (Molitch, 2015). In contrast, a small cohort of pregnancies (n = 25), the frequency of neural tube defects was increased (Rastogi et al., 2017). The Swedish Birth Defects Registry reported no increased frequency of birth defects among 152 infants whose mother used cabergoline during embryogenesis (Kallen, 2019).

### Quinagolide

Quinagolide is a non-ergot-derived selective dopamine D2 receptor agonist. It is used to treat elevated prolactin levels (hyperprolactinemia) associated with gonadal dysfunction, including reduced libido, infertility, and osteoporosis.

Among 150 infants exposed to quinagolide, the frequency of birth defects appeared increased with 9 infants who had major birth defects (Webster, 1996). However, two of the 9 infants had chromosomal abnormalities. Among 253 infants in the Swedish Birth Defects Registry, the frequency of birth defects was not increased (Kallen, 2019).

### ACROMEGALY

Overproduction of growth hormone (GH) characterizes acromegaly, resulting in the overgrowth and thickening of bones and soft tissues. Pituitary adenoma is the most common cause. Therapy usually consists of surgery, radiation, medical therapy, or some combination of the three. Amenorrhea is frequent and fecundity is low in acromegalic women because an estimated 50 percent of women with acromegaly are anovulatory and hyperprolactinemic. Acromegaly during pregnancy is extremely rare (van der Spuy and Jacobs, 1984; Cheng *et al.*, 2012; Dias *et al.*, 2013; Motivala *et al.*, 2011). Symptomatic tumor expansion may occur during gestation because maternal estrogen levels increase (Yap *et al.*, 1990). Optimal management is conservative, and similar to prolactinoma therapy using dopamine agonists. Definitive therapy outside of pregnancy is transsphenoidal resection, but is preferably postponed until after delivery. Treatment with octreotide (somatostatin ligand) and pegvisomant (growth hormone blocker) has been used during pregnancy.

The placenta also normally produces a growth hormone variant (placental GH) in increasing amounts up to delivery (Frankenne *et al.*, 1987). GH secretory patterns in pregnant acromegalic women suggests that the increased insulin-like growth factor (IGF-I) level present in late pregnancy is not pituitary-GH-dependent. The major difference between normal and acromegalic pregnancy is that growth hormone secretion normally decreases after ~20 weeks gestation. Among gravidas with acromegaly, growth hormone does not decrease but maintains a plateau well above normal levels, even in late pregnancy. Placental growth hormone does not seem altered in acromegaly in pregnancy (Muhammad *et al.*, 2017). Excess maternal GH apparently does not cross the placenta to achieve any appreciable concentration in the fetal compartment. When treatment is necessary, bromocriptine is used to treat acromegaly.

## CUSHING SYNDROME AND CUSHING'S DISEASE

Cushing syndrome is rare, and is characterized by elevated cortisol secretion regardless of etiology. The syndrome in pregnancy is described as overproduction of corticotropin-releasing factor (CRF), excessive pituitary adrenocorticotrophic hormone (ACTH) stimulating the adrenals (Cushing's disease), adrenal hyperplasia/adenoma, ectopic sources of ACTH or cortisol, or excessive glucocorticoid therapy. Cushing's disease refers to pituitary-dependent Cushing syndrome. Cushing syndrome's etiology is frequently a pituitary adenoma or hyperplasia. Approximately 40–50 percent of Cushing diagnoses are adrenal adenomas. During pregnancy, the frequency of primary adrenal lesions is apparently somewhat higher than in the non-pregnant state (Gormley *et al.*, 1982). Pregnancy is infrequent among women with Cushing syndrome because most female patients with Cushing are amenorrheic (Gormley *et al.*, 1982; Grimes *et al.*, 1973).

Diagnosis of Cushing is confounded because many of the symptoms (hypertension, weight gain, fatigue, striae, and increased pigmentation) are common in normal pregnancies. Symptoms more specific to Cushing syndrome include thinning of skin, spontaneous bruising, and muscle weakness are symptoms. Increased adrenal androgens cause hirsutism and acne in pregnant women with Cushing syndrome (Grimes *et al.*, 1973). Pregnancy outcomes are usually extremely poor. An estimated 50 percent of recognized pregnancies end in spontaneous abortion, premature delivery or stillbirth (Aaron *et al.*, 1990; Gormley *et al.*, 1982; Grimes *et al.*, 1973).

Treatment of Cushing during pregnancy depends on the etiology of the disorder and the stage of pregnancy at diagnosis. Pituitary and adrenal adenomas should be removed surgically (van der Spuy and Jacobs, 1984), but the recommendations are to wait until pregnancy is completed. When Cushing is diagnosed in the first trimester, pregnancy termination may be considered, especially if adrenal carcinoma is suspected. Cushing in late pregnancy may be treated with metyrapone until delivery of the infant. After delivery, definitive surgery may be done.

## METYRAPONE FOR CUSHING'S DISEASE

An 11-hydroxylase inhibitor, metyrapone (Metopirone), causes a decrease in cortisol production, followed by a subsequent rise of deoxycortisol, the immediate precursor of cortisol. In animal studies, metyrapone crosses the placenta (Baram and Schultz, 1990). Metyrapone is used infrequently during late pregnancy as medical therapy for Cushing's disease to delay surgical intervention until after delivery (Connell *et al.*, 1985b; Gormley *et al.*, 1982). In summary, the ideal therapy for Cushing's disease in pregnancy is surgical intervention. Metyrapone therapy is used to treat Cushing until delivery or fetal maturity. Surgery is postponed until after delivery. In a rat study, pregnant animals were dosed during organogenesis at about seven times the usual human dose; resorptions occurred in 80 percent of pregnancies treated with the drug (Nevagi and Rao, 1970).

### DIABETES INSIPIDUS

True diabetes insipidus (DI) in pregnancy is extremely rare in pregnancy, and occurs in an estimated three per 100,000 pregnancies (Hime and Richardson, 1978). Diabetes insipidus (of hypothalamic or neurogenic origin) is an unusually infrequent disorder caused by deficient arginine vasopressin (AVP) release from the posterior pituitary in response to normal physiologic stimuli. This results in low blood levels of AVP and impaired renal conservation of water.

Clinical characteristics are polyuria, excessive thirst (polydipsia), and low urinary specific gravity. Diabetes insipidus may be idiopathic, autosomal dominant inheritance, or secondary to trauma or tumor. Fertility is not impaired and fetal outcomes are not adversely affected in patients with diabetes insipidus when the disease is successfully treated (Hime and Richardson, 1978; Jouppila and Vuopala, 1971). Therapy includes hormone replacement. The drug of choice in pregnancy is DDAVP (1-deamino-8-D-arginine vasopressin) given as a nasal spray. Other therapeutic regimens in patients with partial diabetes insipidus are not recommended for use during pregnancy (chlorpropamide, clofibrate, and carbamazepine). *Note that DDAVP is not effective for the treatment of nephrogenic diabetes insipidus.*

The frequency of birth defects in 157 infants exposed to DDAVP (desmopressin) was not increased in the Swedish Birth Defects Registry (Kallen, 2019). An earlier study on birth defects in 29 infants who were exposed to desmopressin or vasopressin found one birth defect (Kallen *et al.*, 1995). In a published literature review, 49 infants exposed to desmopressin (DDAVP) during organogenesis were found, and three had one had a major birth defect, and unrelated chromosomal abnormalities (trisomy 21) (Ray, 1998). A recent literature review reported that among 35 infants in 32 different studies exposed to desmopressin during the first trimester, no birth defects occurred. However, the C-section rate was 54 percent (Kyriakos *et al.*, 2021).

## ADRENAL GLAND

### MATERNAL ADRENAL FUNCTION

Maternal adrenal function undergoes a number of changes during the course of normal pregnancy. Estrogen rises during gestation and causes an increased liver production of cortisol-binding globulin (CBG), and thus a rise in plasma cortisol levels while plasma ACTH concentrations are low (Carr *et al.*, 1981).

Plasma-unbound cortisol increases two- to threefold, and there is a twofold increase in free cortisol excretion (Clerico *et al.*, 1980; Nolten *et al.*, 1980). Elevation of free cortisol in pregnancy does not result in cortisol hypersecretion (Gibson and Tulchinsky, 1980). Renin activity increase is associated with elevated aldosterone levels, but this seems not to be clinically significant (Smeaton *et al.*, 1977). Adrenal disorders that may complicate pregnancy include Addison's disease, Cushing syndrome, and congenital adrenal hyperplasia. Cushing syndrome was discussed in the previous section on the pituitary gland.

### MATERNAL ADRENAL INSUFFICIENCY (ADDISON'S DISEASE)

Insufficient ACTH secretion by the pituitary may cause adrenal corticosteroid insufficiency, insufficient adrenal secretion of corticosteroids, or inadequate steroid replacement therapy. Adrenal atrophy secondary to autoimmune disease occurs in about three quarters of diagnosed cases. Addison's disease diagnosis in pregnancy may be difficult because the signs and symptoms (weakness, fatigue, anorexia, nervousness, increased skin pigmentation) parallel those observed in a normal pregnancy. Addison's disease can follow a chronic, indolent course, or progress into a true acute medical emergency characterized by an "Addisonian crisis" (severe nausea, vomiting, diarrhea, abdominal pain hypotension). Pregnancy is known to aggravate Addison's disease. Addison's disease does apparently not affect spontaneous abortion rate, prematurity rate, and neonatal outcome (Brent, 1950; Satterfield and Williamson, 1976). Chronic adrenal insufficiency requires adequate adrenal replacement in the form of cortisone acetate or prednisone and 9-alpha-fluoro-hydrocortisone. During labor, delivery, and the first few days postpartum, the mother should be monitored closely, ensuring a good state of hydration with normal saline and adequate cortisol hemisuccinate replacement. It is common for women with adrenal insufficiency to be diagnosed for the first time during the puerperium when they develop adrenal crisis (Brent, 1950). Treatment involves replacement steroids during an Addisonian crisis including cortisol hemisuccinate (Solu-Cortef), with fluid replacement as isotonic saline, and glucose administration.

Among 186 infants born to women with Addison's disease, the frequency of congenital malformations was not increased compared to controls (Björnsdottir *et al.*, 2010).

## MEDICATIONS FOR ADDISON'S DISEASE

### Cortisone Acetate

Cortisone is a glucocorticoid normally excreted by the adrenal gland. Cortisone is used for replacement therapy and to treat allergic and inflammatory diseases. The Collaborative Perinatal Project included only 34 pregnancies exposed during the first trimester to cortisone, and the frequency of congenital anomalies among the exposed pregnancies was no greater than expected (Heinonen *et al.*, 1977a).

### PREDNISONE AND PREDNISOLONE

Prednisone and prednisolone are synthetic glucocorticoids. Prednisone is biologically inert but is metabolized in first pass through the liver to prednisolone, a biologically active compound. Prednisone and prednisolone are used for replacement therapy and to treat a variety of allergic and inflammatory conditions.

The frequency of birth defects was not increased among infants born to 43 and 204 women in two studies who were treated with prednisone/prednisolone during the first trimester (Heinonen *et al.*, 1977; Kallen, 1998). Among 111 infants exposed to prednisone in the first trimester, the frequency of major birth defects was 4.5 percent (n = 5) (Park-Wylie *et al.*, 2000). In a meta-analysis published with these findings, the odds of cleft palate was significant with calculated as OR = 3.35 based 25 oral cleft cases (Park-Wylie *et al.*, 2000). In the Swedish Birth Defects Registry, the frequency of birth defects in 2374 infants exposed to prednisolone during the first trimester the rate of birth defects in general, or of oro-facial clefts specifically, was not increased (Kallen, 2019). However, the frequency of heart defects and ASD/VSD were significantly increased compared to controls. In another study, no cases of cleft palate were reported among 311 infants born to women who used corticosteroids during the first trimester (Gur *et al.*, 2004).

Perinatal death does not appear to be more frequent than without either drug in most series of infants born to women treated with prednisone or prednisolone, but the risk of fetal growth retardation may be increased (Reinisch *et al.*, 1978).

No such effect on fetal growth was apparent in two smaller studies, one of which also involved women treated throughout pregnancy with prednisone/prednisolone (Lee *et al.*, 1982; Walsh and Clark, 1967). Newborn infants born to women who took prednisone throughout pregnancy usually have normal adrenocortical reserves and no symptoms of adrenal suppression (Arad and Landau, 1984).

Dose-related fetal growth retardation, cleft palate, genital anomalies, and behavioral alterations occur in the offspring of mice treated in pregnancy with prednisone or prednisolone in doses within or above the human therapeutic range (Ballard *et al.*, 1977; Gandelman and Rosenthal, 1981; Pinsky and DiGeorge, 1965; Reinisch *et al.*, 1978). Increased frequencies of cleft palate are also observed among the offspring of pregnant hamsters treated during pregnancy with prednisolone in doses 80–240 times that used in humans (Shah and Kilistoff, 1976).

### CORTICOSTEROIDS IN GENERAL

Among 631 infants whose mothers used therapeutic corticosteroids during the first trimester, the frequency of non-syndromic cleft palate was increased more than six fold (Rodriguez-Pinilla and Martinez-Frias, 1998). However, the absolute risk of orofacial clefts is probably less than 1 percent in pregnancies exposed to corticosteroids in the first trimester, considering the prevalence of the use of corticosteroid drugs and of cleft palate (Shepard *et al.*, 2002), if the association is causal. There is no consensus on whether this relationship is causal.

### Fludrocortisone

There are no epidemiologic studies of malformations in infants born to women treated with fludrocortisone during pregnancy.

### Cortisol Hemisuccinate

No epidemiologic studies have been reported regarding malformations in women treated with this drug during pregnancy. See "Corticosteroids in General."

### 17α-Hydroxyprogesterone Caproate

Among 1,008 offspring, who were diagnosed with cancer, 234 were exposed in utero during embryogenesis to 17α-hydroxyprogesterone caproate. The risk of any cancer was increased 2.6 fold, and the risk increased with the number of injections, indicating a dose–response relationship. Colorectal cancer was increased 5.5 fold and prostate cancer was also increased 5.5 fold. Pediatric bain cancer risk was increased 347 fold (Murphy *et al.*, 2021).

### Congenital Adrenal Hyperplasia

Five principal enzymatic steps are required for the conversion of cholesterol to cortisol in the adrenal gland. An inherited defect in any one of these enzymes may result in congenital adrenal hyperplasia (CAH). In over 90 percent of cases, the deficient enzyme is 21-hydroxylase (New *et al.*, 1983). This enzyme is necessary for the conversion of 17-hydroxyprogesterone to 11-deoxycortisol, and a deficiency results in a decrease in cortisol, and a compensatory rise in ACTH, followed by adrenal hyperplasia with elevated cortisol precursors and adrenal androgens. Classical CAH is the most severe form, and is characterized by a salt-wasting crisis soon after birth because of impaired aldosterone production. Genital virilization is common in female infants, and both sexes manifest electrolyte imbalance and hypotension that can be life threatening if not promptly treated by steroid hormone replacement. Simple virilizing CAH is a less severe form characterized by female virilization, but without the salt-wasting component. Adult-onset CAH may not manifest until adolescence, with (in females) oligomenorrhea, progressive hirsutism, and relatively short stature. Chorionic villus sampling, using DNA probes for HCA genes, when compared to parental chromosomes, will allow an earlier diagnosis. Currently, all known heterozygotes are treated with high-dose glucocorticoids until chorionic villus sampling results are known. If a male fetus is present, treatment stops. If a female fetus is present, treatment is continued because virilization of affected females can be prevented. Once DNA/HLA results are known, medication is discontinued only if the female fetus is unaffected.

Medications used to treat congenital adrenal hyperplasia include prednisone, fludrocortisone (see the section on "Medications" for Addison's disease), and dexamethasone.

# CONTRACEPTION

## ORAL CONTRACEPTIVES

A wide variety of oral contraceptive formulations is available, including estrogen/progestin combinations and progestational agents that suppress ovulation and implantation. If exposure to oral contraceptives during embryogenesis increases the risk of birth defects, the increase is small compared to the risk of malformations in the general population (3.5–5 percent). Congenital anomalies were not increased in frequency among more than 500 infants born to women who took oral contraceptives during the first trimester (Harlap and Eldor, 1980; Heinonen *et al.*, 1977b; Nora *et al.*, 1978; Vessey *et al.*, 1979). A slight increase of congenital anomalies was associated with use of oral contraceptives in the first trimester in several studies, but it is generally accepted that the risk is not real, or extremely small. Among 9986 infants in the National Birth Defects Prevention Study, the frequency of birth defects was not increased (Waller *et al.*, 2010). In the Swedish Birth Defects Registry, the frequency of birth defects was not increased among 4565 infants exposed to oral contraceptive use during organogenesis (Kallen, 2019).

## NORPLANT

The Norplant system is a unique subdermal contraceptive system providing five years of continuous birth control.

No epidemiologic studies have been published regarding malformations in the offspring of women who became pregnant with a Norplant system in place. Levonorgestrel is the progestin component in many oral contraceptive preparations.

## INTRAUTERINE DEVICE

Pregnancy with an intrauterine device (IUD) in place is associated with increased incidence of spontaneous abortion, approximately threefold greater than among women without an IUD (Lewit, 1970; Tatum *et al.*, 1976; Vessey *et al.*, 1974). When the device is removed or expelled spontaneously, spontaneous abortion is reduced to approximately 20–30 percent, which is much closer to the rates of miscarriage in the general population (Alvior, 1973; Tatum *et al.*, 1976). Several studies of women who had copper-containing IUDs in place during pregnancy have found no increase in the rate of abnormalities over the expected rate in the general population (Guillebaud, 1981; Poland, 1970; Tatum *et al.*, 1976). The frequency of congenital anomalies in the offspring of women who had progesterone-containing IUDs in place during pregnancy has not been published.

### New Intrauterine Devices

New IUD devices available ease insertion and removal, and reduce pain, bleeding, and expulsion rates. They include the intrauterine system (IUS) that gradually releases levonorgestrel (Mirena), or progesterone (Progestasert). Rather than T-shaped copper IUDs of the 1980s and 1990s, the frameless IUD devices (e.g., GyneFix) are copper cylinders secured together with a string.

## SPERMICIDAL AGENTS (NONOXYNOLS)

Spermicidal intravaginal sponges, foams, creams, and suppositories contain nonoxynols, surfactants that are extremely toxic to sperm. The risk of congenital anomalies was not increased in frequency among more than 1,200 infants whose mothers used nonoxynol spermicides during embryogenesis (Heinonen *et al.*, 1977a; Mills *et al.*, 1982). Similar results were found in large studies of the frequency of congenital anomalies among infants whose mothers used a multiagent spermicide that contained nonoxynol (Huggins *et al.*, 1982; Polednak *et al.*, 1982; Strobino *et al.*, 1988). The frequency of heterogeneous anomalies (chromosomal abnormalities, hypospadias, limb reduction defects, neoplasms) was statistically increased in more than 700 infants born to women who had used any vaginal spermicide within 10 months of conception (Jick et al., 1981). However, methodological flaws in that study (Cordero and Layde, 1983), combined with simple data errors in classification of spermicidal exposures in the cases, cast doubt on the meaning of this study. It is now widely accepted that neither nonoxynols nor other spermicides are associated with an increased risk for chromosomal abnormalities and congenital anomalies (Bracken, 1985). A case-control study of the use of topical contraceptives among mothers of infants with chromosomal abnormalities or limb reduction defects found no difference in the frequency of spermicide use around the time of conception between the case and the normal control groups (Cordero and Layde, 1983).

Among 11,050 infants born after first trimester exposure to spermicidal compounds, the frequency of birth defects was not increased (Gallaway et al., 2009).

Unfortunately, spermicides led to genesis of the term "litogen." Despite overwhelming scientific data that indicate spermicides are harmless, more than $3 million were awarded to parents of an infant born with multiple congenital anomalies whose mother had used nonoxynol during pregnancy.

### DEPO-PROVERA

This agent is discussed under "Progestational Agents."

## INFERTILITY

### OVULATION INDUCTION AGENTS

### Clomiphene Citrate (Clomid)

This drug has nonsteroidal estrogenic and antiestrogenic activity, and is given orally to stimulate ovulation. Clomiphene is sometimes inadvertently given in an unrecognized early pregnancy. Women using clomiphene should be cautioned that pregnancy is to be excluded before each new course of the drug.

Malformations were not increased in frequency among 1500 infants of women who had clomiphene preconceptionally (Barrat and Leger, 1979; Harlap, 1976; Kurachi et al., 1983). Multiple case-control studies of neural tube defects failed to find a significant association with artificial induction of ovulation and risk of a congenital anomaly (Cornel et al., 1989; Cuckle and Wald, 1989; Czeizel, 1989). In a well-designed, case-control study, the frequency of clomiphene usage was not increased among more than 500 women who delivered children with a neural tube defect compared with a similar number of normal controls (Mills et al., 1990). Among 397 infants born after clomiphene exposure during embryogenesis, the frequency of birth defects was not increased (Tulandi et al., 2006). In another study of 251 infants exposed to clomiphene during the first trimester, the frequency of birth defects was not increased (Sharma et al., 2014).

Analysis of the National Birth Defects Prevention Study, the frequency of birth defects was increased among 90 infants exposed to clomiphene (Reefhuis et al., 2011). The defects include Dandy-Walker, septal heart defects, aortic coarctation, esophageal atresia, cloacal exstrophy, craniosynostosis, and omphalocele. The frequency of neural tube defects was increased in a study of 219 infants exposed to clomiphene during embryogenesis (Benedum et al., 2016). Among 1,872 infants whose mothers took clomiphene during the first trimester, the frequency of birth defects was not increased (Weller et al., 2017).

In the Swedish Birth Defects Registry, the frequency of birth defects was not increased among 1,836 infants were exposed to clomiphene during organogenesis (Kallen, 2019).

In summary, the weight of the evidence indicates clomiphene is not associated with an increased risk of congenital anomalies.

## Human Menopausal Gonadotropins (Pergonal, Metrodin)

Pergonal is an extract of urine from postmenopausal women; it contains follicle-stimulating hormone (FSH) and luteinizing hormone (LH). It is administered by intramuscular injection and is used to stimulate multiple ovarian follicular development in ovulation induction cycles. Metrodin is a purified extract of urine from postmenopausal women and primarily contains FSH. It is similar to Pergonal in its administration protocols. The frequency of birth defects was not increased among 176 and 168 infants born following exposure to follitropin compounds, alpha and beta, respectively, in the Swedish Birth Defects Registry (Kallen, 2019). Among 54 infants exposed to urofollitropin, the frequency of congenital anomalies was not increased (Kallen, 2019). In total, 398 infants were born after FSH treatments, and the frequency of malformations was not increased (Kallen, 2019).

## Gonadotropin-Releasing Hormone Agonists

Gonadotropin-releasing hormone (GnRH) agonists are widely used in clinical gynecologic practice for the treatment of endometriosis and uterine leiomyomas. Leuprolide acetate (Lupron) is an agent that is frequently used for these conditions. Although no epidemiological studies are published of infants born following Lupron therapy, it is unlikely that the risk of congenital anomalies is high following exposure to this drug during pregnancy (Friedman and Polifka, 2006). Chronic administration of agonists down-regulates the pituitary gonadotropin receptors, thereby suppressing release of LH and FSH, leading to a hypoestrogenic state. The likelihood of pregnancy occurring while a woman is given GnRH agonists is extremely low. However, GnRH agonists may also be used prior to HMG therapy in infertile women undergoing *in vitro* fertilization cycles. Typically, administration is begun in the luteal phase of the cycle, when a patient may be in the early stage of a pregnancy. No epidemiologic studies are published on the risk malformations in the offspring of women treated with this drug during pregnancy.

In a large retrospective study of GnRH in 758 infants born with no increased frequency of birth defects, although it was indicated that cardiac and gastrointestinal tract abnormalities were over represented (Wang *et al.*, 2018). Compared to progestin ovarian stimulation in 855 conceptions, GnRH administration was not associated with an increased frequency of birth defects in live-born infants (Wang *et al.*, 2018): "While the relative risk of birth defects among ART pregnancies is increased when compared with spontaneous conceptions, the absolute risk remains low" (Chung *et al.*, 2021). "Because the balance of evidence suggests an association with pooled birth defects, it is reasonable to inform patients of potential increased risk keeping in mind the low absolute risk and limited alternatives to conception" (Kawwass and Badell, 2018). Apparently, assisted reproduction therapy (ART) or fertility treatments are not associated with a large increase in the risk of birth defects, although multiple gestations are associated with an increased frequency of congenital anomalies.

> The absolute risk [for birth defects] remains low at 0.15% in IVF-ICSI conceptions and 0.02% in spontaneous conception . . . Because the balance of evidence suggests an association with pooled birth defects, it is reasonable to inform patients of potential increased risk keeping in mind the low absolute risk and limited alternatives to conception.
>
> (Kawwass and Badell, 2018)

## GENERAL HORMONAL THERAPY

### Estrogens

### Ethinyl Estradiol

Ethinyl estradiol is a synthetic estrogen used to treat menopausal symptoms and menstrual disorders. This drug and progestin are common combinations in oral contraception.

Congenital anomalies were not increased in frequency among infants born to women given ethinyl estradiol during embryogenesis or at any time during pregnancy (Heinonen *et al.*, 1977a). Results from two other studies of ethinyl estradiol use during pregnancy showed that it was not associated with an increased risk of congenital anomalies (Kullander and Kallen, 1976; Spira *et al.*, 1972). Congenital anomalies were not increased in frequency in teratology studies of three species of non-human primates given large doses of ethinyl estradiol during pregnancy (Hendrickx *et al.*, 1987). In the Swedish Birth Defects Registry, the frequency of birth defects was not increased among 1807 infants born to women who used ethinyl estradiol during the first trimester (Kallen, 2019).

An increased frequency of intrauterine deaths was observed at doses that were also maternally lethal in one monkey species studied. Miscarriages occurred more frequently among monkeys given approximately 100 times the amount of ethinyl estradiol included in oral contraceptive dose regimens (Prahalada and Hendrickx, 1983). In rodent teratology studies, no increase in the frequency of congenital anomalies after embryonic treatment was found, but early intrauterine deaths were increased in frequency at the highest doses (Chemnitius *et al.*, 1979; Yasuda *et al.*, 1981).

### Conjugated Estrogens

Conjugated estrogens are a combination of estrogens from natural sources used to treat menopausal symptoms, osteoporosis, and hypothalamic amenorrhea. They are not indicated for use during pregnancy.

Among 614 infants born to women who used estrogenic compounds during gestation, an increase in certain congenital anomalies was found—cardiovascular, eye and ear defects, and Down's syndrome (Heinonen *et al.*, 1977b). However, this association was reevaluated in another report, and the link between estrogens and cardiac malformations was not borne out (Wiseman and Dodds-Smith, 1984). Notably, use of conjugated estrogens during early pregnancy was not reported in the Swedish Birth Defects Registry (Kallen, 2019).

### Diethylstilbestrol

This nonsteroidal synthetic estrogen, approved by the Food and Drug Administration in 1942 for use in pregnancy to prevent miscarriages, is strongly associated with an increased frequency of clear-cell adenocarcinoma of the vagina and cervix among daughters of women treated with diethylstilbestrol (DES) early in pregnancy. Between 500,000 and two million pregnant women took this drug. In a registry including more than 400 cases of clear-cell adenocarcinoma of the vagina and cervix diagnosed in the US since 1971, no less than 65 percent of patients' mothers took DES in early pregnancy (Herbst, 1981). Of the women who took DES early in pregnancy, 80 percent had taken it during the 12 weeks prior to conception. The malignancy was diagnosed among females 7–30 years old, with a median age of 19 years. Estimates suggest that 0.14–1.4 per 1,000 daughters of women treated with DES during pregnancy will develop clear-cell adenocarcinoma of the vagina or cervix by the age of 24.

Nonmalignant abnormalities, especially adenosis, are common among the daughters of pregnant women who were treated with diethylstilbestrol. Gross structural abnormalities of the cervix or vagina are identified in about one quarter and abnormalities of the vaginal epithelium in one-third to one-half of women whose mothers took diethylstilbestrol during gestation (Bibbo, 1979; Herbst *et al.*, 1978; Robboy *et al.*, 1984; Stillman, 1982). T-shaped uterus, constricting bands of the uterine cavity, uterine hypoplasia, or paraovarian cysts also occur with increased frequency among females exposed *in utero* (Kaufman *et al.*, 1984). Among males exposed to DES *in utero*, epididymal cysts, hypoplastic testes, and cryptorchidism are reported with increased frequency (Stillman, 1982). Preterm delivery, spontaneous abortions, and ectopic pregnancy occurred with increased frequency in females whose mothers took diethylstilbestrol during gestation (Barnes *et al.*, 1980; Herbst, 1981).

DES is no longer available in the United States to treat humans.

### PROGESTATIONAL AGENTS

### Progestins: Analogs of Progesterone

Progestins are a group of chemically related hormones with similar actions. Progesterone is the only natural progestin and is not well absorbed by the oral route unless given in micronized form.

Synthetic progestins structurally related to progesterone are more commonly used. Low-dose progestins are used for contraception with an estrogen, and are used in the therapy of menstrual disorders at higher doses. In the 1960s and 1970s much higher doses of progesterones were used for oral contraception (Schardein, 2000), and are currently used to treat threatened abortion.

In a review, female pseudohermaphroditism, including various degrees of clitoral hypertrophy with or without labioscrotal fusion, was reported in several-hundred children born to women treated with progesterone analogs in high doses during early pregnancy (Schardein, 1980, 1985, 2000). The frequency of occurrence of this anomaly varies with different progestins. Fewer than 100 cases of male pseudohermaphroditism have been reported, and the anomaly is usually isolated hypospadias (Aarskog, 1979; Mau, 1981; Schardein, 2000). Exposure to progestational agents during embryogenesis, therefore, seems not to increase substantially the risk for non-genital congenital anomalies in infants born to treated women. Exposure to "unspecified progestins" in 5,333 infants was not associated with an increased frequency of malformations in the Swedish Birth Defects Registry (Kallen, 2019).

## Norethindrone

Norethindrone is a synthetic progestational agent derived from 19-nortesterone, which is used as an oral contraceptive and to treat menstrual disorders. Among more than 100 infants born to women who took norethindrone during the first trimester, congenital anomalies were not increased in frequency, or in more than 100 infants whose mothers took this drug after the first trimester (Heinonen et al., 1977a). Two case-control studies of 365 infants with congenital anomalies yielded similar results (Kullander and Kallen, 1976; Spira et al., 1972).

Norethindrone exposure in 244 infants exposed in the first trimester was associated with an increased frequency of cleft palate (9 cases of cleft palate) in an unpublished PhD thesis (Ahmed, 2017).

Several cases were reported in which use of norethindrone during pregnancy, at doses that were much greater than those used in contemporary practice, was associated with masculinization of the external female genitalia (clitoral hypertrophy with or without labioscrotal fusion), but internal genitalia and subsequent pubertal development were normal (Schardein, 1980, 1985). The genital anomalies observed include various degrees of masculinization (Wilkins et al., 1958). Clitoral hypertrophy may occur in exposures any time after the 8th embryonic week, but labioscrotal fusion is limited to exposure during the 8th to 13th embryonic weeks. The risk for pseudohermaphroditism among female infants born to women who took norethindrone during pregnancy is probably less than 1 percent (Bongiovanni and McPadden, 1960; Ishizuka et al., 1962). No increased risk of fetal sexual malformation was reported in a meta-analysis of published reports of women exposed to sex hormones after conception (Ramin-Wilms et al., 1995).

Masculinized external female genitalia were observed in several species of experimental animals, including nonhuman primates, following maternal treatment with high doses of norethindrone during pregnancy (Hendrickx et al., 1983; Schardein, 2000). Non-genital malformations were not increased in frequency among three species of nonhuman primates given up to 100 times the oral contraceptive dose of norethindrone during pregnancy in combination with ethinyl estradiol (Hendrickx et al., 1987; Prahalada and Hendrickx, 1983). Contemporary low-dose therapy with norethindrone is not a risk factor for genital malformations, and probably poses no increased risk for congenital anomalies in general.

## Norethynodrel

Norethynodrel is a synthetic progestational agent that is a component of oral contraceptive preparations and is used to treat menstrual disorders. Congenital anomalies were not increased in frequency among more than 150 infants born to women who took norethynodrel during the first trimester, or among more than 150 women who took the drug after the first trimester (Heinonen et al., 1977a).

Virilization of female fetuses has not been reported in the human; however, female rat fetuses born to mothers that received several-hundred times the human contraceptive dose had masculinized external genitalia (Kawashima *et al.*, 1977). Treatment of human pregnancy within the low-dose range presently employed for contraception and for menstrual irregularity will not cause female virilization.

### Norgestrel

This synthetic progestational agent is used with estrogen compounds in oral contraceptives and for menstrual disorders. There are no controlled studies of congenital anomalies among infants born to women who used norgestrel during pregnancy. Although no human reports have associated the use of norgestrel during pregnancy with masculinization of external female genitalia, large doses administered in the latter two-thirds of pregnancy would be expected to produce virilization based upon clinical experience with other closely related compounds. The frequency of congenital anomalies was not increased among mouse and rabbit litters born to females treated with very large doses of norgestrel during pregnancy (Heinecke and Kohler, 1983; Klaus, 1983).

### Medroxyprogesterone Acetate

Medroxyprogesterone is the most widely used oral and parenteral progestational agent. It is used to treat menstrual disorders and as an injectable contraceptive. Major congenital anomalies were not increased in frequency among almost 500 infants born to women treated with medroxyprogesterone during the first trimester, or among 217 infants whose mothers took the drug after the first trimester of pregnancy (Heinonen *et al.*, 1977a; Yovich *et al.*, 1988).

Claimed associations between maternal use of high-dose progestins early in pregnancy and masculinization of the genitalia in female children, feminization of the genitalia in male children, a variety of malformations of other organ systems and certain behavioral alterations (Hines, 1982; Schardein, 1980, 1985; Wilson and Brent, 1981) are apparently not true. A large study that included 1274 cases where medroxyprogesterone was taken for first-trimester bleeding failed to reveal an increased rate of malformations when compared to 1,146 control infants (Katz *et al.*, 1985).

The frequency of birth defects was not increased with medroxyprogesterone exposure in the first trimester among 812 infants during the first trimester in the Swedish Birth Defects Registry (Kallen, 2019).

Although ambiguous external genitalia occurred among both sons and daughters of women who were treated with high doses of medroxyprogesterone to prevent miscarriage during pregnancy, these abnormalities were isolated and very rare (Schardein, 2000; Yovich *et al.*, 1988). Growth, sexual maturation, and sexually dimorphic behavior were unaltered among 74 teenage boys and 98 teenage girls whose mothers had taken medroxyprogesterone during pregnancy (Jaffe *et al.*, 1989, 1990). Animal teratology studies in rats, rabbits, and monkeys demonstrated that Non-genital anomalies were not increased in frequency, and genital ambiguity occurred only at very high doses of medroxyprogesterone during pregnancy (Andrew and Staples, 1977; Eibs *et al.*, 1982; Foote *et al.*, 1968; Kawashima *et al.*, 1977; Lerner *et al.*, 1962; Prahalada *et al.*, 1985a, 1985b; Tarara, 1984).

### Megestrol Acetate

Megestrol is a synthetic oral progestational agent. The risk for virilization of female fetuses appears minimal with maternal use of large doses of this agent during pregnancy. No studies of congenital anomalies among infants whose mothers were treated with megestrol during pregnancy have been published. External genitalia of female rats born to mothers treated with very large doses of megestrol during pregnancy were virilized (Kawashima *et al.*, 1977). The Swedish Birth Defects Registry include only two infants exposed to megestrol during the first trimester (Kallen, 2019).

## ANDROGENS

Androgen use during pregnancy is strictly contraindicated, primarily due to the risk of masculinization of a female fetus.

## Danazol

Danazol is a synthetic steroid absorbed by the gastrointestinal tract, metabolized by the liver, and has a half-life of 4.5 hours. The drug has moderate androgenic activity, and is used to treat endometriosis. Inadvertent use during early pregnancy results in virilization of female infants (Duck and Katayama, 1981; Kingsbury, 1985; Peress *et al.*, 1982; Quagliarello and Greco, 1985; Rosa, 1984; Shaw and Farquhar, 1984). A review of fetal exposure to danazol in 129 cases compiled from case reports revealed miscarriages in 12 cases and 23 elective abortions. There were 57 female fetuses whose mothers took danazol during the period of sensitivity to androgenic substances (8th week of embryogenesis and thereafter), and 23 (40 percent) presented with virilization (clitoromegaly, partial fusion of labia majora) (Brunskill, 1992). The lowest daily dose that resulted in virilization was 200 mg (Brunskill, 1992). Androgen influences on development of internal genitalia were present in only two cases (Quagliarello and Greco, 1985; Rosa, 1984). Therefore, the available data strongly indicate that virilization of the female fetus is a risk when there is exposure to danazol during the period of androgen receptor sensitivity (beginning at the 8th week of embryogenesis and continuing through the fetal period). Virilization was not found among any infants exposed before the 8th week of embryogenesis (Rosa, 1984). Only three infants were exposed to danazol during the first trimester in the Swedish Birth Defects Registry (Kallen, 2019).

Danazol is usually prescribed for only a three to six-month course. A patient who becomes pregnant while taking the medication may not be diagnosed until a considerable fetal exposure has occurred because the drug is expected to cause amenorrhea. Therefore, physicians should be aware of the risk of female genital ambiguity occurring in the offspring of women who are prescribed this drug.

## METHYLTESTOSTERONE

Methyltestosterone is a synthetic derivative of testosterone, the primary endogenous androgen. More than a dozen female infants were born to women treated with methyltestosterone during pregnancy, and they all had varying degrees of virilization of the external genitalia (clitoral enlargement and labioscrotal fusion) (Grumbach and Ducharme, 1960; Schardein, 2000). Paralleling other androgenic agents, clitoral enlargement may be induced by exposure to methyltestosterone throughout the postembryonic period, but labioscrotal fusion seems restricted to the period between the 8th and 13th weeks of gestation, and the degree of virilization appears dose related. Successful surgical correction of the defects associated with virilization is available. Sexual maturation seems normal, while menarche in virilized girls seems close to the median, following a healthy course.

Female rats, dogs, and rabbits born to mothers treated with methyltestosterone in doses similar to those used medically had a dose-dependent increased frequency of virilization (Jost, 1947; Kawashima *et al.*, 1975; Neumann and Junkmann, 1963; Shane *et al.*, 1969) similar to humans.

Methyltestosterone and testosterone propionate were associated with clitoromegaly with or without fusion of the labia minora. Hoffman and colleagues (1955) reported a masculinized fetus following administration to the mother of testosterone enanthate from the fourth to the ninth months. Grumbach and Ducharme (1960) summarized the human reports and concluded that masculinization of the female fetus was a significant risk with the use of these drugs.

## Nandrolone

Nandrolone is an androgenic and anabolic steroid administered parenterally to treat metastatic breast cancer. Illicitly, it is used to increase muscle mass and enhance athletic performance. No studies have been published that have analyzed congenital anomalies among infants born to women treated with nandrolone during pregnancy. However, the strong androgenic action of this agent would be expected to cause virilization of the external genitalia in female fetuses. Intrauterine deaths were increased in frequency among rats born to mothers who were given up to twice the medically administered dose (Naqvi and Warren, 1971).

## Stanozolol

No human studies of the use of stanozolol, an anabolic steroid, during pregnancy have been published. In rats, stanozolol during early pregnancy was associated with virilization of female fetuses (Kawashima *et al.*, 1977). As with other androgenic steroids, it is reasonable to expect virilization of the external genitalia of a female fetus with maternal use of stanozolol.

## Oxymetholone

Another anabolic androgen is oxymetholone, which is used to treat anemia. Oxymetholone possesses significant androgenic action, and is expected to cause virilization of the external genitalia of female fetuses.

No human studies are published of oxymetholone exposure during pregnancy. Embryonic loss occurred frequently after injection of about four times the usual human dose of oxymetholone in rats in early pregnancy (Naqvi and Warren, 1971). Significant virilization was found in female rats born to mothers given large doses of oxymetholone during pregnancy (Naqvi and Warren, 1971), and embryonic death was increased in frequency in pregnant rats given several times the medically administered dose (Kawashima *et al.*, 1977).

## Tibolone

Tibolone is an antiandrogenic compound used primarily to treat menopausal symptoms and osteoporosis. It is contraindicated for use during pregnancy. No studies are published of its use during pregnancy.

## SPECIAL CONSIDERATIONS

### MORNING AFTER PILL

The morning after pill, formerly RU-486, contains mifepristone. Other formulations may sometimes contain levonorgestrel. These drugs act by preventing implantation, rather than by preventing conception. The effects of either of these drugs on a post implantation pregnancy are unknown. Friedman and Polifka (2006) state that the risk of congenital anomalies is unknown following a failed attempt at abortion but "this risk may be substantial because the process of attempted abortion may disrupt normal embryogenesis or fetal development."

When emergency contraception does not prevent pregnancy, inadvertent exposure during organogenesis occurs. A prospective study of 332 infants whose mothers took levonorgestrel as "morning after" contraception, only four infants had congenital malformations, of which two were major birth defects (Zhang *et al.*, 2009). In the Swedish Birth Defects Registry, only nine infants were exposed to levonorgestrel during the first trimester. However, among 805 infants were exposed to levonorgestrel plus ethinylestradiol in the first trimester, the frequency of birth defects was not increased (Kallen, 2019).

### BREAST CANCER

Aromatase inhibitors may be used to replace tamoxifen, because of fewer untoward effects, in the treatment of breast cancer. These agents include anastrozole (Arimidex), exemestane (Aromasin), and letrozole (Femara). These drugs are contraindicated for use during pregnancy (see Chapter 7).

## HYPERPROLACTINEMIA

Excess pituitary prolactin secretion can lead to symptoms of galactorrhea, menstrual irregularities, and infertility. Menstrual cycle abnormalities caused by hyperprolactinemia include primary and secondary amenorrhea, oligomenorrhea, and luteal phase defects. Hyperprolactinemia may result from a variety of different causes (pituitary adenoma, hypothyroidism, various pharmacologic agents). Etiology should be established prior to beginning therapy. Primary therapy for idiopathic hyperprolactinemia, or a small pituitary adenoma, is an ergot alkaloid compound, such as bromocriptine. Many physicians prefer to use cabergoline (Dostinex) to treat hyperprolactinemia instead of bromocriptine to avoid side effects.

Cabergoline exposure occurred during the first trimester in 231 pregnancies to 194 women (Sant Anna *et al.*, 2020). Cabergoline was withdrawn in 196 (89 percent) patients when pregnancy was recognized (average EGA at drug discontinuation) 5–6 weeks. 80 percent were discontinued during the first trimester. The rate of birth defects was 4.3 percent, which is not different from the population background rate (Sant'Anna *et al.*, 2020).

Dopamine agonist activity suppresses prolactin release from the pituitary. Surgical therapy is reserved for very large pituitary tumors, and/or ones unresponsive to medical treatment (see earlier sections on "Prolactinoma" and "Bromocriptine").

## ENDOMETRIOSIS

Endometriosis is the presence of endometrial implants (glands and stroma) outside the endometrial cavity. Most frequently implanted sites are the pelvic viscera and peritoneum. Various therapeutic regimens have been used to treat all stages of disease, including surgical ablation and extirpation, drug therapy, or both. Medical therapy for endometriosis includes hormonal regimens of oral contraceptives, danocrine, or gonadotropin-releasing hormone (GnRH) agonists. Pregnancy usually resolves endometriosis; therefore, treatment during pregnancy is probably not an issue. See earlier section on GnRH agonists for birth defects information.

## SUMMARY

Hormonal agents should usually not be administered during pregnancy. Inadvertent oral contraceptive use during embryogenesis is not associated with an increased risk of congenital anomalies. **Diethylstilbestrol, high doses of progestins derived from testosterone, and all androgens are strictly contraindicated during pregnancy**.

# 5 Antiasthma Agents during Pregnancy

Asthma is the most common pulmonary disease in pregnancy is an obstructive pulmonary disease charaterized by reversible chronic airway hyperreactivity to a variety of stimuli (Box 5.1). During an acute asthmatic attack, airway resistance is increased while forced expiratory flow and volume rates are decreased. Asthma complicates approximately 4–8 percent of pregnancies pregnancy (Bracken *et al.*, 2003), and has increased more than fourfold since 1990 (ACOG, 2008). Asthma severity varies over the course of pregnancy, but it is not established that the disease is aggravated during gestation.

---

**BOX 5.1    STIMULI THAT EXACERBATE ASTHMA**

- *Allergies*
  - Poison ivy, pollen
  - Household pets, odors
- *Cold weather drugs*
  - Acetyl salicylic acid
  - Indomethacin
  - Beta-blockers (Inderal)
- *Emotional stress*
- *Environmental pollutants (dust, smog, air pollution)*
- *Exercise*
- *Occupational factors (asbestos, plaster)*
- *Respiratory tract infections (viral, bacterial)*

---

Among more than 1,000 patients reported in nine investigations, about 48 percent of gravid asthmatics experienced no change in clinical severity of their symptoms and approximately 29 percent improved. In approximately 23 percent of pregnant asthmatics, the disease severity worsened. A prospective investigation indicated asthma severity was not associated with preterm delivery, but "controller medications" (oral steroid and theophylline therapy) was associated. IUGR was associated with asthma, and speculated to be due to fetal hypoxia during asthma maternal attacks (Bracken *et al.*, 2003). Earlier studies of asthma during pregnancy reported that asthma severity increased in an estimated ~30 percent of women during pregnancy (Cunningham, 1994; Schatz *et al.*, 1988; Stenius-Aarniala *et al.*, 1988).

It appears that those gravidas who have severe asthma are at greatest risk of exacerbation of symptoms, and should be more closely monitored than mild asthmatics.

*Certain medications, possibly used during labor and delivery, have the potential to worsen asthma. Nonselective β-blockers, carboprost (15-methyl prostaglandin F2 α) and ergonovine may trigger bronchospasm. Magnesium sulfate is a bronchodilator, but indomethacin can induce bronchospasm in patients who are sensitive to aspirin. Prostaglandin E2 or prostaglandin E1 can be used for cervical ripening, the management of spontaneous or induced abortions, or the management of postpartum hemorrhage* (ACOG, 2008).

DOI: 10.1201/9780429160929-5

Most severe asthma occurred among 1,396 of 36,985 (3.8 percent) pregnancies (Kallen *et al.*, 2000). Asthma during pregnancy is associated with a doubling in the rate of preterm labor, low birth weight, and preeclampsia (ACOG, 2008; Kircher *et al.*, 2002; Kallen *et al.*, 2000). In contrast, no differences in the frequency of prematurity, low birth weight, and perinatal mortality were found among 182 pregnancies complicated by asthma compared to 364 nonasthmatic controls, however, an increased complication rate was observed among gravidas with severe uncontrolled asthma (Jana *et al.*, 1995). The overall rates of rates of worsened asthma, hospitalizations, IUGR, and prematurity are increased by severity. Levels of severity are classified by frequency and rate of asthma symptoms (Box 5.2).

### BOX 5.2   EFFECTS OF PREGNANCY ON ASTHMA

| Asthma Severity Rate | Exacerbation Rate | Hospitalization |
|---|---|---|
| Intermittent (well controlled) | — | — |
| Mild–Persistent (not well controlled) | 12.6% | 2.3% |
| Moderate–Persistent (not well controlled) | 25.7% | 6.8% |
| Severe (very poorly controlled) | 51.9% | 26.9% |

## TREATMENT REGIMENS

*Treat [pregnant] women with pharmacological step therapy for chronic asthma.*

(Cunningham *et al.*, 2017)

Most medical treatments for asthma are safe during pregnancy. The first-line treatments include antihistamines, decongestants, and intranasal glucocorticoids. The clinical goals of asthma treatment are to: (1) control or decrease the frequency and number of asthmatic exacerbations, to protect mother and fetus, (2) avoid status asthmaticus (severe obstruction persisting for days to weeks), (3) prevent respiratory failure, and (4) to prevent death. Additional treatment objectives during pregnancy include: (1) assure adequate fetal oxygenation, and (2) decrease or prevent fetal effects of asthma pharmacotherapy (ACOG, 2008).

Available antiasthma agents accomplish these goals without added risk to either mother or fetus (Bracken *et al.*, 2003; ACOG, 2008; Schatz *et al.*, 2004). Several categories of medical treatments for asthma are available (Box 5.3):

### BOX 5.3   MEDICATIONS AND INDICATIONS USED FOR THE TREATMENT OF ASTHMA DURING PREGNANCY

**MEDICATIONS**

**Anti-inflammatory agents**

- Beclomethasone
- Cromolyn sodium
- Prednisone

**Beta adrenergic agonists**

- Albuterol, Epinephrine, Isoetharine, Isoproterenol, Metaproterenol, Terbutaline
- **Methylxanthines**: Aminophylline, Theophylline
- **Antihistamines**: Chlorpheniramine, Tripelennamine

- **Decongestants**: Oxymetazoline, Pseudoephedrine
- **Cough medications**: Dextromethorphan, Guaifenesin
- **Other**: Antibiotics, Anticholinergics

## INDICATION: PATIENT UNRESPONSIVE TO BRONCHODILATORS

- Hydrocortisone: 4 mg/kg body weight IV loading dose followed by 3 mg/kg IV q 6 h for 2–3 days. Switch to oral prednisone
- Methylprednisolone: 0.5–1 mg/kg (approximately 125 mg) IV bolus followed by 60 mg IV q 6 h Prednisone 30–60 mg PO daily
- Beclomethasone: 2 puffs (100 · g) tid—qid
- Patients on maintenance dose of steroids Hydrocortisone: 100 mg IM or IV q 6–8 h · 24 h
- Methylprednisolone: 125 mg IV bolus followed by 60 mg IV q 6 h

*Sources:* Adapted in part from the National Asthma Education and Prevention Program, Cloutier *et al.*, 2020; ACOG, 2008.

One medical authority has indicated that inhaled corticosteroids are the most efficacious of anti-asthma agents (Dombrowski, 1997; see also "Antihistamines and Expectorants" later in this chapter).

### METHYLXANTHINES

Xanthines and methylxanthines have unusual pharmacokinetics during pregnancy, and it important to note their unusual behavior. Xanthines tend to increase their steady-state concentration during pregnancy, and this effect is magnified during the third trimester. Accordingly, maintaining desired plasma concentrations requires different doses throughout pregnancy, and physicians should anticipate a decrease in doses required as the pregnancy advances because plasma concentrations increases.

---

### TABLE 5.1
### Medication Dosages for Treatment of Asthma during Pregnancy

| Drug | Dosage |
| --- | --- |
| Beclomethasone | 2–6 puffs bid to qid |
| Budesonide | 1–3 puffs |
| Cromolyn sodium | 2 puffs qid |
| Epinephrine | 0.3–0.5 mL of 1:1000 solution q 20 min |
| Flunisolide | 2–4 puffs |
| Fluticasone | 2–6 puffs |
| Mometasone | 1 puff |
| Prednisone | Burst for acute symptoms, 40 mg/day for 7 days, and then taper for 7 days |
| Theophylline | 400–600 mg/day initial and increase to therapeutic level of 8–12 g/mL |
| Terbutaline (inhaled) | 2–3 puffs q 4–6 h prn |
| Terbutaline (subcutaneous) | 250 g q 15 min |
| Triamcinolone | 4–10 puffs |

*Source:* ACOG, 2008.

---

## THEOPHYLLINE

A xanthine derivative, theophylline, has potent diuretic effects and is commonly used for bronchodilation actions. It is a competitive inhibitor of phosphodiesterase, which inactivates cAMP (Feldman and McFadden, 1977). Increased intracellular cAMP levels stimulates bronchodilation. Theophylline salts were previously the first line of therapy for asthma control during pregnancy. The frequency of congenital anomalies was not increased among 606 infants whose mothers used theophylline during the first trimester. Similarly, birth defects were not increased in frequency in 1294 infants whose mothers used the drug any time during pregnancy (Heinonen *et al.*, 1977; Schatz *et al.*, 1997; Stenius-Aarniala *et al.*, 1995).

Theophylline crosses the placenta, and high maternal doses may result in toxicity in the neonate (Arwood *et al.*, 1979; Horowitz *et al.*, 1982; Labovitz and Spector, 1982; Omarini *et al.*, 1993; Yeh and Pildes, 1977) because an estimated 100 percent of the maternal dose reaches the fetus. Adverse effects of theophylline in the neonates includes tachycardia, jitteriness, vomiting, and occasional apneic episodes during theophylline clearance (Arwood *et al.*, 1979; Horowitz *et al.*, 1982; Spector, 1984; Turner *et al.*, 1980; Yeh and Pildes, 1977).

## AMINOPHYLLINE

Aminophylline and theophylline are available for parenteral use, and there are numerous oral theophylline preparations. The range for therapeutic plasma concentrations of theophylline is between 10 and 20 mg/mL. It is important to consider the wide variation in dosage required to achieve this plasma concentration in pregnant patients because of differences in pregnancy stage, CYP-1A2, and volume of distribution. Caution must be used because of potential maternal and neonatal toxicity. Parenteral aminophylline is given as a loading dose of 5–6 mg/kg body weight infused over 20–30 min followed by a continuous infusion of 0.2–0.9 mg/kg/h. Loading dose should be reduced by half or completely omitted for patients already taking oral theophylline preparations. Aminophylline was used in the past for initial asthma therapy and as polytherapy with beta-adrenergic agonists.

Aminophylline use was supplanted by corticosteroids (Dombrowski, 1997), but oral theophylline derivatives are still prescribed by many clinicians (Neame *et al.*, 2015). Intravenous aminophylline for the acute treatment of asthma in pregnant women "offers no therapeutic advantages" and may be associated with toxicity (Wendel *et al.*, 1996).

Aminophylline has been associated with uterine activity at higher dosages than those required to treat asthma, but it was not an effective agent for the treatment of premature labor.

Theophylline may have an additional benefit in the pregnant asthmatic because it may be associated with a decreased frequency of preeclampsia in these women (Dombrowski *et al.*, 1986), but this association has not been replicated. Aminophylline should no longer be "the mainstay of therapy for severe asthma," and the primary role of theophylline derivatives is for chronic outpatient therapy (ACOG, 2008).

# BETA-ADRENERGIC AGENTS

Epinephrine, isoetharine, isoproterenol, metaproterenol, and terbutaline are included in the beta-adrenergic class of drugs.

## EPINEPHRINE

Epinephrine has alpha and beta-adrenergic actions. It is used to relieve bronchospasm and other allergic reactions. Acute asthma attacks are treated with 0.3–0.5 mL of 1:1000 epinephrine subcutaneously every 30 min, up to three times (Table 5.2). Epinephrine use is contraindicated in those with severe hypertension, cardiac arrhythmias, and a heart rate of more than 140 beats per minute. Epinephrine is

**TABLE 5.2**
**Adrenergic Drugs Used for the Treatment of Asthma**

| Drug | Receptor | Administration | Recommended Dosages |
|------|----------|----------------|---------------------|
| Epinephrine | a, $b_1$, $b_2$ | Subcutaneous | 0.3–0.5 mL 1:1000 solution q 20 min |
| Isoetharine | $b_1$ | Inhaled<br>Inhaled metered dose<br>Aerosolized | 200–300 ⌠g/puff, 1–2 puffs q 4 h 340 ⌠g/puff, 3–7 puffs q 3–4 h 0.5 mL of 1% solution, diluted 1:3 with saline |
| Isoproterenol | $b_1$, $b_2$ | Inhaled | 1:100 solution, 3–7 inhalations q 4–6 h1:200 solution, 5–15 inhalations q 4–6 h |
| Metaproterenol | $b_2$ | Intravenous<br>Inhaled metered dose<br>Nebulizer | 0.5–5 ⌠g/min by infusion 650 ⌠g/puff, 2–3 puffs q 3–4 h 0.3 mL of 5% solution q 4 h |
| Terbutaline | $b_2$ | Subcutaneous<br>Oral | 250 ⌠g q 15 min 2.5 mg q 4–6 h |

not associated with an increased frequency of congenital anomalies or adverse fetal effects. Congenital anomalies were increased in frequency among 189 women who used epinephrine during the first trimester, but not among 508 who used the drug only during the first and second trimesters (Heinonen *et al.*, 1977). Birth defects (i.e., inguinal hernia) that were increased were not of clinical significance, and probably not causally related to the drug exposure but rather the disease being treated (i.e., inguinal hernia and preterm delivery). Maternal treatment with epinephrine readily crosses the placenta. Epinephrine is endogenous, and is released from the adrenal medulla as a stress response. Therefore, it seems reasonable to conclude that it is unlikely that epinephrine is associated with an increased risk of malformations in the fetus when used in usual therapeutic adult doses.

Epinephrine causes congenital anomalies in animal species, but only at doses hundreds to thousands of times greater the usual human dose.

## ISOPROTERENOL

A stimulant acting on beta-adrenergic receptors, isoproterenol is the most potent drug in the group. Used to treat asthma and cardiac arrhythmias, isoproterenol is by inhalation, but can be used parenterally to treat status asthmaticus (Table 5.2). There are no reports of an association of isoproterenol and birth defects following first trimester exposure. Congenital anomalies were not increased in frequency among 31 offspring exposed during the first trimester (Heinonen *et al.*, 1977). It is a FDA category C under the old system.

## ISOETHARINE

Isoetharine, an oral sympathomimetic drug used orally or intranasally (1-percent solution) to treat bronchospasms. Isoetharine is the most selective beta agent of this class. It has weak bronchodilation properties, but does not stimulate the heart as other beta agents do. No published studies are available on congenital anomalies in infants of mothers exposed to isoetharine during pregnancy. No animal teratology studies in animals have been published. Isoproterenol is a closely related drug. Under the old system, it is a FDA category C.

## METAPROTERENOL AND ALBUTEROL

Resorcinol drugs include metaproterenol and albuterol. Their effects are due to (1) manipulation of the catecholamine molecule, (2) more beta$_2$ selectivity, and (3) longer duration of action than other beta-adrenergic agents. Metaproterenol and albuterol are given orally, parenterally, or inhalationally. Maternal systemic concentrations are lower when the drug is given by inhalation, thus lowering any theoretical risk to the embryo or fetus.

The resorcinol agents available in the US include metaproterenol, albuterol, and terbutaline. Beta sympathomimetics, metaproterenol and albuterol, are used as a bronchodilator and to arrest premature labor. Among 361 infants with first trimester exposure to metaproterenol, the frequency of birth defects was not increased (Rosa, personal communication, cited in Briggs et al., 2002). First trimester exposure to albuterol did not increase the frequency of congenital anomalies among 1090 infants (Rosa, personal communication in Briggs et al., 2017). In another series of 1753 pregnancies exposed to albuterol during the first trimester, the frequency of birth defects was not increased (Schatz et al., 2004). Fetal tachycardia has been reported with maternal albuterol therapy in the third trimester, but has not been associated with any adverse neonatal effects (Hastwell et al., 1978; Ryden, 1977). The drugs metaproterenol and albuterol are FDA category C under the old classification system.

## TERBUTALINE

A potent bronchodilator, terbutaline is also been used to prevent or treat premature labor, although it does not have FDA approval for this purpose.

For tocolysis, terbutaline carries a "Black Box" warning. Oral terbutaline is 2.5–5 mg three or four times daily. It can be given subcutaneously (0.25–0.5 mg), but has less activity.

The frequency of birth defects was not increased among 149 infants exposed to terbutaline during the first trimester (Rosa, personal communication, cited in Briggs et al., 2017). Terbutaline crosses the placenta (Ingemarsson et al., 1981). It has been associated with fetal tachycardia and transient neonatal hypoglycemia when used as a tocolytic agent (Epstein et al., 1979; Ingemarsson, 1976; Wallace et al., 1978).

In summary, based on available data, metaproterenol, albuterol, and terbutaline are unlikely to be associated with an increased risk of congenital anomalies, with first trimester exposure.

## ANTI-INFLAMMATORY AGENTS

### GLUCOCORTICOIDS

Glucocorticoids are a mainstay of asthma treatment. Inhaled glucocorticoid adrenal glucocorticoids are given to severely asthmatic pregnant women (Box 5.3). A meta-analysis of systemic corticosteroid use in 535 infants exposed to the drugs during the first trimester in four studies, the frequency of birth defects was not increased, expect for cleft palate (Park-Wyllie et al., 2000). However, a recent large case-control study of first trimester exposure to systemic corticosteroids found no increased risk for oral clefts in 2,372 cases (Skuladottir et al., 2014). Steroids are used in acute asthmatic exacerbations with persistent severe airway obstruction, or when asthma symptoms worsen even with optimal bronchodilator therapy. Asthma is dangerous to the mother, and the disease must be managed to maintain oxygenation.

Chronic glucocorticoid use is the first line of treatment of asthma control during pregnancy (ACOG, 2008). It is of greatest benefit in patients with frequent recurrences and those with worsening disease despite a prior optimal regimen. Steroids act by inducing protein lipocortin production, which inhibits phospholipase and decreases arachidonic acid release (Townley and Suliaman, 1987). Bronchodilation enhanced by beta agonists occurs as with steroid use, accompanied by decreased mucous gland secretions and an inflammatory response.

Among 503 pregnant acute asthmatic patients followed prospectively, the odds of an attack while maintained on an inhaled steroid (n = 257) was reduced fivefold compared to those who did not receive an inhaled steroid (Stenius-Aarniala et al., 1996). Glucocorticoids effects usually take about six to eight hours after first dose administration. Therefore, it is of utmost importance to maintain uninterrupted bronchodilator therapy to avoid troughs in drug concentration.

## Prednisone and Prednisolone

Two synthetic glucocorticoids used to treat asthma are prednisone and prednisolone are biologically inert and the active metabolite forms of the drug, respectively. Maternal-to-fetal ratio of prednisone/prednisolone is approximately 10:1, indicating that the fetus is exposed to only approximately 10 percent of the active drug (Beitins et al., 1972; Levitz et al., 1978). Prednisone is the glucocorticoid of choice for asthma treatment.

Details of prednisone and prednisolone use during pregnancy are discussed in Chapter 4. It is important to reiterate that it is unlikely that prednisone or prednisolone exposure during the first trimester is associated with an increased risk of congenital anomalies, particularly cleft palate. Analyses in available studies suggest the risk of cleft palate was less than 1 percent in humans following exposure during organogenesis to glucocorticosteroids (Carmichael et al., 1999; Shepard and Lemire, 2010), if it is increased at all (Hviid et al., 2011).

Infants born to mothers who received prednisone throughout gestation usually had normal adrenocortical reserves and lacked symptoms of adrenal suppression (Arad and Landau, 1984), although there are case reports of adrenal insufficiency. Additionally, in two other reports, no evidence of neonatal adrenal insufficiency was found in newborn infants of women who took prednisone daily (as much as 60 mg in one study) throughout pregnancy (Schatz et al., 1975; Weinberger et al., 1980).

## Beclomethasone

One of the first-lines therapies, beclomethasone (a synthetic glucocorticoid) is given by inhalation for bronchial asthma (ACOG, 2008). Hospital readmissions for asthma decreased 55 percent in pregnant women using inhaled beclomethasone (Wendel et al., 1996). Animal models have found an increased frequency of cleft in rodents models with steroids used in pregnancy for asthma, including, beclomethasone (Esaki et al., 1976; Furuhashi et al., 1977; Nomura et al., 1977; Tamagawa et al., 1982). However, beclomethasone was not associated with an increased frequency of congenital anomalies in 395 infants exposed to this class of drug (beclomethasone, budesonide, flunisolide, fluticasone, triamcinolone) during the first trimester (Rosa, personal communication, cited in Briggs et al., 2017; Schatz, 2001). In one prospective study of this agent in pregnancy, it was not associated with an increase in the frequency of malformations in 45 pregnancies in 40 women (Greenberger and Patterson, 1983). Among 277 infants whose mothers used beclomethasone during the first trimester, the frequency of congenital anomalies was not increased (Nemazy et al., 2004). A review that included more than 1000 first trimester exposed pregnancies, the frequency of malformations was not increased (de Aguiar et al., 2014). The frequency of birth defects was not increased among 200 infants whose mothers used beclomethasone during embryogenesis in the Swedish Birth Defects Registry (Kallen, 2019).

The risk of an asthma attack when maintained on a beclomethasone (n = 214) was significantly reduced compared to those who did not receive an inhaled steroid. No reduction in birth weight or increase in the frequency of birth defects was found in the treated group compared to the untreated group (Stenius-Aarniala et al., 1996). Fetal growth retardation and pregnancies complications were not increased in frequency in a review of 1,000 beclomethasone-exposed pregnancies (de Aguiar et al., 2014).

## Budesonide

Budesonide, a corticosteroid prevents bronchial inflammation, lessening the severity of an asthma attack. Inhaled budesonide may be used in conjunction with other asthma treatments (e.g., bronchodilators). It prevents symptoms of asthma when used daily to decrease attack frequency and severity, but provides no relief when an asthma attack that has already started.

Among 2014 pregnancies exposed to budesonide during organogenesis, the frequency of congenital anomalies was not increased (Kallen *et al.*, 2000). A study from the Swedish Birth Defects Registry reported 5070 infants born following first trimester exposure to budesonide reported an increased frequency of cardiovascular defects (Kallen, 2019). However, the frequency of orofacial clefts was not increased (Van Zutphen *et al.*, 2015).

Inhaled fluticasone was detected in cord blood, with a fetal: maternal ratio of 1 percent and 10 percent (Battista *et al.*, 2016).

## FLUNISOLIDE

No birth defects were reported among 25 infants exposed to flunisolide in the first trimester (Namazy *et al.*, 2004). Rat and rabbit offspring exposed to 10 and 20 times the usual; human dose had increased frequencies of congenital anomalies (Manufacturer Package Insert). Dose related increased frequencies of congenital anomalies (cleft palate) and maternal mortality was reported after flunisolide exposure at high doses during embryogenesis produced in mice and rats (Tamagawa *et al.*, 1982; Itabashi *et al.*, 1982).

## FLUTICASONE

Fluticasone is an inhaled corticosteroid used to treat asthma. First trimester exposure to fluticasone in 62 infants resulted in no increased frequency of congenital anomalies (Howley *et al.*, 2020). Among 5,362 infants born to women who used fluticasone during organogenesis, the frequency of birth defects was not increased (Charlton *et al.*, 2016). Analysis of the risk for congenital heart defects was done for fluticasone and first trimester use. Among 65 infants exposed to fluticasone, the frequency of congenital heart defects was not increased (Van Zutphen *et al.*, 2015). The Swedish Birth Defects Registry included 946 infants whose mothers used fluticasone during embryogenesis, and the frequency of birth defects was not increased (Kallen, 2019).

## TRIAMCINOLONE

Triamcinolone is a synthesized fluorinated corticosteroid administered orally, parenterally, topically, or by oral inhalation used to treat asthma. No birth defects were reported among 27 infants exposed to triamcinolone during organogenesis (Howley *et al.*, 2020). In the Swedish Birth Defects Registry, 82 infants were exposed to triamcinolone during embryogenesis, and there were two severe malformations (cleft palate, branchial fistula), or approximately 2.4 percent for major congenital anomalies, and 3.7 percent for all birth defects (Kallen, 2019).

## CORTISONE

An inactive precursor of hydrocortisone, cortisone is secreted by the adrenal cortex and is converted by the liver to the active compound. Four of 27 newborns whose mothers were treated with cortisone had congenital anomalies, but no distinct patterns of malformations were found (Wells, 1953). No increase in the frequency of congenital anomalies was found among the small number of infants (n = 34) exposed to this steroid in the first trimester (Heinonen *et al.*, 1977). Among 662 infants with cleft palate and 734 controls mothers, there was no association between cortisone/hydrocortisone exposure and oral clefts (Carmichael *et al.*, 1999). In a large Swedish registry study, the frequency of birth defects was not increased among 81 infants whose mothers used hydrocortisone during embryogenesis (Kallen, 2019).

In a small number (n = 36) of infants exposed to cortisone during pregnancy, the frequency of cleft palate was increased, based on four infants with the birth defect (Rodriguez-Pinilla *et al.*, 1998).

A number of mouse and other rodent studies have associated cleft palate with cortisone and hydro-cortisone during organogenesis dating back 70 years (Baxter and Fraser, 1950). The teratogenic effects of cortisone (i.e., cleft palate) has been shown in several animal species (Loevy and Roth, 1968).

The relevance of these findings to the clinical use of cortisone in human pregnancy remains unknown. It seems unlikely that cortisone therapy substantially increases the risk of cleft palate in infants born to women who used the drug during the first trimester, and if it does, the risk is probably less than 1 percent. **Analyses across available studies suggest the risk of cleft palate was less than 1 percent after first trimester exposure for corticosteroids** (Carmichael et al., 1999; Shepard and Lemire, 2010), **if it is increased at all** (Hviid et al., 2011).

## BETAMETHASONE

A synthetic glucocorticoid that crosses the placenta readily, betamethasone use during the first trimester of pregnancy and the frequency of birth defects has not been published.. Betamethasone has been used to accelerate fetal lung maturation in pregnant women with premature labor. No alterations in growth or intellectual function were noted among children exposed to betametha-sone treatment during the first trimester, followed up at ages 4, 6, and 10–12years-old (MacArthur et al., 1981, 1982; Schmand et al., 1990; Smolders-de Haas et al., 1990). Among 28 infants exposed to betamethasone during the first trimester, no birth defects were reported (Kallen, 2019) in the Swedish Birth Defects Registry.

Betamethasone was associated with cleft palate, as has been found in studies of other cortico-steroids. An increased frequency of cleft palate was reported among the offspring of pregnant rats, mice, and rabbits exposed to betamethasone during organogenesis (Ishimura et al., 1975; Mosier et al., 1982; Walker, 1971; Yamada et al., 1981). The frequency of omphaloceles was increased in frequency among the offspring of pregnant rats betamethasone-exposed during early gestation (Mosier et al., 1982; Yamada et al., 1981).

## DEXAMETHASONE

Dexamethasone is to treat asthma during pregnancy and to stimulate fetal lung maturation. The drug crosses the placenta reaching fetal serum levels comparable to maternal levels (Osathanondh et al., 1977). As with other steroids, use of dexamethasone to treat pregnant asthmatics was not associated with adverse maternal or fetal effects (Schatz et al., 1975). The Collaborative Group on Antenatal Steroid Therapy (1984) observed no adverse effects of in utero exposure to dexametha-sone in infants in a long-term follow-up.

The teratogenic effects of dexamethasone in animal species are similar to those of cortisone. For example, neural tube defects were induced in rabbits (Buck et al., 1962) and cleft palates in mice (Pinsky and DiGeorge, 1965). Also, Jerome and Hendrickx (1988) administered 10 mg/kg dexamethasone daily between days 22 and 50 in six pregnant rhesus monkeys and observed cra-nium bifidum and aplasia cutis congenital in one and three fetuses, respectively. The Swedish Birth Defects Registry reported 75 infants whose mother used dexamethasone during pregnancy, and the frequency of birth defects was not increased (Kallen, 2019).

As discussed with prednisone previously, first trimester exposure may be associated with a very small risk of oral clefts (see Chapter 4, and earlier in this chapter).

## CHROMONES

### CROMOLYN/ NEDOCROMIL

The mechanisms of cromolyn sodium nedocromil are inhibition of mast cell degranulation and thus the release of the chemical mediators of anaphylaxis, and is taken by inhalation for asthma prophylaxis. Among 296 infants whose mothers took cromolyn sodium during the first trimester, the frequency of birth defects was not increased (Wilson, 1982a, b). Among infants born to 151 and 191 women who used cromolyn sodium during the first trimester, the frequency of congenital anomalies was not increased (Rosa, personal communication) (Schatz *et al.*, 1997). The frequency of birth defects was not increased in an unpublished study that included 191 infants born to women who used cromolyn during the first trimester (Rosa, unpublished, Briggs *et al.*, 2017).

Older reports of its use during pregnancy indicate no adverse fetal effects, and included more than 300 first-trimester exposed pregnancies (Dykes, 1974; Wilson, 1982).

## MISCELLANEOUS AGENTS

### MONTELUKAST

Montelukast is a leukotriene inhibitor, which relieves inflammation and bronchospasm asthma symptoms. The drug is used to prevent asthma attacks in individuals as young as 12 months old, and to prevent exercise-induced bronchospasm in asthmatics as young as 6 years.

Among 185 infants exposed to montelukast during organogenesis, the frequency of birth defects was not increased (Merck, 2007). Several investigations have reported on use of montelukast in early pregnancy. A Danish registry analysis of 1827 infants exposed to montelukast the first trimester, the frequency of birth defects was not increased (Cavero-Carbonell *et al.*, 2017). In another study, data collected for insurance billing purposes identified 1187 women who took montelukast during the first trimester and indicated the frequency of congenital anomalies was not increased in frequency (Nelsen *et al.*, 2012). It is relevant to know that the Nelsen *et al.* study targeted limb reduction/transverse limb reduction defects as follow-up to a cluster of 7 such defects in their surveillance system, and Nelsen *et al.* (2012) used infants exposed to inhaled corticosteroids as the control group. The frequency of limb reduction defects was not increased either (Nelsen *et al.*, 2012). Montelukast use during the first trimester in 160 pregnancies was not associated with an increased frequency of birth defects (Sarkar *et al.*, 2009). Among 633 infants exposed to montelukast, birth defects were not increased in frequency (Kallen, 2016, 2019).

No difference in the frequency of birth defects was found in a comparison of leukotriene receptor antagonists (montelukast or zafirlukast) in the manufacturer's registry of 74 infants born after first trimester exposure to compared to asthmatics who did not take either drug during gestation (Bakhirena *et al.*, 2007).

Birth weight was 304 g lighter in montelukast exposed pregnancies matched to asthmatic pregnant women who had not taken the drug during gestation (Sarkar *et al.*, 2009).

### OMALIZUMAB

Omalizumab is a recombinant DNA-derived humanized IgG1k monoclonal antibody that, unlike an ordinary anti-IgE antibody, does not bind to IgE already bound by the high affinity IgE receptors on mast cells, basophils, and dendritic cells.

Among 160 infants born to women reported to the manufacturer's pregnancy registry there were seven major birth defects; the frequency of congenital anomalies was not increased compared to the general populations rate of ~3.5 percent (Namazy *et al.*, 2014).

### ANTICHOLINERGICS

Anticholinergics, such as atropine, produce bronchodilation in asthmatics. Their systemic side effects limited their use (Van Arsdel and Paul, 1977). Atropine readily crosses the placenta to the fetal circulation and may cause fetal vagal blockade with subsequent fetal tachycardia (Hellman and Fillisti, 1965; Kanto *et al.*, 1981; Kivalo and Saarikoski, 1977). No increase in congenital defects among 401 offspring of women with exposure to atropine during early pregnancy, or 1198 infants whose mothers used the drug anytime during pregnancy was reported found (Heinonen *et al.*, 1977).

The Swedish Birth Defects Registry reported 61 infants whose mothers used anticholinergics during embryogenesis, among whom the frequency of birth defects was not increased (Kallen, 2019).

### ANTIBIOTICS

Upper respiratory infections should be treated aggressively in the pregnant asthmatic patient, as in the non-pregnant patient (see Chapter 2). Penicillins are considered safe for use during pregnancy. Erythromycin is probably a safe alternative in the patient who is allergic to penicillin. If initiating erythromycin, it may be prudent to monitor for possible hepatotoxicity of the estolate salt of erythromycin (McCormack *et al.*, 1977). Tetracyclines should be avoided during pregnancy (Table 5.3) because of their adverse effects on fetal teeth (permanent staining) and bones (abnormalities in bone formation) (Anthony, 1970; Cohlan *et al.*, 1967; Harcourt *et al.*, 1962; Rendle-Short, 1962; Swallow, 1964).

### ANTIHISTAMINES AND EXPECTORANTS

Chapter 11 covers antihistamine and expectorant use during pregnancy. The following relevant medications are included in Chapter 11: brompheniramine, cetirizine, chlorpheniramine, dexchlorpheniramine, diphenhydramine, hydroxyzine, loratadine, oxymetazoline, pheniramine, phenylephrine, pseudoephedrine, tripelennamine and triprolidine are generally considered safe for use during pregnancy. Some literature suggests that expectorants and mucolytics have efficacy for asthma treatment.

It is of utmost importance that **iodide-containing agents**, including theophylline mixtures that contain iodides, **not be used during pregnancy**. The iodine blocks the fetal thyroxine synthesis, resulting in fetal hypothyroidism or congenital goiter (Carswell *et al.*, 1970; Galina *et al.*, 1962; Briggs *et al.*, 2021). Other drugs used to treat asthma are also contraindicated for use during pregnancy (Table 5.3).

## RISK SUMMARY

The FDA Pregnancy Risk Rating is compared to the Teratogen Information System (TERIS) risk rating in Table 5.4. Generally, the TERIS risk rating provides greater information than the FDA rating. However, the FDA rating is an aggregate risk of not only birth defects, but also of possible

---

**TABLE 5.3**

**Drugs That Should Be Avoided in the Treatment of Asthma during Pregnancy**

| Agent | Effects |
|---|---|
| Beta-blockers | Bronchospasm |
| Cyclopropane | Bronchoconstriction |
| Iodide-containing mixtures | Fetal goiter |
| | Congenital hypothyroidism |
| Opiates, sedatives, tranquilizers | Depressed alveolar ventilation |
| Prostaglandin $F_{2a}$ | Bronchoconstriction |
| | Stained fetal teeth |
| Tetracyclines | Abnormalities in fetal bone formation |

**TABLE 5.4**
**Summary of Drugs Used to Treat Asthma**

| Drug | TERIS Risk | FDA Risk Rating |
|---|---|---|
| Albuterol | Undetermined | C |
| Atropine | Unlikely | C |
| Beclomethasone | Unlikely | C |
| Betamethasone | Undetermined | C* |
| Chlorpheniramine | Unlikely | B |
| Cortisone | Unlikely | C* |
| Cromolyn | Unlikely | B |
| Dexamethasone | Minimal | C* |
| Ephedrine | Unlikely | C |
| Epinephrine | Unlikely | C |
| Erythromycin | None | B |
| Hydrocortisone | Unlikely | C* |
| Isoetharine | Undetermined | C |
| Isoproterenol | Unlikely | C |
| Metaproterenol | Undetermined | C |
| Methylprednisolone | Unlikely | See parent drug, prednisone |
| Penicillin | None | B |
| Pheniramine | Unlikely | C |
| Prednisone | Oral clefts: Small | C* |
| | Other congenital anomalies: Unlikely | |
| Terbutaline | Unlikely | B |
| Tetracycline | Unlikely | D |
| Theophylline | None | C |

*Abbreviations:* NA, not available; TERIS, Teratogen Information System; FDA, Food and Drug Administration.
*Sources:* Compiled from Friedman *et al.*, *Obstet Gynecol*, 1990; 75: 594; Briggs *et al.*, 2021; Friedman and Polifka, 2006.

adverse events during the second and third trimester. The TERIS risk rating is directed toward the risk for birth defects (i.e., teratogenicity).

## SPECIAL CONSIDERATIONS

### ACUTE ASTHMA

Patients with an acute asthma attack should have a clinical assessment, including evaluation for symptoms suggestive of complications such as pneumonia or pneumothorax and for the presence of agitation, pulse paradoxus, severe wheezing, or cyanosis (Box 5.5). Beta-adrenergic agonists are a critical element of first-line pharmacological therapy (ACOG, 2008; Robin and Felder, 2021). The guidelines for management of asthma during pregnancy are given in Box 5.6. These actions include the medications listed in Table 5.2. During an acute asthma attack, 0.3–0.5 mL of epinephrine in a 1:1000 dilution is administered subcutaneously every 30 min. Alternatively; 0.25 mg of terbutaline in two to three doses can be given subcutaneously every 20–30 min. Some physicians advocate the use of inhaled beta agonists initially. Each dose should be followed by spirometry. Evaluation should include forced expiratory volume in 1 s (FEV) and peak expiratory flow rate (PEFR) (ACOG, 2008;

Robin and Felder, 2021). Supplemental oxygen should be administered, as needed, to maintain a $pO_2$ greater than 60 mmHg. Intravenous hydration is also important, along with respiratory care to remove the tenacious secretions.

---

### BOX 5.4    MANAGEMENT OF ACUTE ASTHMA ATTACK IN PREGNANCY

- Brief medical history
- Physical examination
- FEV1 or PEFR and oxygen saturation
- Continuous electronic fetal monitoring and/or biophysical profile
- Repeat assessments of the patient and fetus → need for continuing care.
- **Discharge:** FEV1 or PEFR measurements ≥ 70 percent sustained for 60 minutes after last treatment
  - No distress and reassuring fetal status → discharge
- **Incomplete Response:** FEV1 or PEFR measurements ≥ 50 percent and < 70 percent, mild or moderate symptoms), then disposition (continued treatment in the emergency department, discharge home, or hospitalization) will need to be individualized.
- **Poor response:** For patients with a poor response (FEV1 or PEFR measurements less than 50 percent), hospitalization is indicated. For patients with a poor response and severe symptoms, drowsiness, confusion, or $PCO_2$ level greater than 42 mm Hg, intensive care unit admission is indicated and intubation should be strongly considered.

*Source:* Dombrowski *et al.*, 2010; ACOG, 2008.

---

### BOX 5.5    STEP THERAPY MEDICAL MANAGEMENT
### OF ASTHMA DURING PREGNANCY

*Mild Intermittent Asthma*

- No chronic medication regimen
- Albuterol *prn*

*Mild Persistent Asthma*

- First-line treatment: Low-dose inhaled corticosteroid (e.g., beclomethasone)
- Failed first-line therapy: Cromolyn, leukotriene receptor antagonist, or theophylline (target serum level 5–12 μ g/mL, decrease maternal dose in 3rd trimester)

*Moderate Persistent Asthma*

- First-line treatment
  - Preferred: Low-dose inhaled corticosteroid and salmeterol
  - Second preference: Medium-dose inhaled corticosteroid
  - Third preference: If needed, medium-dose inhaled corticosteroid and salmeterol are indicated
- Alternative: Low dose or (if needed) medium dose inhaled corticosteroid and either leukotriene receptor antagonist or theophylline (serum level 5–12 mcg/mL, decrease maternal dose in 3rd trimester)

> ### *Severe Persistent Asthma*
>
> - First-line treatment: High-dose inhaled corticosteroid and salmeterol and (if needed) oral corticosteroid
> - Second-line treatment: High-dose inhaled corticosteroid and theophylline (serum level 5–12 mcg/mL, decrease maternal dose in 3rd trimester) and oral corticosteroid if needed
>
> *Source:* Modified from Dombrowski *et al.*, 2010.

If initial spirometry indicates severe obstruction, an intravenous bolus of 125 mg methylprednisolone should be considered. Methylprednisolone is indicated in patients who are on chronic corticosteroids. It has been recommended that corticosteroids should be part of the initial therapy for women with severe, acute asthma (National Heart, Lung and Blood Institute, 1991).

After two or three doses of epinephrine or inhaled beta-agonists, if the wheezing is not corrected, then intravenous theophylline may be indicated. Dosing should be based on theophylline serum levels, if the patient has been receiving oral theophylline. *It should be noted that theophylline requirements decrease as pregnancy advances because pharmacokinetic parameters are counterintuitively altered in pregnancy*. The patient should be admitted to the hospital if she demonstrates a poor spirometric response to therapy, has no symptom improvement, or has pneumonia or pneumothorax.

Endotracheal intubation and mechanical ventilation should be considered when signs of respiratory failure are present. Specifically, PaCO greater than 40 mmHg, PaO less than 70 mmHg and pH less than 7.38 are indicators of impending respiratory failure. Immediate endotracheal intubation should be performed when (1) a PaCO of greater than or equal to 55 mmHg or (2) a PaO of less than or equal to 65 mmHg is obtained. Patients who respond quickly to such therapy should be discharged on an intensified regimen. A tapering schedule of oral corticosteroids should be given if intravenous steroids were used. Close follow-up should be arranged to reassess their clinical condition and possible adjustments in medication. In addition, precipitating factors (Box 5.1) should be avoided.

Opiates, sedatives, and tranquilizers are contraindicated in asthmatics because they cause alveolar ventilatory depression, and are associated with respiratory arrest immediately after use (Table 5.3). Beta-adrenergic blockers and parasympathetic agents should also be avoided in asthmatics because they can cause bronchospasm. Additionally, if prostaglandins are needed for labor induction or termination of pregnancy, prostaglandin E (PGE), a bronchodilator, should be administered, **rather than prostaglandin F (PGF)**, because it has **potent bronchoconstricting** effects and may precipitate status asthmaticus (Fishburne *et al.*, 1972a, 1972b; Hyman *et al.*, 1978; Smith, 1973).

## CHRONIC ASTHMA

To prevent adrenal crisis, chronic asthma patients require additional steroid therapy for asthma control during the stress of labor if they have received oral steroid therapy for more than 2 weeks within the previous year. The usual regimen is hydrocortisone, 100 mg IM or IV every six to eight hours for 24 hours. Corticosteroids should be given in cases of severe or mild asthma with wheezing that is unresponsive to bronchodilators. Initially, prednisone, 30–60 mg daily is given to prevent status asthmaticus. Beclomethasone dipropionate is effective and safe when prolonged steroid use is necessary.

Beta-agonist by inhalation every three to four hours as needed is used for outpatient management of chronic asthma, along with inhalation steroids such as beclomethasone. Cromolyn sodium can be given chronically by inhalation, and is effective in improving the symptoms of an asthmatic. An added benefit with cromolyn use is a decreased requirement for other antiasthma agents. Cromolyn therapy is best begun during remissions because it requires several days to reach an effective dosing regimen. Medications that cause bronchospasm or depress alveolar ventilation should be avoided in the pregnant woman with asthma (Table 5.3).

# 6 Anesthetic Agents and Surgery during Pregnancy

Non-obstetrical surgery occurs in approximately 1–2 percent of pregnant women in the US some-time during gestation (Brodsky, 1983; Friedman, 1988; Tolcher *et al.*, 2018), and the rate seems consistent across time. A considerable proportion of surgeons are reluctant to perform operative procedures on women known to be pregnant because of the possible untoward outcomes. However, emergency procedures are unavoidable.

Elective or indicated surgical procedures may occur before pregnancy is recognized.

Obstetrical surgery (i.e., cesarean section) is increasingly common with a steady rise in the cesarean section (C-section) rate from 4–5 percent in the 1960s to rates exceeding 20 percent (Gilstrap *et al.*, 1984; Notzon *et al.*, 1987) in the 1980s, to the current recommended level of 25 percent (ACOG, 2016). C-section rate in the United States was 31.7 percent in 2019 (Hamilton *et al.*, 2020).

Diagnostic imaging (modalities, dosimetry, contrast agents) are beyond the scope of this chapter, which is focused on anesthetic agents and surgery per se.

General clinical principles demand the surgeon's attention include physiological differences between gravid and non-pregnant women (Box 6.1). Non-obstetricians must keep in mind that two patients are involved in the surgery: *the mother and her fetus*. It is a fact that ***all anesthetic agents and 98 percent of medications cross the placenta***, exposing the fetus to medically significant levels of any anesthetic or adjuvant given to the mother. A high priority during surgery is cardiopulmonary function because even mild changes in maternal cardiopulmonary status (i.e., changes in blood pressure or oxygen saturation) can have physiologically important sequelae for the fetus, and need separate maternal and fetal monitoring.

---

### BOX 6.1  GENERAL PRINCIPLES FOR SURGERY AND ANESTHESIA DURING PREGNANCY

- Two patients: Mother and embryo-fetus
- Assume that all anesthetics and 98 percent of medications cross the placenta, resulting in therapeutically active fetal levels
- Minor maternal cardiopulmonary status changes may have profound effects on the fetus
- Numerous maternal physiological changes occur during pregnancy (Table 6.1)
- Aspiration pneumonitis risk is increased during pregnancy
- Laboratory and radiologic procedures should be performed as indicated
- Indicated surgery during pregnancy should be performed stat because delays increase risks of maternal or fetal morbidity and mortality

---

Placental hypoperfusion and fetal hypoxemia may result from even a minimal degree of maternal hypotension and hypoxia, and, therefore, must be avoided. Surgery preparation for pregnant women should include being placed on their left side (left lateral tilt), adequately hydrated, and pre-oxygenated prior to induction of anesthesia.

DOI: 10.1201/9780429160929-6

Anesthetic agent pharmacokinetics have been reported for only pancuronium, and its disposition was a pregnancy-associated decreased half-life, which was apparently due to significantly increased renal clearance (Little, 1999).

Several maternal physiologic changes occur during pregnancy (Table 6.1), and the most marked is expansion of the maternal blood volume by up to 50 percent. Increased blood volume is caused by a plasma volume increase of approximately 1000 cc and a 300–500 cc increase in red cells. This usually results in lower hematocrit compared to the non-pregnant woman, and is commonly known as physiologic anemia of pregnancy. Increased renal blood flow is a result of the increase in blood volume. Accordingly, the glomerular filtration rate increases (as measured by the endogenous creatinine clearance) because of increased blood volume. Serum creatinine and blood urea nitrogen

**TABLE 6.1**
**Physiologic Changes during Pregnancy**

| System | Effect |
| --- | --- |
| *Cardiovascular* | |
| Cardiac output | Increase |
| Blood volume | Increase |
| Heart rate | Increase |
| Blood pressure | Initial decrease[a] |
| Peripheral resistance | Decrease |
| Hematocrit | Decrease |
| Proportion of blood to uterus | ~10% |
| *Hematologic* | |
| Leukocytes | Increase |
| Fibrinogen (I) | Increase |
| Factors VII–X | Increase |
| Factor II | Slow increase |
| Factors XI, XIII | Decrease |
| Platelets | Unchanged |
| Prothrombin time/ | |
|   partial thromboplastin time | Slow decrease |
| *Respiratory* | |
| Tidal volume | Increase |
| Vital capacity | Unchanged |
| Functional residual capacity | Decrease |
| Compliance | Unchanged |
| Minute ventilation | Increase |
| $pCO_2$ | Decrease |
| $HCO_3$ | Decrease |
| *Renal* | |
| Serum creatinine | Decrease |
| Serum blood urea nitrogen | Decrease |
| Creatinine clearance | Increase |
| *Gastrointestinal* | |
| Gastric emptying | Decrease |
| Cardiac valve competency | Decrease |
| Regurgitation | Increase |

[a] Returns to pre-pregnancy levels by term.
*Sources:* From Little, 1999; Gilstrap and Hankins, 1988.

decrease because of dilution by increased plasma volume. Other changes in the renal system include dilatation of the ureters and a relative stasis of urine, resulting in a "relative" hydronephrosis. The relative hydronephrosis is frequently more pronounced on the right than on the left side.

Cardiopulmonary changes during pregnancy include a slight increase in heart rate and decreased systolic and diastolic blood pressures in the second trimester as maternal physiology adapts to expanded volume. Blood pressure gradually returns to pre-pregnancy levels by the third trimester. Most women have a mild systolic flow murmur by mid-pregnancy.

Respiratory rate increases slightly during pregnancy with a decrease in physiologic 'dead space' as pregnancy progresses. Tidal volume is increased during pregnancy, but minute ventilation and compliance do not change during pregnancy. Blood $pCO_2$ and $HCO_3$ decrease during pregnancy, while pH is slightly increased during pregnancy. Hence upper normal range $pCO_2$ for non-pregnant women likely indicates $CO_2$ retention. Gastrointestinal system changes during gestation affect pregnant women that require anesthesia and/or surgery. Aspiration pneumonitis risk in surgery on the gravid patient is increased because of pregnancy-associated reductions in intestinal motility and gastric emptying. Hepatic function is also altered e.g., alkaline phosphatase levels are increased) during pregnancy.

Hepatic cytochrome P-450 (CYP) 3A4 and CYP2D6 activities increase during pregnancy. In contrast, the enzyme responsible for metabolism of >50 percent of pharmacologic agents (CYP1A2) is downregulated, signaling that non-pregnant doses may be too high during gestation. Anesthesia dose management in the pregnant patient indicates that lower doses than in the non-gravid patient may achieve the desired anesthetic effect. CYP2C19 activity is upregulated in pregnant compared to non-pregnant women, but even during pregnancy, its activity does not exceed normal adult male levels. Extrahepatic enzymes (e.g., cholinesterase) also metabolize some anesthetics, and cholinesterase activity is diminished during pregnancy.

Liver fibrinogen production is increased during pregnancy with serum levels rising to as high as 400 mg/dL during the third trimester. This causes increased red cell sedimentation rates in pregnant women late in pregnancy. Hematocrit is decreased during pregnancy because of expanded volume, and accompanied by a relative leukocytosis (white blood cell count greater than or equal to 10,000–12,000 or even higher during labor). Other hematologic measures are unchanged during pregnancy such as relative percent of immature forms (i.e., "bands"), lymphocytes, eosinophils, and platelet count. INR, whole blood clotting time, prothrombin time, and partial thromboplastin time are within normal ranges during pregnancy.

When it is indicated for life-threatening maternal conditions, surgery should be performed immediately. Indicated laboratory tests and radiologic procedures should be performed without hesitation when properly guided life-saving surgical procedures are needed.

## ANESTHETIC AGENTS

Secondary effects of anesthetic agents (hypotension, hypoxia) are important to avoid in the gravid patient because they may cause adverse fetal effects. Anesthetic adjuncts, or other 'non-anesthetic' drugs and medications during the pre-, intra-, and post-operative periods may also adversely affect the fetus. It is important to know which anesthetic agents carry risk of possible untoward fetal and maternal effects.

## LOCAL ANESTHETICS

Local anesthetics may be injected in subdural or epidural spaces for regional anesthesia (Table 6.2). Topical application results in negligible fetal exposure and minimal risk because systemic concentrations usually remain very low, if detectable. Importantly, regional techniques (spinal and epidural procedures, paracervical and pudendal blocks) result in physiologically important fetal exposure to clinically significant anesthetic levels.

**TABLE 6.2**
**Anesthetic Agents Used in Non-Obstetric Surgery Gravid Patients**

| Agent | Class | Principal Use |
|---|---|---|
| Benzocaine | Ester | Topical |
| Bupivacaine | Amide | Local and epidural blocks |
| Chloroprocaine | Ester | Local and epidural blocks |
| Etidocaine | Amide | Epidural block |
| Lidocaine | Amide | Local, epidural, and spinal blocks |
| Mepivacaine | Amide | Local and epidural blocks |
| Procaine | Ester | Local block |
| Tetracaine | Ester | Spinal |

Local anesthetics have an aromatic ring with an intermediate alkyl chain with either (1) an amide or (2) an ester linkage. Protein-bound fraction is directly related to anesthetic potency, and duration of action is determined by the amount of binding. Anesthetics that are highly protein bound are lipid soluble and readily cross the placenta (Morishima et al., 1966; Pedersen and Finster, 1987). The frequency of birth defects among offspring of women who used lidocaine (n = 293), benzocaine (n = 47), or tetracaine (n = 23) during the first trimester, showed there were no adverse fetal effects when these agents were used any time during pregnancy (Heinonen et al., 1977). The Swedish Birth Defects Registry reported 20 infants whose mothers used tetracaine during the first trimester for local anesthesia, and no birth defects were reported (Kallen, 2019). The meaning of these small sample sizes is unclear. No animal teratology studies of these agents have been published.

No studies of bupivacaine, chloroprocaine, or prilocaine have been published regarding the use of the drugs during pregnancy. Transient neurobehavioral changes in infants whose mothers received local anesthetic agents have been reported, and vary from moderate for regional blocks (Rosenblatt et al., 1981; Scanlon et al., 1974; Standley et al., 1974) to minimal for epidural anesthesia on newborn behavior (Tronick et al., 1976).

## EPINEPHRINE

A naturally occurring sympathomimetic, epinephrine is added to local anesthetics to prolong action by causing local vasoconstriction. The frequency of inguinal hernia was increased following first trimester exposure of 189 infants, to epinephrine (Heinonen et al., 1977), which may be associated with preterm birth. However, it is unlikely that epinephrine is a teratogen, although in some animal models the drug has been associated with birth defects (Nahsimura and Tanimura, 1976; Shepard and Lemire, 2010). Among 102 women who used epinephrine for asthma in the Swedish Birth Defects Registry, the frequency of birth defects was not increased (Kallen, 2019). Epinephrine is also used as a test agent to detect intravascular injection of local anesthetics.

Certain local anesthetics (e.g., lidocaine), especially those used in combination with epinephrine, when used for paracervical block anesthesia during labor have been associated with fetal heart rate bradycardia. Fetal bradycardia is thought to occur secondary to vasoconstriction of the uterine artery caused by the anesthetic agent (Fishburne et al., 1979). Paracervical block is not recommended in the presence of fetal heart rate variability abnormalities, or in compromised uterine blood flow (Carlsson et al., 1987). Bupivacaine is contraindicated for paracervical block anesthesia in pregnancy because of potential fetal bradycardia; lidocaine or chloroprocaine are preferred agents for paracervical block.

## GENERAL ANESTHETICS

The preferred approach for pregnant women undergoing obstetrical procedures is regional anesthetic techniques. General anesthesia is frequently used for non-obstetrical surgery, or emergency procedures in pregnant women. Under general anesthesia, fetus exposure to a variety of agents occurs, and includes narcotics, paralyzing agents, and inhalational anesthetic agents.

### THIOPENTAL AND KETAMINE

Thiopental is no longer available. Propofol is the primary agent used to induce general anesthesia. Ketamine is a narcotic anesthetic administered intravenously for rapid induction of anesthesia prior to the intubation and initiation of inhalational anesthetic agents. Propofol is the most often used agent for this purpose. The frequency of congenital malformations was not increased in human or animal studies exposed to ketamine (Heinonen *et al.*, 1977; Friedman, 1988). Ketamine is rarely used in obstetrics, except for rapid anesthesia in emergency operative vaginal deliveries. Ketamine presents two problems when used during pregnancy: (1) clinically important increases in blood pressure and (2) significant maternal hallucinations. Ketamine was not teratogenic in one animal study (Friedman, 1988), but in another the fetal rat prefrontal cortex development was abnormal following ketamine exposure (Zhao *et al.*, 2016).

## NEUROMUSCULAR BLOCKING AGENTS

Succinylcholine is the most commonly used agent for inducing paralysis prior to intubation and the initiation of actual surgical procedures. An estimated 10–20 percent of patients may have lowered cholinesterase activity. Reduced cholinesterase activity pregnancy is part of the physiological changes during pregnancy. Therefore, pregnant patients usually require a lower dose of succinylcholine than non-gravid women do. Newborns may be exposed to sufficient drug to induce neuromuscular blockade, which will necessitate supportive therapy. Other common agents used for neuromuscular blockade are vecuronium bromide, pancuronium bromide, and atracurium besylate (Box 6.2). Succinylcholine is a depolarizing agent, while the other three neuromuscular blocking agents (vecuronium bromide, pancuronium bromide, and atracurium besylate) are non-polarizing.

---

### BOX 6.2   NEUROMUSCULAR BLOCKING AGENTS

- *Depolarizing agents:* Succinylcholine (Anectine)
- *Non-depolarizing agents:* Atracurium besylate (Tracrium), Pancuronium bromide (Pavulen), Vecuronium bromide (Norcuron)

---

This neuromuscular agent class may require a dose increase as gestation progresses because of a reduced half-life (higher metabolic clearance) and increased renal clearance (Little, 1999). No reports of use of these agents during pregnancy are published for use of these neuromuscular blocking agents. According to the manufacturer's package insert, atracurium is teratogenic in rabbits. However, its high molecular weight (>1000) and high polarity suggest atracurium should not cross the placenta in substantial quantities.

## INHALED ANESTHESIA AGENTS

Inhalation general anesthesia agents used in pregnancy: Nitrous oxide, halothane, methoxyflurane, enflurane, and isoflurane.

Ether, cyclopropane, and chloroform are not routinely used in present-day anesthesia. No adequate human studies regarding potential teratogenicity of either of these agents are published (Friedman, 1988).

### Halothane and Other Halogenated Agents

Halogenated agents are used frequently to supplement the standard nitrous oxide, propofol and muscle relaxant regimens for balanced general anesthesia. Halogenated agents decrease maternal awareness and recall, allow for a higher percentage of oxygen inspiration, and result in higher fetal oxygen concentrations (Shnider *et al.*, 1979).

Halothane is the prototype halogenated anesthetic agent. It was not associated with an increased frequency of birth defects among 26 infants whose mothers received halothane in the first trimester (Heinonen *et al.*, 1977). Increased fetal loss, growth retardation, malformations, and behavioral abnormalities were reported in animal studies of halothane in pregnancy (Friedman, 1988). A case-control study of birth defects in infants born to female nurses exposed to anesthetic drugs during the first trimester found an increased frequency of birth defects associated with halothane, isoflurane, sevoflurane, and nitrous oxide compared to 1,026 infants born to women not exposed to anesthetic gases during pregnancy (Table 6.3). It is important to note that the sample sizes are small, and the data are based entirely on self-report. Women with an infant with a birth defect are more likely to report exposures than women who had an infant without a birth defect (Teschke *et al.*, 2011).

Notably, the type of birth defects analyzed included only genitourinary organs, musculoskeletal system, and integument (skin disorders). Specifically, the birth defects were minor skin anomalies, while the frequency of major birth defects was not increased (Teschke *et al.*, 2011).

No epidemiologic investigations of the frequency of human birth defects and the use of methoxyflurane or isoflurane during the first trimester are published. Halogenated anesthetic agents were reported to cause a variety of malformations in animal studies at doses many times those used in humans (Friedman, 1988).

## TABLE 6.3
## Birth Defects among Infants Born to Nurses Exposed to Anesthetic Gases during Embryogenesis

| Control:<br><br>Drug Exposure | Anomalies | OR | Children without Birth Defects |
|---|---|---|---|
| Any halogenated anesthetic gas | 11/66 | 2.6 | 1026** |
| Desflurane | 4/26 | 2.4 | 1026 |
| Enflurane | 3/20 | 2.3 | 1026 |
| Halothane | 4/18 | 3.8 | 1026** |
| Isoflurane | 10/56 | 2.8 | 1026** |
| Sevoflurane | 8/30 | 4.7 | 1026** |
| Nitrous oxide | 21/153 | 1.8 | 1026** |

** Significantly increased.
*Source:* Modified from Teschke *et al.*, 2011.

Enflurane and halothane cross the placenta (Abboud *et al.*, 1985), reaching up to 60 percent of maternal concentrations. Infants born to women delivered by cesarean section did not differ from unexposed controls on Apgar scores, umbilical cord acid-base status, and neonatal neurobehavioral scores.

Increased blood loss in the mother during cesarean section, reported in some studies, was associated with halogenated agents (Gilstrap *et al.*, 1987). The association was not observed in other studies (Abboud *et al.*, 1985; Lamont *et al.*, 1988; Warren *et al.*, 1983).

Uterine relaxation is associated with increased blood loss, particularly with prolonged use of high doses. Otherwise, it seems apparent that halogenated agents are safe for both mother and fetus, although the data are not conclusive.

## NITROUS OXIDE

The most commonly used inhalation anesthetic agent in obstetrics, nitrous oxide, is usually part of a balanced general anesthetic regimen that includes a fast-acting anesthetic (e.g., use of propofol instead of thiopental), a muscle relaxant (e.g., succinylcholine), and a halogenated agent (e.g., isoflurane). The frequency of congenital anomalies was not increased among more than 650 infants exposed to nitrous oxide during the first trimester (Heinonen *et al.*, 1977; Crawford and Lewis, 1986; Teschke *et al.*, 2011). As with many other agents, nitrous oxide was reported to be associated with increased fetal loss, growth retardation, and congenital anomalies in animal studies (Friedman, 1988; Mazze *et al.*, 1984).

Certain anesthetists use high concentrations (e.g., 70-percent nitrous oxide, 30-percent oxygen). Lower nitrous oxide concentrations (50 percent) have been used with higher oxygen concentrations (50 percent), responding primarily to concerns that higher nitrous oxide concentrations may be associated with neonatal neurobehavioral alterations. Neonatal neurobehavioral abnormalities associated with nitrous oxide and halothane were also found in animal studies (Koeter and Rodier, 1986; Mullenix *et al.*, 1986). Recommendations are to use lower concentrations of nitrous oxide (e.g., 50 percent) higher concentrations of oxygen (e.g., 50 percent) with an halogenated agent to the anesthesia regimen (ACOG, 2017). Nitrous oxide may be used safely with other analgesia forms.

## SYSTEMIC ANALGESICS

Systemic analgesics are used for analgesia for women in labor (meperidine, morphine, pentazocine, butorphanol, alphaprodine) (see Chapter 8). Three very potent synthetic opioid analgesics (fentanyl, sufentanil, and alfetanil) (Box 6.3) are often used as (1) premedication prior to surgery, (2) an adjunct for induction of anesthesia, and (3) an adjunct in maintaining general anesthesia. Fentanyl is used in combination with a neuroleptic agent (droperidol) for the same indications. However, analgesic use near term is not plausibly related to birth defects as congenital anomalies arise from exposures during organogenesis (i.e., first trimester).

---

**BOX 6.3   AGENTS UTILIZED FOR GENERAL ANESTHESIA OR AS ADJUNCTS**

*Inhalational agents*

- Enflurane (Ethrane)
- Halothane (Fluothane)
- Isoflurane (Forane)
- Methoxyflurane (Penthrane)

> ### Narcotic
>
> - Alfentanil (Alfenta)
> - Fentanyl (Sublimaze)
> - Fentanyl + Droperidol (Innovar)
> - Sufentanil (Sufenta)
>
> ### Other
>
> - Ketamine (Ketalar)

Nonetheless, recently published investigations indicate that some narcotic analgesics agents are associated with birth defects in human and animal studies when exposure occurs during embryogenesis. While the risk of birth defects is increased, the absolute increase in risk is small (Brussard *et al.*, 2011; see Chapter 8).

Maternal meperidine use during the first trimester was not associated with an increased frequency of birth defects in 268 infants (Heinonen *et al.*, 1977). Among 39 infants with birth defects, the frequency of meperidine exposure was not increased (Brussard *et al.*, 2011). Morphine use during the first trimester was associated with an increased frequency of birth defects in 70 infants born following exposure (Heinonen *et al.*, 1977). Intravenous fentanyl was not associated with low Apgar scores or neonatal respiratory depression compared to controls in one study (Rayburn *et al.*, 1989), but other studies found depressed Apgar scores and respiratory depression (ACOG, 2019).

Three synthetic narcotic analgesics (fentanyl, sufentanil, alfetanil) have been used as an adjunct to epidural analgesia during labor. Neonatal respiratory depression is a risk with use of these agents during labor (ACOG, 2018).

A summary of estimated risks for birth defects in anesthetic exposed pregnancies is shown in Table 6.4.

## SPECIAL CONSIDERATIONS

### NON-OBSTETRIC SURGERY

During pregnancy, non-obstetric surgery is sometimes necessary, ranging from approximately one in 500 to one in 635 births (Affleck *et al.*, 1999). In a large Danish health registry, the frequency of non-obstetric surgery was 1.5 percent in 1996 and 1.6 percent in 2015 (Rasmussen *et al.*, 2019). The major change noted was a transition to laparoscopic surgery. Maternal mortality related to non-obstetric surgery is no greater than mortality in the non-pregnant patient. Adverse fetal effects from surgery are probably related more to the specific condition requiring the surgery than to the surgery itself, given an uncomplicated course. For example, compared to controls, the frequency of spontaneous abortion among 2,565 women undergoing surgery during the first or second trimester with general anesthesia was greater for gynecologic procedures compared to surgery in other anatomic regions. However, the frequency of congenital anomalies was not increased among gravidas who had surgery in the first trimester (Duncan *et al.*, 1986). The most frequent nontrauma indication for non-obstetric surgery during pregnancy is appendicitis, which occurs among approximately one in 3,000 births (Affleck *et al.*, 1999), and is apparently distributed equally across the three trimesters (Black, 1960; Rasmussen *et al.*, 2019). Importantly, laparoscopic surgery for appendicitis during pregnancy increased from 4.2 percent in 1996 to 79.2 percent in 2015 (Rasmussen *et al.*, 2019).

Biliary tract disease and cholecystitis are the second most common surgical conditions after appendicitis, and occurs in approximately one to 10 per 10,000 pregnancies (Affleck *et al.*, 1999;

**TABLE 6.4**

**Summary of Cardiovascular Anesthetic Drugs: Teratogen Information System (TERIS) and Food and Drug Administration (FDA) Risk Estimates**

| Drug | Risk | Risk Rating |
|------|------|-------------|
| Atracurium | Undetermined | C |
| Benzocaine | Unlikely | NA |
| Bupivacaine | Undetermined | NA |
| Cyclopropane | Undetermined | NA |
| Diazepam | Minimal | D |
| Droperidol | Undetermined | C |
| Enflurane | Undetermined | NA |
| Epinephrine | Unlikely | C |
| Ether | Undetermined | NA |
| Fentanyl | Undetermined | C * |
| Halothane | Undetermined | NA |
| Isoflurane | Undetermined | NA |
| Ketamine | Undetermined | B |
| Lidocaine | Local administration: None | B |
| | Intravenous administration: Unknown | |
| Meperidine | Unlikely | B* |
| Methoxyflurane | Undetermined | NA |
| Morphine | Congenital anomalies: Unlikely | C * |
| | Neonatal neurobehavioral effects: Moderate | |
| Nitrous | Occupational exposure: Unlikely | NA |
| | Anesthesia: Unlikely | |
| Pancuronium | Undetermined | C |
| Prilocaine | Undetermined | NA |
| Procaine | None | NA |
| Succinylcholine | Unlikely | C |
| Tetracaine | Undetermined | NA |
| Thiopental | Unlikely | NA |
| Vecuronium | Undetermined | NA: Not available |

*Sources:* Compiled from: Friedman *et al.*, *Obstet Gynecol*, 1990; 75: 594; Briggs *et al.*, 2021; Friedman and Polifka, 2006; Kallen, 2019.

Hill *et al.*, 1975). Closed (laparoscopic) surgery morbidity and mortality was not different from the open surgery cholecystectomy (Affleck *et al.*, 1999; Barone *et al.*, 1999).

Intestinal obstruction, inflammatory bowel disease, breast disease, and ovarian diseases are the third most frequent need for surgical procedures in pregnancy. Cardiovascular disease surgery during pregnancy is less common, and affects approximately 1–4 percent pregnancies in the US (ACOG, 2019). Common procedures (mitral valvulotomy, valve replacement, cardiopulmonary bypass are routinely done in gravid patients with good outcomes (ACOG, 2019). Anesthesia for non-obstetrical surgery may be general endotracheal or regional methods. Anesthetic technique is chosen based on (1) type of procedure to be performed, (2) emergent need for the procedure, (3) patient fasting time, and (4) patient and surgeon preferences.

General anesthesia is done using a balanced technique employing nitrous oxide, oxygen, propofol, succinylcholine, and a halogenated agent. Preparation of gravidas for surgery includes antacid prophylaxis to prevent aspiration pneumonia. In the ideal situation, the patient should also fast for

10–12 hours prior to scheduled surgery, but this may not be possible in all cases (e.g., emergency procedures). With timely extubation when reflexes have returned, endotracheal intubation will help prevent complications of aspiration. High-concentration oxygen should be used during general anesthesia; hypotension in the pregnant surgical patient must be avoided.

Anesthetic choice depends on (1) procedure length, (2) and anesthesiologist's preference. Adequate patient preload with a balanced salt solution is recommended prior to actual block initiation. This prevents maternal hypotension and protects from decreased uteroplacental blood flow. Complications of regional anesthesia (Box 6.4) can be minimized using preventative techniques to decrease hypotension incidence and severity associated with regional blocks (Box 6.5).

---

### BOX 6.4   POTENTIAL COMPLICATIONS OF REGIONAL ANESTHESIA

**Subarachnoid block**

- Arachnoiditis
- Bladder dysfunction
- Headaches
- Hypotension
- Meningitis

**Total spinal block/ Epidural block**

- Hematoma or infection
- Hypotension
- Subarachnoid or intravascular injection

*Source:* ACOG, 2017.

---

### BOX 6.5   HYPOTENSION: PREVENTION AND TREATMENT FROM REGIONAL ANESTHESIA

| Positioning | Ephedrine |
|---|---|
| Left lateral position | 25–50 mg IM prophylactically |
| Left uterine displacement | 10–15 mg IV for hypotension |
| **Preanesthetic Hydration (Loading)** | |
| 500–1000 cc balanced salt solution | |

---

### ANESTHESIA FOR CESAREAN SECTION: THE UNCOMPLICATED PATIENT

The preferred anesthesia method for uncomplicated gravidas undergoing cesarean section is regional anesthesia. Subarachnoid (spinal) or epidural block, or a combination of anesthetic techniques, are used routinely for uncomplicated C-section patients.

Regional anesthetic agents for use in cesarean section are given in Box 6.6. The most common complication of regional anesthesia is hypotension, and it can have the most serious effect on the fetus (Box 6.5).

---

**BOX 6.6   CESAREAN SECTION REGIONAL ANESTHETIC**

**Subarachnoid block**

- Bupivacaine (Marcaine, spinal)                                         7.5–10.5 mg
- Lidocaine (Xylocaine) 5 percent in 7.5 percent glucose   60–75 mg
- Tetracaine (Pontocaine) 1 percent                                   8–10 mg

**Epidural block**

- Bupivacaine (Marcaine) 0.5 percent
- Chloroprocaine (Nesacaine) 2–3 percent
- Lidocaine (Xylocaine) 1–2 percent

---

Central nervous system (CNS) toxicity is a potentially serious complication of unintentional intravascular injection of local anesthetic. During pregnancy, epidural veins are engorged and large, making them vulnerable to inadvertent puncture with a needle or catheter. CNS toxicity symptoms include slurred speech, dizziness, metallic taste in the mouth, ringing in the ears, facial paresthesia, seizures, and syncope. It is recommended that doses of peripheral and central neuraxial local anesthetics be reduced during pregnancy (El-Boghdadly *et al.*, 2018). In the past three decades, evidence has accumulated that indicates clinical use of certain local anesthetics in pregnancy may cause irreversible conduction blockade to occur (Datta *et al.*, 2010).

CNS toxicity treatment is primarily supportive care: airway and ventilation support, oxygen, prevention and treatment of seizures (diazepam), and treatment for hypotension (fluid, ephedrine, and lateral uterine displacement) (Gilstrap and Hankins, 1988).

General anesthesia is used for uncomplicated cesarean section. An estimated 21–26 percent of uncomplicated C-sections are performed under general anesthesia (Shroff *et al.*, 2004). As previously described, the balanced general technique of nitrous oxide, oxygen, propofol, succinylcholine and a halogenated agent provides satisfactory anesthesia for uncomplicated cesarean sections. General anesthesia gravid patients should be preoxygenated and placed in the lateral position with left lateral uterine displacement to relieve pressure on the uterine artery. General anesthesia provides reliable and expeditious anesthesia if hypotension is avoided. The major maternal risk is aspiration pneumonitis, and the major fetal risk is neonatal cardiorespiratory depression. All gravidas undergoing cesarean section should be managed assuming they have "full stomachs," emphasizing the importance of endotracheal intubation.

## ANESTHESIA FOR CESAREAN SECTION: THE COMPLICATED PATIENT

Cesarean section patients often have other medical complications (e.g., hypertension, diabetes, heart disease). Communication between obstetrician and anesthesiologist is of great importance. This is a critical point where communication frequently breaks down, and leads to poor patient outcomes (Shroff *et al.*, 2004).

An estimated 5 percent of gravidas have pregnancy-induced hypertension (PIH), which is a clinical challenge for anesthesia in cesarean section (Lopez-Jaramillo *et al.*, 2005). Severe PIH (chronic blood pressure >160/110 mmHg) is associated with increased blood volume that normally increases ~40–50 percent above non-pregnant volume by term. In women with severe PIH, blood volume usually does not expand appreciably above the non-pregnant state, unlike the normotensive pregnant woman whose volume increases to 40–50 percent above the non-gravid state. Typically low colloidal osmotic pressures and 'leaky vessels characterize severe PIH patients. These patients are more likely to develop pulmonary edema after intravenous infusion of crystalloid solutions.

Hematologic abnormalities (thrombocytopenia, hemolytic anemia) are observed in a small percentage of PIH patients. Anesthetic choice is controversial for cesarean section in women with severe PIH. General anesthesia, preferred by some, is not risk-free. During intubation or extubation, clinically important hypertension may develop, and with it attendant risks of cerebral hemorrhage or cardiac failure. Endotracheal intubation for general anesthesia may develop a hypertensive response that can be dampened by using antihypertensives such as nitroglycerin (Hodgkinson *et al.*, 1980; Snyder *et al.*, 1979). A very short-acting narcotic, remifentanil, used during general anesthesia for cesarean deliveries resulted in good maternal hemodynamics and perinatal outcome (Heesen *et al.*, 2013). General anesthesia efficacy and safety in these patients is shown in one study of 245 cases of eclampsia in which no cases of cerebral hemorrhage, pulmonary edema, or mortality were observed when hypertension is properly managed (Pritchard *et al.*, 1984).

A major problem with conduction anesthesia (spinal or epidural) is hypotension, secondary to sympathetic blockade. Hypotension is difficult to treat in women with severe PIH because they may be overly sensitive to pressor agents, increasing the likelihood of exaggerated untoward effects. Great caution must be used when preloading with crystalloid solutions to prevent fluid overload in vasoconstriction. Spinal block is contraindicated in women with severe PIH, Many authorities advocate use of epidural anesthesia for these women (Jouppila *et al.*, 1982; Moir *et al.*, 1972; Newsome and Branwell, 1984). If epidurals are used in pregnancy woman with PIH, it is important to carefully manage fluid preload, closely monitor blood pressure and prevent hypotension, and test coagulation status. For women with mild PIH, either epidural or general anesthesia is effective.

Pregnant women with diabetes mellitus (~2 percent of pregnancies), often require cesarean section. When necessary, cesarean sections for pregnant diabetics should be scheduled as the first case in the morning with blood glucose well controlled prior to surgery. General anesthesia or regional techniques (including spinal) may be used, if there are no other pre-existing conditions. A non-dextrose (sugar free) solution should be used to prevent neonatal hypoglycemia if preload is required for regional techniques.

General anesthesia is indicated for certain cardiac lesions. Pregnant women with aortic stenosis are at clinically important increased risk for hypotension and hypovolemia, and are best managed by general anesthesia when cesarean section is required. Gravidas with pulmonary hypertension and diminished venous return to the heart are especially at increased risk for hypotension and hypovolemia. Hence, they do not receive regional anesthesia when surgery is required. For women with recent myocardial infarctions, epidural or general anesthesia is efficacious.

Anesthetic technique choice depends on the specific type of maternal heart lesion present and the patient's functional cardiac status (New York Heart Association Classification; Dolgin *et al.*, 1994; Dunselman *et al.*, 1988). Epidural anesthesia is preferred in pregnant women requiring surgery with most types of heart disease. However, close attention must be given to preload and hypotension.

# 7 Antineoplastic Drugs during Pregnancy

Any type of cancer is uncommon during pregnancy, and occurs in approximately one in 1,000–6,000 pregnant women (Haas, 1984; Kennedy *et al.*, 1993; Pepe *et al.*, 1989; Smith *et al.*, 2003; Alpuim Costa *et al.*, 2020). An estimated 12.8 percent of all cancers in women occur in the 15–44 age group. Approximately one in 118 women with cancer (0.085 percent) will be pregnant, (Third National Cancer Survey, 1975). Population- and hospital-based studies show that the most frequently occurring cancers that present during pregnancy are those of the cervix, breast, and ovary (Haas, 1984; Pepe *et al.*, 1989).

The frequencies of non-genital type cancers during pregnancy are shown in Figure 7.1 with expanded detail in Table 7.1. The frequencies of the various forms of genital cancers in pregnancy are shown in Table 7.2, with cervical cancer being the most common.

Cancer during pregnancy presents several dilemmas: Whether or not to continue pregnancy or to terminate, or how to treat the specific cancer should the choice be to continue the pregnancy. Four major factors must be considered in the (1) gestational age of the pregnancy, (2) patient's desire to continue the pregnancy, (3) whether pregnancy per se alters the cancer's course, and (4) ultimate prognosis for the mother and infant.

## TABLE 7.1
### Frequencies of Non-Genital Cancers in Pregnancy

| Malignancy Type | Incidence (per number of gestations) |
|---|---|
| Any malignancy, all sites | 107.9–111.3 in 100,000 |
| Malignant melanoma | 1:1000–10 000 to 5.2–15.5 in 100,000 |
| Breast carcinoma | 1:3000–1:10 000 to 23.6–33 in 100,000 |
| Lymphoma | 1:1000–1:6000 |
| Leukemia | 1:75 000–1:100 000 |
| Colon cancer | 1:13 000 |
| Hodgkin's lymphoma | 1 in 6000 or 5–8 in 100,000 |
| Non-Hodgkin's lymphomas | Extremely rare (< 1 in 100 000) |
| Acute leukemia | 1 in 75 000 to 1 in 100 000 |
| Gastric cancer | 0.25 to 0.01 in 100,000 |
| *Gastrointestinal* | |
| Colon | 2–3.7 in 100,000 |
| Pancreatic | Only 21 cases reported 1954 to 2017 |
| Carcinoid | Rare |
| Hepatic cancer | 1 in 100,000 |
| Renal cell | Rare |
| Thyroid | 10.9–27.3 in 100,000 |
| Other Cancers | |

*Sources:* Compiled from Doll *et al.*, 1989; Pavlidis, 2002; Maggen *et al.*, 2019, 2020; Cottreau *et al.*, 2019; Norouzi *et al.*, 2012.

DOI: 10.1201/9780429160929-7

## TABLE 7.2
## Frequency of Genital Cancers in Pregnancy

| Type of Genital Cancer | Frequency | Proportion of Diagnosed Neoplasms in Gestation |
|---|---|---|
| Cervical cancer | — | 13.5 |
| | Carcinoma *in situ* | 1.3 in 1,000 to 1 in 770 |
| | Carcinoma of cervix | 1 in 2,000–10,000 |
| | Invasive carcinoma | 0.5 in 1,000 to 1 in 2200 |
| | Cervix/Uterus | 9.5 to 12.7 in 100,000 (2019) |
| Ovarian cancer | 1 in 18,000–1 in 25,000 | 10.5 |
| Ovarian cancer | 5.7 to 11.6 in 100,000 (2019) | |
| Ovarian carcinoma | 1 in 10,000 to 1 in 100,000 | |

*Sources:* Compiled from Smith *et al.*, 2003; Pavlidis *et al.*, 2002; Cottreau *et al.*, 2019; Franciszek Dłuski *et al.*, 2020.

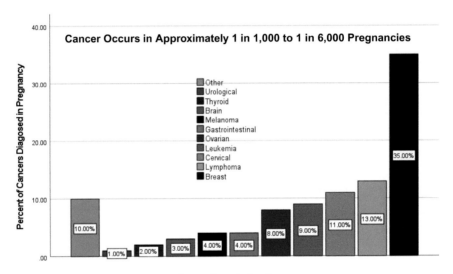

**FIGURE 7.1**   Frequency of types of cancer during pregnancy.

(Compiled from data in Maggen *et al.*, 2020.)

Pregnancies with gestational ages close to viability (i.e., 24–28 weeks) may usually be continued with only mild to moderate adverse effects on the fetus. Various therapeutic modalities are available, but none are known to be safe for use during pregnancy because **pregnancy is a time of rapid cell hyperplasia and hypertrophy, and the goal of cancer treatment is to inhibit both forms of cell growth**. Gravidas with pregnancies less than 24 weeks gestational age may best be termination, depending upon the patient's preference after discussion of the possible adverse outcomes. Pregnancy termination decisions between 24 and 28 weeks are more difficult because the discussion is then concerning termination of a viable fetus. Most frequently, terminations decisions depend upon the patient's wishes, the type of neoplasm and stage of maternal cancer.

Available data suggest that pregnancy affects neither the progression nor prognosis for most cancers. However, pregnancy may interfere with the diagnostic procedures for some types of malignancies, especially cancer located near the uterus.

Pharmacokinetics of antineoplastic medications are poorly studied. Information available are sufficient only to speculate regarding the effects of pregnancy on metabolism and renal clearance of cyclophosphamide, for example. Of the five cytochrome P-450 enzymes that metabolize cyclophosphamide (Matalon *et al.*, 2004), the activity of one, CYP3A4 (Little, 1999), is significantly increased during pregnancy. This implies that dose level and/or dose frequency must be adjusted for pregnant women throughout pregnancy by monitoring drug levels, and adjusting level and frequency schedules to maintain therapeutic levels.

The most difficult consideration in cancer treatment during pregnancy is optimal regimen formulation. The optimal regimen must include maternal and fetal effects of: (1) diagnostic tests, (2) surgical procedures, (3) radiotherapy, and (4) chemotherapy (Box 7.1). Limited data indicate the pregnant pharmacokinetics of certain antineoplastics (docetaxel, paclitaxel, doxorubicin, epirubicin) do not differ from non-pregnant adults (Janssen *et al.*, 2021b).

---

**BOX 7.1   CANCER DURING PREGNANCY:
BASIC PRINCIPLES OF MANAGEMENT**

- A multidisciplinary approach is mandatory.
- Patients should be informed in detail about the risks and benefits of treatment. Patient beliefs and wishes should be acknowledged.
- The treatment of pregnant patients should take into consideration the physiologic changes in pregnancy.
- Many diagnostic radiographic procedures do not cause harm to the fetus when used with proper shielding.
- Open or laparoscopic surgery may be safe in experienced hands.
- Systemic chemotherapy should not be started during the first trimester, if possible.
- Most chemotherapeutic agents are safe during the 2nd and the 3rd trimester, except for fetal growth retardation.
- Chemotherapy is not recommended after 35 weeks EGA. This allows a 3-week window between the last cycle of chemotherapy and delivery to allow maternal and fetal bone marrow to recover.
- Anti-VEGF (vascular endothelial growth factor) and other antiangiogenic drugs (i.e., inhibition of blood vessel growth factors) are contraindicated during pregnancy.
- No robust data exist regarding targeted therapies.
- The dosage should be the same as for non-pregnant patients based on actual height and weight of the patient. Increased volume of distribution changes as pregnancy advances must be included in dose calculations. That is, the same dose/m2 or dose/kg should be used.
- Radiation therapy should preferably be given post-partum, if possible.
- Termination of pregnancy may be considered in case of need for immediate treatment during the first trimester.
- No difference in maternal prognosis has been shown after termination of pregnancy.
- However, differences at the survival rates between pregnant and non-pregnant cancer patients may exist.
- No evidence exists that subsequent pregnancies increase the risk for neoplastic disease recurrence.

*Sources:* Modified from Voulgaris *et al.*, 2011; Amant *et al.*, 2019.

The **MOST IMPORTANT** risk to manage is minimization of embryo-fetal exposure to ionizing radiation. Many diagnostic tests can be performed safely during pregnancy because most diagnostic X-ray procedures expose the fetus to no or very low-dose radiation (i.e., < 1 rad per procedure). The general guideline applies to pelvic neoplasms. The general "rule of thumb" has been that fetal or embryonic radiation exposure of less than 5 "skin" rads is associated with little to no risk. **The exception to this is the critical period of neural plate development (days 10–18 post-conception)**, with the threshold for significant risk being as high as 15–20 "skin" rads (Brent, 1987). Skin rads are the amount of radiation delivered to the mother's skin surface. Therefore, procedures that involve little to no radiation exposure to the pelvic region can be safely performed. Specifically, barium enemas, pyelography, chest films, and non-pelvic computerized tomography may safely be performed, if deemed necessary during the initial diagnosis of malignancies during pregnancy. Diagnostic modalities such as magnetic resonance imaging and ultrasonography are often able to provide the same diagnostic information as X-ray studies and carry no known risk to the fetus or embryo. Diagnostic techniques such as cystoscopy and sigmoidoscopy may be performed safely until the end of the second trimester. (Pentheroudakis and Pavlidis, 2006).

Surgical oncology procedures can be done during pregnancy to treat life-threatening disease, especially if they do not involve the pelvis or pelvic organs (Miller and Bloss, 1995). After 10 weeks gestational age (8 weeks post conception), ovaries can usually be removed without apparent adverse effects on pregnancy. However, progestational agents for replacement therapy should be used if oophorectomy is necessary prior to this time. Most antineoplastic agents employed in chemotherapy are used because they impede or halt normal cell division, and this affects the exposed conceptus. Chemotherapy usually impedes embryo-fetal cell division, differentiation, replacement, increase in size (hypertrophy), and migration in the embryo. Antineoplastic agents are, therefore, capable of inducing growth retardation and structural, physiological, and functional abnormalities. Any agent that is used to stop or impede cell proliferation in size and/or number is potentially teratogenic (i.e., congenital abnormalities) and may cause fetal growth retardation. The frequency of birth defects was 25 percent for polytherapy chemotherapeutic regimens and 17 percent for single-agent exposure in the first trimester in an early review of 163 pregnancies exposed (Doll et al., 1989) (Table 7.3). A recent international study that included 779 pregnancies exposed to chemotherapy during pregnancy found that only 4 percent of fetuses exposed to antineoplastics during pregnancy had birth defects (de Hahn et al., 2018).

The frequency of malformations in 131 pregnancies with second-trimester exposure was 1.5 percent, below the background risk for the human population (Doll et al., 1988), but one would not expect structural anomalies to be induced outside the first trimester. It is expected that antineoplastic agent exposure after the period of embryogenesis (i.e., second and third trimesters of pregnancy) to increase only the risk of fetal growth retardation. Potential immediate fetal and neonatal effects are summarized in Box 7.2.

---

**TABLE 7.3**

**Frequency of Congenital Anomalies Associated with First-Trimester Use of Chemotherapy**

| Class | Congenital Anomalies (%) |
| --- | --- |
| Alkylating agents | 6 in 44 (14%) |
| Antimetabolites[a] | 15 in 77 (19%) |
| Plant alkaloids | 1 in 14 (7%) |
| Other Amsacrine Cisplatin Daunorubicin Procarbazine | |
| Total | 24 in 139 (17%) |

[a] 13 (24%) exposed to aminopterin or methotrexate.
*Sources:* Compiled from Doll et al., 1989; de Hahn et al., 2018.

---

## BOX 7.2  POTENTIAL EFFECTS OF ANTINEOPLASTIC AGENTS ON THE FETUS AND NEWBORN

**Immediate effects**

| | |
|---|---|
| Spontaneous abortion | Premature birth |
| Teratogenic effects | Growth retardation |
| Organ toxicity | |

**Long-term or delayed effects**

| | |
|---|---|
| Carcinogenesis | Developmental retardation |
| Sterility | Mutation |
| Growth retardation | Teratogenic in future offspring |

*Sources:* Adapted from Doll *et al.*, 1989; Koren and Lishner, 2011.

Long-term or delayed effects of prenatal exposure to chemotherapy for cancer include, for example, sterility or carcinogenesis for the child (Box 7.2). However, for the benefit of the mother, treatment for some neoplasms (for example, for acute leukemia) must begin immediately upon diagnosis, including the first trimester (Koren *et al.*, 1990).

Transplacental metastasis is a fetal risk from maternal cancer. It is well documented that certain cancers may spread to the developing fetus, yielding a grave fetal prognosis (Read and Platzer, 1981). Malignant melanoma is the most common cancer to metastasize to the fetus and placenta (Anderson *et al.*, 1989; Eltorky *et al.*, 1995; Read and Platzer, 1981).

Management and treatment of specific types of cancers are discussed under "Special Considerations." Specific chemotherapeutic agents, considered later, can be divided into several classes: alkylating agents, antibiotics, antimetabolites, plant alkaloids, and miscellaneous (Boice, 1986). Antineoplastic agents can also be classified as cycle-specific and cycle-nonspecific agents. Cycle-specific agents (antimetabolites, antibiotics, and plant alkaloids) arrest cell division only during specific phases of the replication cycle. In contrast, cycle-nonspecific agents (alkylating agents) are cytotoxic during all phases of cell replication (Caliguri and Mayer, 1989).

## ALKYLATING AGENTS

Alkylating agents available for use include drugs poorly studied for use during pregnancy (Box 7.3). These agents act by transferring alkyl groups to such biological substrates as nucleic acids and proteins. Alkyl groups block replication of DNA via the cross-linking bioactive molecules (i.e., polymerases) needed for cell division. The basis for suspecting that this group of drugs is associated with birth defects is limited to a few case reports or small case series.

## BOX 7.3  ALKYLATING AGENTS

| | |
|---|---|
| Bendamustine | |
| Busulfan (Myleran) | Melphalan (Alkeran) |
| Cyclophosphamide (Cytoxan, Neosar) | Triethylene |
| Thiophosphoramide (Thiotepa) | Chlorambucil (Leukeran) |
| Mechlorethamine (Mustargen) | Carmustine (BCNU) |

## BUSULFAN

Busulfan (Myleran) is an FDA-approved alkylating agent for the palliative treatment of chronic myelogenous leukemia. It is a primary treatment for acute non-lymphocytic leukemia. A summary of 16 different reports of 22 infants born to busulfan-exposed patients found two infants with major congenital anomalies (2/22, 9.1 percent) (Doll *et al.*, 1989). Six (14 percent) of 44 infants exposed to alkylating agent (30 different reports) had major congenital anomalies. In a more recent analysis, 6/31 (19.4 percent) infants exposed to busulfan was found (Nicholson *et al.*, 1968; Lee *et al.*, 1962; Diamond *et al.*, 1960; Abarmovici *et al.*, 1978; Gililland *et al.*, 1983; Ozumba *et al.*, 1992; Boros *et al.*, 1977; Dugdale and Fort, 1967; Zuazu *et al.*, 1991). The frequency of birth defects in animals whose mothers were given busulfan during organogenesis was increased in rodents.

## CYCLOPHOSPHAMIDE

Cyclophosphamide (Cytoxan, Neosar), an alkylating agent, is metabolized mainly by the liver to several active alkylating metabolites (phosphoramide mustard and acrolein) that cause tumor cell DNA crosslinking. Cyclophosphamide is used to treat several types of cancer, including (1) certain forms of acute and chronic leukemia, (2) ovarian, (3) multiple myeloma, (4) mycosis fungoides, and (5) breast carcinoma. It has also been used in treatment of cancers of the bladder, cervix, colorectum, endometrium, Ewing's sarcoma, head and neck, lymphomas, kidney, lung, osteosarcoma, pancreas, and trophoblastic tumors.

*In vitro* studies of cyclophosphamide metabolism with rat embryos demonstrated that the teratogenic effects of the drug are metabolites of a mono-functional liver oxygenase system (Fantel *et al.*, 1979; Kitchen *et al.*, 1981; Mirkes *et al.*, 1981, 1985) because morphologic changes *in vitro* were very similar to those seen *in vivo* (Greenway *et al.*, 1982).

Cyclophosphamide is associated with an increased frequency of skeletal and central nervous system anomalies when exposed during organogenesis in rats (Chaube *et al.*, 1968), mice (Gibson and Becker, 1968), rabbits (Fritz and Hess, 1971), and monkeys (McClure *et al.*, 1979).

Human data are limited to several case reports. Three case reports and one case series include a set of twins (one normal infant and one malformed exposed during organogenesis was reported). The twin with birth defects had multiple congenital abnormalities and subsequently developed thyroid cancer and neuroblastoma, while the other twin was normal (Zemlickis *et al.*, 1993). An infant with multiple anomalies (cleft palate, absent thumbs, and multiple eye defects) whose mother was treated with cyclophosphamide in the first trimester is reported in another case report, (Kirshon *et al.*, 1988). Bilateral absence of the big toe, cleft palate, and hypoplasia of the fifth digit was reported in an infant whose mother took cyclophosphamide throughout pregnancy (Greenberg and Tanaka, 1964). Among 10 infants whose mothers took cyclophosphamide during the first trimester, no birth defects were observed (Blatt *et al.*, 1980). No ill effects have been reported in association with second and third trimester exposure to cyclophosphamide (Matalon *et al.*, 2004).

Pancytopenia and other hematologic abnormalities have been observed in infants whose mothers were treated with cyclophosphamide and other agents during pregnancy (Pizzuto *et al.*, 1980) However, hematologic abnormalities do not occur in all neonates exposed to the drug, even if their mothers had severe pancytopenia (Meador *et al.*, 1987). Importantly, use of multiple agents appears more closely associated with pancytopenia in the fetus and newborn than does cyclophosphamide monotherapy.

## CHLORAMBUCIL

An oral bifunctional alkylating agent, chlorambucil (Leukeran), is a nitrogen mustard-type agent used to treat chronic leukemia and lymphomas. Chlorambucil has been used to treat breast, trophoblastic, and ovarian carcinomas. Two case reports of this agent used in pregnancy reported unilateral (left) renal and ureter agenesis in the infants whose mothers used the drug during pregnancy (Shotton and Monie, 1963; Steege and Caldwell, 1980). However, causal inferences cannot be made based on case reports.

No epidemiological studies of chlorambucil during pregnancy have been published. In a review, one of five fetuses exposed in the first trimester had a birth defect (Doll *et al.*, 1989). A normal infant was born after maternal treatment with chlorambucil (conception through 20 weeks gestation) for chronic lymphocytic leukemia (Ali *et al.*, 2009).

Central nervous system anomalies, postcranial skeleton, and palatal closure were increased in frequency among rodents whose mothers were given large doses of chlorambucil during pregnancy (Chaube and Murphy, 1968; Mirkes and Greenaway, 1982; Monie, 1961). Urogenital malformations, including absence of a kidney, were found in fetuses of rats given chlorambucil (National Toxicology Program, 1992).

## IFOSFAMIDE

Ifosfamide (Ifex) is a prodrug (requires metabolic activation by microsomal liver enzymes to active drug) chemotherapeutic that is a synthetic analog, chemically related to nitrogen mustards. As is the typical mechanism of action for alkylating agents, ifosfamide action is mediated by formation of DNA adducts. Ifosfamide is particularly toxic to the urinary epithelium and must be given with mesna (Mesnex, Uromitexan). It is a third-line chemotherapy of germ cell testicular cancer. Ifosfamide is also used to treat acute leukemias and lung, pancreas, breast, cervix, and endometrium cancers, as well as Ewing's sarcomas, lymphomas, osteosarcoma, soft tissue sarcoma, and ovarian cancer.

The frequency of congenital anomalies in fetuses whose mothers used this agent during pregnancy has not been analyzed and published. Two case reports are published of fetuses exposed *in utero* to ifosfamide-containing combination chemotherapy, of which one developed oligohydramnios (Barrenetexa *et al.*, 1995; Fernandez *et al.*, 1989). Exposure of 9 fetuses during the third trimester was reported in a case series, and no untoward sequelae were noted (Mir *et al.*, 2012). The manufacturer reports that it is embryotoxic and associated with birth defects in mice, rats, and rabbits exposed to ifosfamide during organogenesis.

## MECHLORETHAMINE

A nitrogen mustard alkylating agent, mechlorethamine (Mustargen), is used to treat Hodgkin's disease, polycythemia vera, mycosis fungoides, chronic leukemia, lymphomas, and lung carcinoma. Mechlorethamine is also used to treat brain, breast, and ovarian cancers. Data on its use during pregnancy is limited to two case reports of congenital anomalies after first-trimester polydrug chemotherapy (Garrett, 1974; Mennuti *et al.*, 1975) are published, No epidemiological studies of the use of mechlorethamine during pregnancy are published. Chemotherapy with mechlorethamine and other drugs that were discontinued prior to conception did not increase the frequency of congenital anomalies among more than 40 infants above the 3.5–5 percent background rate expected in the general population (Andrieu and Ochoa-Molina, 1983; Schilsky *et al.*, 1981; Whitehead *et al.*, 1983). However, prior exposure is probably not relevant to exposure to this drug during gestation.

Among 12 children born to women treated with mechlorethamine and other antineoplastic agents during pregnancy in one series there were no birth defects (Aviles *et al.*, 1991; Aviles and Neri, 2001). However, the significance of these findings is not clear because most exposures were outside the first trimester, and this is a very small number of cases.

The frequency of congenital anomalies was increased among the offspring of pregnant rodents given mechlorethamine at doses several times in the usual human dose (Beck *et al.*, 1976; Gottschewski, 1964; Murphy *et al.*, 1957; Nishimura and Takagaki, 1959).

Chromosome breaks in somatic cells were reported among embryos of pregnant animals given mechlorethamine during organogenesis (Soukup *et al.*, 1967). The relevance of this finding to human reproduction is unknown because only gonadal cell lines are relevant to reproduction, and they were not analyzed.

## MELPHALAN

Melphalan (Alkeran) is a phenylalanine derivative of nitrogen mustard, and a bifunctional alkylating agent. It is an FDA-approved antineoplastic agent for treatment of multiple myeloma, ovarian, and breast carcinomas. Melphalan may also be used to treat chronic myelocytic leukemia, melanoma, osteosarcoma, soft tissue sarcoma, and thyroid cancers. The manufacturer reports that oral melphalan caused an increased frequency of congenital anomalies and embryonic death in rat models (Manufacturer product information). No studies of the use of this drug during pregnancy in humans are published. Melphalan is an alkylating agent with chemical effects (strong mutagenic and cytotoxic action) that strongly suggest it may be associated with an increased frequency of birth defects, and it should be avoided during pregnancy, especially during the first trimester.

## TRIETHYLENE THIOPHOSPHORAMIDE

Triethylene thiophosphoramide (Thiotepa) is another alkylating agent, and is FDA-approved to treat ovarian, bladder and breast carcinomas, and malignant effusions. No epidemiological studies are published of the frequency of congenital anomalies exposure to this drug during organogenesis. None of four fetuses exposed to triethylene thiophosphoramide in the first trimester had congenital anomalies (Doll *et al.*, 1989). In another case report, one infant born following exposure to the drug in the last half of pregnancy had fetal growth retardation (Stevens and Fisher, 1965). Animal models of exposure to triethylene thiophosphoramide exposure during pregnancy showed an increased frequency of birth defects and fetal growth retardation among the offspring of pregnant rodents (Korogodina and Kaurov, 1984; Murphy *et al.*, 1958; Tanimura, 1968).

## CARMUSTINE

Carmustine (BCNU) is an alkylating agent, FDA-approved for chemotherapy of a variety of neoplasms including multiple myeloma, lymphomas, and brain tumors. In a case report, one patient took carmustine throughout pregnancy and delivered a normal neonate (Schapira and Chudley, 1984). Carmustine must be suspected of being teratogenic because of its biochemical action (an alkylating agent) on substrates such as nucleotides. Rodents exposed to carmustine at several times the usual human dose during embryogenesis had increased frequency of birth defects (Wong and Wells, 1989). Otherwise, little information is published about the use of this agent during pregnancy in humans or animals.

## BENDAMUSTINE

Another alkylating agent, bendamustine is a bifunctional mechlorethamine related antineoplastic used to treat chronic lymphocytic leukemia, B cell non-Hodgkin lymphoma. Pregnant mice given the drug during organogenesis had an increased frequency of embryonic losses, decreased fetal weight, and birth defects (exencephaly, cleft palate, and spinal deformities) (Manufacturer's product information).

## ANTIMETABOLITES

Three types of antimetabolite neoplastics are in use—folate antagonists, purine antagonists, and pyrimidine antagonists (Box 7.4). Aminopterin is one of the original antimetabolites, and is a folate antagonist. This antineoplastic agent was previously used as an abortifacient, but is no longer widely used as an antineoplastic or abortifacient. Aminopterin is a well-known teratogen that causes the *fetal aminopterin syndrome*. Importantly, the teratogenicity of aminopterin is relevant to other commonly used folate antagonist antineoplastics, indicating a high potential for causing birth defects similar to the syndrome. Notably, methotrexate is currently used to treat rheumatoid arthritis, which can occur among women of reproductive age.

---

### BOX 7.4  ANTIMETABOLITES

| | |
|---|---|
| *Folate antagonists*<br>Methotrexate (Folex, Mexate) | *Pyrimidine antagonists*<br>Cytarabine (Cytosar)<br>Fluorouracil (Efudex, Fluoroplex) |
| *Purine antagonists*<br>Mercaptopurine (Purinethol)<br>Thioguanine (Thioguanine) | |

---

### AMINOPTERIN/METHYLAMINOPTERIN

A synthetic derivative of pterin, aminopterin inhibits enzyme activity at the folate-binding site for dihydrofolate reductase, blocking tetrahydrofolate synthesis.

A "constellation" of birth defects observed among offspring whose mothers used aminopterin or methylaminopterin throughout pregnancy was characterized by short stature, craniosynostosis, hydrocephalus, micrognathia, hypertelorism, limb anomalies, and neural tube defects (Char, 1979; Reich *et al.*, 1977; Thiersch, 1952; Thiersch and Phillips, 1950; Warkany, 1978). The aminopterin syndrome is characterized based upon case reports, consequently, even an estimated risk of these birth defects following maternal exposure to this agent is unknown, **but is likely high** (Warkany, 1978).

Increased frequencies of skull, face, eye, and abdominal wall birth defects of were reported among rodents born to mothers given large doses of aminopterin during pregnancy (Baranov, 1966; Puchkov, 1967). Doses lower than usual human dose produced the same congenital anomalies in rabbits in one study (Goeringer and DeSesso, 1990), and embryo-fetal death in an early rat study (Thiersch and Phillips, 1950). Folate antagonists as a class of antimetabolite drugs have an apparent markedly higher risk of congenital anomalies than other antineoplastic agents. **Folate antagonists are uniformly contraindicated for use during pregnancy** (Doll *et al.*, 1989).

### METHOTREXATE

Methotrexate is a folate antagonist (Folex, Mexate) that inhibits dihydrofolic acid reductase, interrupting DNA synthesis and repair, including trophoblastic cells. Methotrexate is used to treat a several cancers, including acute leukemia, lymphoma, trophoblastic tumors, and breast, cervix, ovary, bladder, kidney, prostate, lung, and testicular carcinomas. The drug is also used to treat non-neoplastic diseases: rheumatoid arthritis, psoriasis, and ectopic pregnancy. Methotrexate is particularly toxic to trophoblastic cells and is used frequently as an abortifacient. It has been used successfully to treat ectopic pregnancies (Grainger and Seifer, 1995; Schink, 1995) and to induce abortion (Hausknecht, 1995).

A spectrum of congenital anomalies similar to the aminopterin syndrome is associated with methotrexate (Warkany, 1978). More than a dozen children with first-trimester exposure to methotrexate exhibited skeletal defects, ocular hypertelorism, craniosynostosis, and occasional mental retardation (Adam *et al.*, 2003; Chapa *et al.*, 2003; Diniz *et al.*, 1978; Milunsky *et al.*, 1968; Nguyen *et al.*, 2002; Powell and Ekert, 1971; Sosa-Munoz *et al.*, 1983; Wheeler *et al.*, 2002; Zand *et al.*, 2003). The frequency of birth defects is apparently dose-related. It has been suggested by some authorities that the risk of birth defects is lower than for aminopterin (Kozlowski *et al.*, 1990; Roubenoff *et al.*, 1988). A finding unrelated to exposure is pregnancy is that the frequency of birth defects was not increased among more than 350 infants whose mothers used it prior to conception (Rustin *et al.*, 1984; Van Thiel *et al.*, 1970). While this finding is unrelated to exposure during embryogenesis or other times in pregnancy, it may be reassuring to women who were concerned about conception following cessation of methotrexate use. The frequency of congenital anomalies was increased among the rodents whose mothers were given methotrexate during embryogenesis (Darab *et al.*, 1987; Jordan *et al.*, 1977; Skalko and Gold, 1974; Wilson *et al.*, 1979).

## MERCAPTOPURINE

An antimetabolite purine antagonist antineoplastic, mercaptopurine (Purinethol, 6-MP), is FDA-approved and used mainly used to treat acute leukemias. It is also used in the treatment of lymphomas. Data regard the use of mercaptopurine during pregnancy is limited to case reports. No controlled studies of human pregnancies exposed to mercaptopurine are published. Two case reports are published that document congenital anomalies in 2 infants whose mothers used mercaptopurine during early gestation (Diamond *et al.*, 1960; Sosa-Munoz *et al.*, 1983). No birth defects were reported among 20 infants born to women exposed to mercaptopurine during pregnancy in a collective review of 12 case reports (Doll *et al.*, 1989; Perucca *et al.*, 1995). One out of 34 infants had a congenital anomaly (1/34, 2.9 percent) in a case series born to women treated with mercaptopurine early in pregnancy. Compared to expected background birth defects rate of 3.5–5 percent, the 2.9 percent does not seem like an increased risk (Francella *et al.*, 2003). Note that the one birth defect was attributed to a chromosomal abnormality, not drug exposure. Eight infants born to women treated with mercaptopurine and other antineoplastic agents during pregnancy had no birth defects (Aviles *et al.*, 1991). Exposure to mercaptopurine is frequently part of a polydrug antineoplastic regimen. This seriously confounds the ability to separate effects of other drugs from those of mercaptopurine. The optimal risk estimates are possible only with monodrug therapies. Neonatal pancytopenia was associated with prenatal mercaptopurine exposure in several case reports (McConnell and Bhoola, 1973; Okun *et al.*, 1979; Pizzuto *et al.*, 1980), but a polydrug regimen was used in most instances. Birth defects (central nervous system, facial, limb) and) were increased in frequency among rodent pups whose mothers were dosed with several times the usual human therapeutic dose of mercaptopurine during organogenesis (Mercier-Parot and Tuchmann-Duplessis, 1967; Puget *et al.*, 1975; Shah and Burdett, 1976).

## THIOGUANINE

Thioguanine (Tabloid), is another purine antagonist, and is FDA-approved to treat acute nonlymphocytic leukemia. Thioguanine was part of a multiple drug regimen to which a fetus was exposed in the first trimester. The newborn had multiple abnormalities similar to Baller-Gerald syndrome (Artlich *et al.*, 1994). An increased frequency of malformations was found in offspring of pregnant rats that were given thioguanine during embryogenesis (Thiersch, 1957).

## CYTARABINE

A pyrimidine antagonist antimetabolite that inhibits DNA polymerase, cytarabine (cytosine arabinoside) (Cytosar-U, Ara-C, Tarabine) is approved to treat leukemia (acute and chronic) and lymphomas. A few reports of monotherapy with this agent during early pregnancy are published. In one report, an infant with limb and ear anomalies was born to a mother received who used cytarabine monotherapy in early pregnancy (Wagner *et al.*, 1980). One review of leukemia treatment during pregnancy reviewed 46 infants published in 24 case reports born to women who received cytosine arabinoside (Ara-C) during pregnancy, and several had received it during the first trimester (Caliguri and Mayer, 1989). Among exposed pregnancies, there were two spontaneous and six therapeutic abortions. Of the remaining 38 pregnancies, four intrauterine deaths (apparently grossly normal) occurred, and one infant with polydactyly and one with adherence of the iris to the cornea were born. One newborn presented with neonatal pancytopenia (Caliguri and Mayer, 1989). Anecdotal reports seem to indicate an increased risk of birth defects following first trimester exposure to cytarabine. However, anecdotal (case reports) information cannot be used to attribute risk. However, findings from animal studies parallel those in humans, which increases suspicion that cytarabine may be associated with birth defects. In addition, treatment of leukemia during pregnancy *after* the first trimester is not associated with a high frequency of congenital abnormalities. Importantly, the folate antagonist methotrexate was a component of the polydrug therapy in several of these gravidas.

Cytarabine was associated with an increased frequency of congenital anomalies in two rodent teratology studies when given during embryogenesis (Chaube and Murphy, 1965; Percy, 1975).

## FLUOROURACIL

Fluorouracil (Adrucil, 5-FU, Efudex, Fluoroplex) is a fluorinated pyrimidine analog. It is approved for treatment of colon, rectum, breast, stomach, and pancreas neoplasms. Other uses include bladder, cervix, endometrium, esophagus, head and neck, liver, lung, ovary, prostate, and skin cancers. Fluorouracil inhibits thymidine synthesis blocking DNA and protein synthesis.

Twenty-four infants born without birth defects were born to mothers treated with intravenous fluorouracil as part of polytherapy with doxorubicin and cyclophosphamide for breast cancer during the second and third trimesters of pregnancy, no congenital anomalies occurred (Berry *et al.*, 1999). It must be noted that these exposures occurred outside the period of embryogenesis, and indicate nothing about the risk of birth defects. This risk can only be assessed from first trimester exposure to the drug. Multiple congenital anomalies was reported in the abortus of a mother treated with 5-fluorouracil during 11 and 12 weeks of gestation (9–10 weeks post-conception) (600 mg IV five times weekly) with colon malignancy (Stephens *et al.*, 1980). **Importantly**, the patient had bowel resection with multiple diagnostic X-ray procedures during late embryogenesis. The anomalies (bilateral radial aplasia, absent thumbs, abnormal fingers, a single umbilical artery, hypoplastic aorta, and esophageal atresia, imperforate anus, and renal dysplasia) were not plausibly related to fluorouracil because of the gestational timing of the exposure (i.e., **exposure occurred outside the period of morphogenesis of these organs**). In a report on 295 infants born to women treated for cancer during pregnancy, 54 had monotherapy with fluorouracil (Song *et al.*, 1988). Timing of exposure during pregnancy is not stipulated, but it is stated that 3 birth defects occurred. In the worst-case scenario which is not true, the rate of birth defects (hydrocephalus, anencephaly, heart malformation) would be 5 percent, which is not elevated. The important aspect of this study is that follow-up at one to 25 years indicated no growth deficits in height or weight (Song *et al.*, 1988).

Two normal infants were born following first-trimester maternal treatment with intravaginal 5-fluorouracil (Odom *et al.*, 1990); the drug is known to be absorbed systemically by this route (Markman, 1985). Skeletal and other major anomalies (cleft palate, central nervous system) were increased in frequency among offspring of pregnant rats, mice, and hamsters born to mothers exposed to this antineoplastic during pregnancy (Chaube and Murphy, 1968; Dagg, 1960; Shah and Mackay, 1978; Wilson *et al.*, 1979).

## ANTIBIOTICS

These agents work through a variety of mechanisms, including alkylation DNA breakage to prevent DNA replication in neoplasias but also affect inhibit replication other cells (Box 7.5).

---

### BOX 7.5   ANTIBIOTIC ANTINEOPLASTIC AGENTS

| *Anthracyclines* | *Other* |
|---|---|
| Daunorubicin (Cerubidine) | Bleomycin (Blenoxane) |
| Doxorubicin (Adriamycin) | Dactinomycin[a] (Cosmegen) |
|  | Mitomycin (Mutamycin) |

[a] Also known as Actinomycin-D.

---

### BLEOMYCIN

An antibiotic, bleomycin (Blenoxane) inhibits DNA synthesis and, to a lesser extent, other protein transcription, including RNA. It is approved to treat carcinomas (renal, cervical, penile, testicular, vulvar, and neck), lymphomas, and sarcomas. **No reports regarding the use of bleomycin mono-therapy during organogenesis are published**. Bleomycin polytherapy after the first trimester reported two normal infants following maternal therapy for a malignant ovarian germ cell tumor during the second trimester with bleomycin in combination with cisplatin and vinblastine (Christman *et al.*, 1990; Kim *et al.*, 1989). Other reports of bleomycin polytherapy with second-trimester exposure to bleomycin-containing combinations for maternal lymphoma resulted in normal infants (Nantel *et al.*, 1990; Rodriguez and Haggag, 1995). Profound but transient neonatal leukopenia (resolved day 13) was reported in one infant following maternal therapy for metastatic adenocarcinoma (early in the third trimester) with bleomycin, etoposide and cisplatin (Raffles *et al.*, 1989). Among rats exposed to bleomycin during organogenesis, birth defects (limb, tail anomalies) were reported in nine rat teratology experiments with bleomycin (Nishimura and Tanimura, 1976).

### DACTINOMYCIN

Also known as actinomycin-D, dactinomycin (Cosmegen), is one of a group of antibiotics produced by various species of streptomyces (the actinomycins). Dactinomycin is approved to treat chorio-carcinoma, Ewing's and Wilms tumors, rhabdomyosarcoma, and testicular and uterine cancers. Dactinomycin is indicated in obstetrics to treat gestational trophoblastic tumors.

No studies are published on the use of dactinomycin use during pregnancy, but it is an FDA category C drug. Four normal infants (one set of twins) were born following Dactinomycin treatment in the second and/or third trimesters of pregnancy (Gililland and Weinstein, 1983); no exposures occurred during embryogenesis. Dactinomycin exposure was associated with an increased frequency of malformations in rodents born to mothers given doses several times the usual human dose (Manufacturer information). However, details of the congenital anomalies were not made available and the manufacturer's product information is unpublished.

### MITOMYCIN

Mitomycin (Mitomycin-C) is an antineoplastic antibiotic that blocks DNA synthesis. Similar to Dactinomycin, mitomycin is isolated from the broth of *Streptomyces caespitosus*, and is approved as a component of polytherapy therapy for pancreatic and stomach cancers. Mitomycin is infrequently used also used to treat hypercalcemia secondary to malignancy.

No reports are published of mitomycin use during human pregnancy and infant outcome (Shepard and Lemire, 2010; Schardein, 2000). The frequency of congenital anomalies was increased in several mouse teratology studies that employed several times the usual human therapeutic dose of the drug during pregnancy (Tanimura, 1968; Friji and Nahatsuka, 1983; Gregg and Snow, 1983; Snow and Tam, 1979). Approximately 6 percent of mitomycin crossed the placenta in pregnant rats (Boike *et al.*, 1989). Unpublished embryo studies in mice suggest that at the four-cell embryo stage, mitomycin may have epigenetic effects that was expressed in future generations.

## ANTHRACYCLINE ANTIBIOTICS

Anthracycline antibiotic antineoplastics include daunorubicin (Cerubidine), doxorubicin (Adriamycin, Rubex), and inhibit nucleic acid synthesis and are nonspecific cell cycle phase agents. Daunorubicin is approved to treat neuroblastoma and acute leukemias. Doxorubicin is approved to treat acute leukemias, lymphomas, Wilms tumor, sarcomas, and carcinomas (bladder, breast, ovary, gastric, thyroid, and small-cell cancers).

No studies of the use of daunorubicin or doxorubicin use during pregnancy are published, but there are a number of case reports. In reviews from 18 reports of 28 pregnancies, daunorubicin use during pregnancy was published in 29 patients. Only four were exposed during the first trimester. Eight pregnancies were exposed at <16 weeks' gestation, and with one exception, all received polytherapy. Twenty-four normal infants (one set of twins) were born following *in utero* anthracycline exposure, there were two spontaneous abortions, one therapeutic abortion and two fetal deaths (Turchi and Villasis, 1988; Wiebe and Sipila, 1994). Notably, fetal deaths were secondary to maternal deaths. In another case report, one infant exposed to doxorubicin and daunorubicin at conception was reported with multiple birth defects, similar to Baller-Gerold syndrome (Artlich *et al.*, 1994). In another summary of case reports, the frequency of birth defects was not increased among 43 infants published in 26 reports with two malformed infants (2/43 = 4.7 percent) (Friedman and Polifka, 2006), but the true rate of ascertainment nor actual denominator is not known.

These drugs are highly toxic and their mechanism of action is to inhibit cell division, which suggests embryonic exposure may not be without risk, depending upon the timing of the exposure. Adverse fetal effects do appear to be appreciably increased, and this aligns with the expected effects of a drug that inhibits cell division. Daunorubicin exposure during embryogenesis was associated with multiple defects in rabbits. Prematurity and low birth weight were found in mice exposed to the drug during embryogenesis (Manufacturer's product information). Published data indicate increased frequencies of birth defects (heart, digestive system, eye, genitourinary [GU] defects) in rats, but not rabbits (Menegola *et al.*, 2001).

## PLANT ALKALOIDS

Antimitotic *Vinca* alkaloids include vinblastine (Velban) and vincristine (Oncovin) that inhibit microtubule formation, producing arrest of the mitotic cell cycle in metaphase (Box 7.6). Etoposide's action is similar.

### BOX 7.6    PLANT ALKALOID ANTINEOPLASTICS

- Vinblastine (Velban, Velsar)
- Vincristine (Oncovin, Vincasar, Vincrex)
- Etoposide (VePesid)

## VINBLASTINE

Vinblastine (Velban, Velsar) is approved to treat lymphoma, Hodgkin's disease, chronic myelocytic leukemia, and several carcinomas (breast, bladder, lung, and testis). Review of five case reports of pregnant women with Hodgkin's disease gave details of 13 normal infants born after prenatal exposure to vinblastine. Eleven infants were exposed to vinblastine during the first trimester while two were exposed in the second trimester. Among the offspring exposed to vinblastine during the first trimester, congenital anomalies were observed in two infants, one spontaneous abortion occurred, and two normal infants were born at term (Metz *et al.*, 1989). In one cohort of 27 infants exposed to vinblastine anytime during pregnancy, no anomalies were reported. Among 17 infants exposed only during the first trimester, no birth defects were noted (Aviles and Neri, 2001; Wiebe and Sipila, 1994). In another case report, there was one normal infant whose mother was exposed to vinblastine, bleomycin, and cisplatin therapy during the second trimester to treat malignant teratoma (Christman *et al.*, 1990). It is important to note there is considerable overlap in the published reports included in the different reviews. Among 134 women treated with doxorubicin, bleomycin, vinblastine, and dacarbazine during pregnancy, no congenital anomalies were reported. However, only seven were exposed during the first trimester (Maggen *et al.*, 2019). Vinblastine was associated with an increased frequency of congenital anomalies in rats, mice, hamsters, and rabbits exposed during embryogenesis (Manufacturer's information).

## VINCRISTINE (ONCOVIN)

Vincristine is an antimitotic antineoplastic used to treat leukemia (acute and chronic), lymphomas, Hodgkin's disease, neuroblastoma, rhabdomyosarcoma, and Wilms tumor, and has been used to treat melanoma, trophoblastic tumors, and some carcinomas (breast, cervical, lung, ovarian). Like other antineoplastics, vincristine is highly cytotoxic because it interrupts cell division. Therefore, it has a high potential to cause birth defects in exposed embryos because cell division and differentiation are the predominate events during embryogenesis and fetal growth and development. For vincristine, no published studies document an association of birth defects with vincristine use during human organogenesis. Among 35 infants born to women who received vincristine, 29 of 35 live-born infants were born with no gross anomalies after exposure at various stages of gestation to vincristine as part of polydrug antineoplastic regimens (Caliguri and Mayer, 1989). Five abortions (two spontaneous, two therapeutic), and two intrauterine deaths (without anomalies) were reported. Importantly, only 11 of 29 infants were exposed to vincristine in the first trimester, and none was malformed. Notably, the vincristine-polytherapy exposed newborns had severe but transient pancytopenia. One infant had polydactyly (highly likely not drug-related). Two major birth defects occurred among 31 infants exposed to vincristine polytherapy regimens in another review (Wiebe and Sipila, 1994). One study included 20 infants born to pregnant women treated for breast cancer included one conceptus exposed in the first trimester that resulted in a spontaneous abortion (Giacalone *et al.*, 1999). An increased frequency of birth defects was found in nonhuman primates and in rats born after their mothers were treated during organogenesis with vincristine and vinblastine (Courtney and Valenio, 1968; Demeyer, 1964, 1965). First trimester exposure has not been studied sufficiently in humans, but it is clear that normal infants are born following exposure in the second and third trimesters with the caveat that low birth weight and pancytopenia is frequent.

## ETOPOSIDE

A semisynthetic derivative of podophyllotoxin, etoposide (VePesid, VP-16VPP), inhibits DNA synthesis. The closely related molecule, podophyllum, has been used to treat condylomas, but is avoided because of its toxicity. It is approved to treat testicular and small-cell lung cancer, acute leukemia, lymphomas, gestational trophoblastic tumors, and a variety of carcinomas. One infant whose mother was treated with etoposide polytherapy during pregnancy was normal at birth (Rodriguez and Haggag, 1995). In another case report, one infant was born with cerebral atrophy following first trimester exposure to etoposide (Elit *et al.*, 1999), but 16 infants in another case report had no congenital anomalies. Etoposide was given in one of 13 pregnancies in the second and third trimesters, the infant was alive and normal at birth (Song *et al.*, 2019).

This agent was teratogenic in animals according to the manufacturer, but details of these studies are not available and the results are not peer reviewed.

## MISCELLANEOUS AGENTS

Antineoplastic agents that do not belong to the categories previously discussed are classified as miscellaneous in this text (Box 7.7).

---

### BOX 7.7    MISCELLANEOUS ANTINEOPLASTIC AGENTS

| | |
|---|---|
| Asparaginase (Elspar) | Hydroxyurea (Hydrea) |
| Altretamine (Hexalen) | Paclitaxel (Taxol) |
| Cisplatin (Platinol) | Procarbazine (Matulane) |
| | Vismodegib |

---

### ASPARAGINASE

Asparaginase (Elspar) is the enzyme L-asparagine amidohydrolase; an *Escherichia coli* derivative approved to treat acute lymphocytic leukemia, and sometimes chronic leukemias and lymphomas. Asparaginase mechanism of action is thought to be asparagine catabolism.

No studies are published about use of asparaginase drug during the first trimester of pregnancy. Pancytopenia was associated with asparaginase treatment during the second and third trimesters. It is classified as FDA fetal risk category C under the old system, and is not yet classified in the new FDA system. No reports of asparaginase monotherapy are published. No birth defects were reported among seven infants whose mothers took L-asparaginase as part of polydrug therapy regimen for leukemia (Caliguri and Mayer, 1989). It is important to note that none was exposed to the drug during the first trimester.

Asparaginase was associated with an increased frequency of congenital anomalies in the offspring of rats, rabbits, and mice given the drug during organogenesis (Adamson and Fabro, 1970; Lorke and Tettenborn, 1970; Ohguro *et al.*, 1969).

### CISPLATIN

A heavy-metal complex, cisplatin (Platinol), inhibits cancer cell growth by inducing interstrand crosslinks in DNA. Cisplatin is approved to treat testicular, ovarian, and bladder cancers. It is used to treat numerous carcinomas, including adrenal, head and neck, lung, neuroblastoma, osteosarcoma, prostate, stomach, cervical, endometrial, and breast.

The only data on cisplatin use in pregnancy are 36 case reports (Mir *et al.*, 2008), which suggest that cisplatin use in the second and third trimesters was not associated with untoward fetal effects (Christman *et al.*, 1990; King *et al.*, 1991). None of the 36 reported cases of cisplatin exposure occurred during the first trimester. However, case reports cannot adequately address safety.

Only one case of exposure to cisplatin during the first trimester was reported, and the infant did not have any birth defects. The child was normal at 10 months old (Kim *et al.*, 2008). Two cases of cisplatin exposure during the first trimester are also published but with no details of outcome

Caution is recommended for its use in the first trimester because platinol interferes with neurulation (neural tube organogenesis) in experimental animals, and corresponds to the 3rd to 4th weeks post conception in humans (Wiebe and Sipila, 1994).

An increased frequency of growth retardation but not birth defects after exposure to cisplatin during embryogenesis has been reported in mice, rats, and rabbits (Anabuki *et al.*, 1982; Kopf-Maier *et al.*, 1985; Nagaoka *et al.*, 1981).

## CARBOPLATIN

Carboplatin (Paraplatin) is a platinum compound whose action is similar to cisplatin, producing predominantly interstrand DNA crosslinks rather than DNA protein crosslinks. Its FDA-approved indications are for the primary and secondary treatment of advanced ovarian cancer. It is also used to treat other types of cancer: bladder, brain, breast, endometrium, head and neck, lung, neuroblastoma, testis, and Wilms tumor. No studies have been published of use of this agent during pregnancy in humans.

Seven case reports of carboplatin treatment during the second and third trimesters with no untoward effects were reported (Mir *et al.*, 2008). Carboplatin was embryotoxic and teratogenic in one rat study of offspring of rats exposed to carboplatin during embryogenesis; fetal weight was reduced, but there were no congenital anomalies (Manufacturer Product information; Kai *et al.*, 1988).

## PROCARBAZINE

A hydrazine derivative, procarbazine (Matulane), inhibits RNA, DNA, and other protein synthesis, and is approved to treat Hodgkin's disease, lymphomas, lung and brain carcinomas, and melanoma.

No studies are published of infants born to women who were exposed to procarbazine during embryogenesis. Six pregnancies exposed to procarbazine in the first trimester (four in combination with other agents) are published.

Among these infants, two were normal, one infant had limb hemangiomas, one elective abortion occurred, and two miscarriages were reported. Of the miscarriages, one had malpositioned, hypoplastic kidneys and the other had four toes on each foot, with bilateral webbing (Gililland and Weinstein, 1983), thus four of six first trimester-exposed pregnancies had birth defects.

In a review of collected cases, the authors summarized their findings, stating that procarbazine use 'in early pregnancy, particularly during the period of fetal neurulation and morphogenesis (third to twelfth weeks menstrual in humans) *does* appear to be associated with the risk of teratologic effects' (Wiebe and Sipila, 1994). However, this is based on two first trimester exposures in two case reports. One infant had a congenital heart defect, and the other had a congenital heart defect and a renal malformation. Among rats whose mothers were given procarbazine during embryogenesis an increased frequency of eye defects was found (Chaube and Murphy, 1968; Tuchmann-Duplessis and Mercier-Parot, 1967).

## HYDROXYUREA

Hydroxyurea (Hydrea) inhibits DNA synthesis. It is approved to treat chronic myelocytic leukemia, ovarian carcinoma, head and neck cancers, and melanoma. No studies have been published on the use of hydroxyurea during pregnancy in humans.

A case report of two infants exposed to hydroxyurea during the second and third trimesters as part of polydrug therapy had no congenital anomalies in the fetus (therapeutic abortion) or the live-born infant (Caliguri and Mayer, 1989). Three subsequent case reports of fetuses exposed in the first and second trimesters revealed no anomalies (Fitzgerald and McCann, 1993; Jackson *et al.*, 1993; Patel *et al.*, 1991).

In a case series of 28 pregnancies with 24 infants (including one set of twins) exposed during the first trimester, there were seven conceptuses that did not result in a live birth (four elective terminations, one therapeutic abortion, and two intrauterine deaths. Of the 21 live-born infants there were no major birth defects, but three had minor anomalies (hip dysplasia, unilateral renal dilation, pilonidal sinus) (Thauvin-Robinet *et al.*, 2001).

Among seven women treated from conception to delivery, one stillborn premature infant and one fetal death occurred (Koh *et al.*, 2002; Koh and Kanagalingam, 2006). Five apparently normal infants were born after exposure to hydroxyurea throughout gestation.

Hydroxyurea is a possible human teratogen based upon mechanism of action, DNA, and essential protein synthesis inhibition.

## Paclitaxel

Paclitaxel (Taxol) is a taxoid, extracted from the bark of the Pacific yew tree, acts as an antimicrotubule agent through prevention depolymerization, thus, halting mitosis. Paclitaxel is approved to treat ovarian and breast cancers, and is used to treat endometrial and non-small-cell lung cancer. No studies of paclitaxel in pregnant women have been published.

Paclitaxel was toxic at therapeutic doses in pregnant rabbits. Experiments at 20 percent of the usual human therapeutic dose was embryolethal and fetotoxic. At 7 percent of the usual human dose, paclitaxel was not associated with an increased rate of birth defects (Unpublished data, manufacturer product information).

## Tamoxifen

Tamoxifen, a non-steroidal selective estrogen receptor modulator, has an anti-estrogenic effect in breast tissue because it competitively binds to estrogen receptors. (Schuurman *et al.*, 2019). It has been reported as contraindicated during pregnancy (Koca *et al.*, 2013). Among 167 pregnant women treated with tamoxifen during pregnancy, the rate of birth defects was 12.6 percent, comparted to 3.9 percent in the general population (Schuurman *et al.*, 2019). However, this literature review only included five congenital anomalies in conceptuses that were exposed during the first trimester and 59 first trimester exposures. The result is a rate of 5/59 or 8.4 percent. However, this study was not of primary data, and its significance is unknown.

## Vinorelbine

Similar to vinblastine and vinblastine, vinorelbine is synthesized from a vinca alkaloid that has been used to treat breast cancer, lung cancer and other neoplasms. Three reports including 3, 20, 1, 1, and 1 pregnancies. Of the three infants exposed, in the first report, treatment began in the second trimester and three were apparently normal at 2 to 3 years of age (Cuvier *et al.*, 1997). Among 20 pregnancies exposed to vinorelbine, two first trimester exposures resulted in spontaneous abortion, and one treated during the second trimester resulted in a fetal death. The findings were mainly limited to second and third trimester exposures, and 95 percent of those who survived (n = 17) had low birth weight and two had complications related to prematurity but were normal at >3 years of follow-up (Giaclone *et al.*, 2000). In three case reports, multiple antineoplastic agents were used to treat breast and lung cancer with exposures beginning in the second trimester. Infants were normal at several years' follow-up (De Santos *et al.*, 2000; Janne *et al.*, 2001; Fanale *et al.*, 2005). Manufacturer's information indicated IUGR in rats exposed during gestation at doses 25–33 percent of the usual human dose.

### VISMODEGIB

Vismodegib is an antineoplastic for which there is no human studies for use during pregnancy. The manufacturer reports that the drug is highly embryotoxic. In rat models, 100 percent of conceptuses were resorbed early during gestation after exposure to this drug.

## SPECIAL CONSIDERATIONS

### NON-GENITAL CANCERS

Melanoma and breast carcinomas are the most frequent forms of non-genital cancers observed in pregnant patient (Table 7.1 and Figure 7.1).

### BREAST CARCINOMA

The most common cancer in women is breast carcinoma, and the lifetime risk indicates it will affect one in eight women, or ~12 percent, at some time (Maggen *et al.*, 2019). Breast carcinoma occurs in an estimated 23.3 to 30 of 100,000 pregnancies (3 percent of all breast carcinomas) (Cottreau *et al.*, 2019). Breast cancer complicates an estimated one in 3,000 pregnancies, and is associated with and accounts for approximately one-third of maternal deaths during gestation. The average delay in diagnosis of breast cancer during pregnancy is an estimated 5–10 months, but is 1 to 4 months in non-pregnant patients. The mean gestational age at breast cancer diagnosis is ~21 weeks. It is controversial in whether or not pregnancy per se influences breast cancer prognosis, but data on prognosis use small, retrospective cohorts confounded by heterogeneous treatment approaches.

Regardless, available data suggest that in pregnant patient with breast cancer, tumors are larger, of worse histological grade, and have greater lymph node involvement than in non-pregnant women. In addition, the risk of metastatic breast cancer is increased 2.5-fold in pregnant versus non-pregnant women (Eastwood-Wilshire *et al.*, 2019). As part of patient history, a family history of any genetic relative of the patient who has had breast cancer is an indication for screening for genetic markers for breast carcinoma.

The treatment plan should be contingent on (1) carcinoma stage and (2) gestational age at diagnosis. Generally, breast surgery may be performed during any stage of gestation (Eastwood-Wilshere *et al.*, 2019; also see Chapter 6). Should the procedure be planned close to term, fetal exposure can be eliminated if the infant is delivered first (Bloss and Miller, 1995). The usual accepted surgical technique for breast carcinoma in the pregnant patient is modified radical mastectomy with axillary node dissection (Liberale *et al.*, 2019; Marchant, 1994). "Lumpectomy" and sampling of axillary nodes followed by radiotherapy has not been satisfactorily evaluated in the pregnant patient: "Some guidelines still suggest that SLNB should not be performed during pregnancy, but mounting clinical and pre-clinical data suggest that the procedure can be performed safely" (McCartan and Gemignani, 2016). Concerns that radiotherapy may present a significant risk to the fetus (Petrek, 1994) Studies have demonstrated that the doses absorbed by the fetus are substantially less than the recommended fetal radiation doses. To minimize radiation exposure, it is advisable to inject the technetium radiocolloid on the morning of surgery as opposed to the preceding day (McCartan and Gemignani, 2016). These guidelines are consistent with the recommendations made in 2005 (Pentheroudakis and Pavlidis, 2006).

Either adjunctive chemotherapy therapy or treatment is often recommended in advanced cases. Women with axillary lymph node metastases appear to be the best candidates for adjunctive chemotherapy (Barnavon and Wallack, 1990; Liberale *et al.*, 2019). Chemotherapy the first trimester with currently available antineoplastic agents is associated with an increased risk of birth defects. Fetal growth retardation is the major risk with chemotherapy during the second and third trimesters, but long-term effects are unknown.

Therapeutic abortion and prophylactic oophorectomy apparently do not improve breast carcinoma treatment outcome during pregnancy (Donegan, 1986). Therapeutic abortion might be a consideration if radiotherapy is deemed necessary or if chemotherapy is necessary during the first trimester. Proper shielding and focused radiotherapy above the maternal diaphragm make it possible to minimize the adverse effects of radiation on the fetus in breast cancer (Pentheroudakis and Pavlidis, 2006).

## Leukemia

Acute leukemia is extremely rare during pregnancy, occurring in approximately one in 75,000 to 100,000 pregnancies (Nolan *et al.*, 2019). However, it is among the most common neoplasms in young women (Caliguri and Mayer, 1989; Catanzarite and Ferguson, 1984; Koren *et al.*, 1990).

Physiological changes during pregnancy may mask the leukemia diagnosis. Non-specific leukemia signs and symptoms (i.e., weakness, fatigue, pallor, anemia, leukocytosis) are sometimes ascribed to pregnancy. It is not known whether there is a delay in the diagnosis of leukemia in pregnant patients compared to non-pregnant controls because no evidence is available (Krashin and Lishner, 2016). One hundred thirty-eight cases of leukemia during pregnancy (13 separate reports published 1955–2013) included 93 recognized pregnancies treated during gestation, and 45 treated after abortion or pregnancy completions. Of the 93 pregnancies that continued, nine were treated during the first trimester, 65 in the second trimester, and 19 in the third trimester (Horowitz *et al.*, 2018). All treatments after 1977 were anthracycline-cytarabine-based regimens (ACBR). Nine pregnancies were treated during the first trimester with 6 normal infants delivered at term or preterm. There was a therapeutic abortion, one intrauterine death and a fetal death at 22 weeks due to previable preterm delivery (Horowitz *et al.*, 2018). Four congenital anomalies (hydrocephalus, VSD, patent ductus, and one unspecified) were noted among the live births, but all were exposed to chemotherapy in the second and/or third trimesters. Therefore, any association with chemotherapy is spurious because organs are formed during the first trimester.

Acute myelocytic leukemia (AML) was the most common malignancy encountered, and most cases (60 percent) were recognized in the latter two thirds of pregnancy (see Table 7.4). Estimated survival rate was 75 percent in one report (n = 45 pregnant women with acute leukemia) (Reynoso *et al.*, 1987), similar to the rate among non-pregnant patients with acute leukemia (Caliguri and

## TABLE 7.4
## Cases (n = 72, 138, and 180) of Leukemia in Pregnancy (1975–1988, 1955–2013, and 2001–2013)

| Trimesters | 1975–1988[1] (n = 72) | 1955–2013[2] (n = 138) | 2001–2013[3] (n = 180) | Average Percent |
|---|---|---|---|---|
| First | 22% | 25.8% | 44.4% | 30.2% |
| Second | 36% | 53.8% | 25.9% | 38.3% |
| Third | 42% | 20.4% | 33.3% | 35.1% |
| Types of leukemia | | | | |
| Acute lymphoblastic | 28% | — | | |
| Acute myelocytic | 61% | — | | |
| Chronic myelocytic | 7% | | | |
| Hairy cell | 1.3% | | | |
| Not specified | 2.7% | 100% | 100%* | |

[1] Caliguri and Mayer, 1989.

[2] Horowitz *et al.*, 2018.

[3] Cottreau *et al.*, 2019.

* Rounding error.

Mayer, 1989). There was no significant difference in survival rates between patients diagnosed at different gestational stages (first trimester, 17 percent, second trimester, 35 percent, third trimester 20 percent). Survival did differ among those who not receive therapy during pregnancy (36 percent versus 28 percent, respectively, p<0.85), but this is based on only 28 patients. Therefore, pregnancy per se does not affect the course of leukemia.

Antineoplastic drugs most commonly used to treat chronic leukemia include antimetabolites (methotrexate, thioguanine, mercaptopurine, and cytarabine), anthracycline antibiotics (daunorubicin and doxorubicin), and plant alkaloids (vincristine). Alkylating agents are also used as antileukemic drugs. Notably, all of these drugs are cytostatic, although mechanisms differ (cytotoxicity, DNA, and protein synthesis suppression). **Therefore, all antineoplastics have a very high potential for causing birth defects with exposure during embryogenesis** because this period is characterized by the highest rate of cell division (hyperplasia) and increase in size (hypertrophy) during human life.

Survival prognosis in the untreated gravida is extremely poor, with life expectancy of less than 3 months (Catanzarite and Ferguson, 1984; Hou and Song, 1995; Kawamura *et al.*, 1994; Koren *et al.*, 1990). **Therefore, chemotherapy should be initiated immediately (even during the first trimester) once the diagnosis of acute leukemia is made.** However, folate antagonists (e.g., methotrexate) should be avoided in the first trimester, if possible.

In 58 infants born to pregnant women who had either acute myelocytic or lymphoblastic leukemia, there were 31 (53 percent) premature births (including five stillbirths), and 23 (43 percent) full-term infants (two of whom were of low birth weight) (Caliguri and Mayer, 1989). No birth defects were reported among 13 fetuses exposed to chemotherapy for leukemia during the first trimester (Caliguri and Mayer, 1989). No congenital anomalies were observed among 21 infants born to women with acute myelocytic leukemia who were who were treated during the first trimester (Abruzzese *et al.*, 2019).

## LYMPHOMAS AND HODGKIN'S DISEASE

Approximately one in 6,000 pregnancies will be complicated by incident malignant lymphoma (Hodby and Fields, 2009).

Approximately 40 percent of lymphoma malignancies are the Hodgkin's type, and are the most frequently encountered lymphoma among pregnant women. The incidence is estimated to be one in 6,000 pregnancies. Non-Hodgkin's lymphoma is "very rare" in pregnancy (Lishner *et al.*, 2016). Similar to breast carcinoma, pregnancy apparently does not change the prognosis for Hodgkin's disease (Lishner *et al.*, 2016). Leukemias and lymphomas can metastasize to the placenta, but the actual risk is unknown. Hodgkin's lymphoma management during pregnancy depends on the disease stage and gestational age at which the disease is diagnosed, as with most other malignancies (Table 7.5). Staging is of utmost importance. Pregnancy may confound or limit types of diagnostic studies that can be safely performed. The majority of diagnostic procedures not involving the abdomen or fetus can be performed safely, if necessary, with minimal risk to the conceptus. Importantly, a single abdominal X-ray and computed tomography (CT) scan usually expose the fetus to less than 1 rad of actual radiation. An alternative to ionizing radiation is magnetic resonance imaging (MRI), and it may be useful in early to mid-pregnancy. Laparotomy lymphoma staging is somewhat controversial and difficult, if not impossible, to accomplish in the latter half of pregnancy because the large uterus obstructs the operating field (Bloss and Miller, 1995).

Early-stage lymphomas in the first half of pregnancy can be approached several ways. Therapeutic abortion is one consideration, although it is not always necessary. Use of modified radiotherapy done at an acceptable distance from the shielded pelvis (i.e., in supradiaphragmatic disease, head and neck, etc.) (Woo *et al.*, 1992). Should chemotherapy be necessary, the most conservative approach is to delay therapy until after the first trimester (i.e., after the ninth week).

**TABLE 7.5**

**Therapeutic Approach to Treatment of Gravidas with Hodgkin Lymphoma or Non-Hodgkin Lymphoma**

| Hematologic Malignancy | Pregnancy Stage | Therapeutic Recommendation |
|---|---|---|
| Indolent non-Hodgkin | Early and Late | Watch and wait.<br>If symptomatic, or disease progresses, use monoclonal antibodies (with/without chemotherapy).<br>Steroids may be used in first trimester to transition to second trimester. |
| Aggressive lymphomas | Early and Late | Consider pregnancy termination and administer therapy. Treat with monoclonal antibodies (R-CHOP). |
| Highly aggressive lymphoma | Up to 20 weeks EGA | Pregnancy termination and therapy CNS prophylaxis. |
| Highly aggressive lymphoma | After 20 weeks EGA | Combination regimen including high dose methotrexate. |
| Hodgkin lymphoma | Early | Postpone treatment to second trimester, if possible.<br>If not possible, consider pregnancy termination. |
| | Late | Treat as non-pregnant woman. |

*Source:* Modified from Lishner *et al.*, 2015.

Patients with early stage disease during the latter half of pregnancy, treatment may reasonably be delayed until after delivery, especially if the patient is asymptomatic. Chemotherapy after the first trimester causes little known risk to the fetus except for pancytopenia and mild to moderate growth retardation. Early treatment of advanced disease during early pregnancy is a concern. Some physicians recommend therapeutic abortion if the advanced-stage lymphoma is diagnosed in the first trimester (Lishner *et al.*, 2016). For advanced disease after the first trimester, chemotherapy should be initiated as soon as possible. If the patient is near term, early delivery is usually indicated, delaying chemotherapy (Table 7.5).

Among nineteen pregnancies (reported in 15 publications) published with first-trimester exposure to chemotherapeutic agents for treatment of lymphomas, 15 (79 percent) of 19 pregnancies resulted in normal infants (three were exposed to mechlorethamine, two to thiotepa, and 10 to vinblastine). One patient who received mechlorethamine had a therapeutic abortion. Unilateral renal agenesis occurred in one infant whose mother took chlorambucil. One patient who received procarbazine gave birth to an infant with multiple hemangiomas. Another patient who received polydrug therapy during pregnancy had an infant with an atrial septal defect (Jacobs *et al.*, 1981). In a review of another case series of 19 patients, three patients were exposed in the first trimester, but two had therapeutic abortions (Vanazzi *et al.*, 2019). Thirteen of 19 patients are alive and had normal infants after being treated during second and third trimesters. Four patients were lost to follow-up, and one infant was born with IUGR.

The largest series reported to date of pregnant women with Hodgkin lymphoma included 134 gravidas, with 22 exposed during organogenesis. Of these 72 (54 percent) were treated during gestation 56 (42 percent) did not receive treatment during pregnancy, and 15 (11 percent) were lost to follow-up (Maggen *et al.*, 2019). Birth defects occurred in 3 percent of the total group, but congenital anomalies were not tabulated by trimester of exposure. The authors stated that birth defects were not increased in frequency, but did note that obstetric complications and prematurity were increased in frequency (approximately 30 percent for complications and prematurity).

## MELANOMAS

The most common cancers during pregnancy are melanomas, occurring among approximately three to five per 1,000 deliveries (Eastwood-Wilshire *et al.*, 2019; Cottreau *et al.*, 2019). Importantly, melanoma tumor type carries the highest risk of metastasis to the placenta and fetus (Anderson *et al.*, 1989; Read and Platzer, 1981). Apparently, pregnancy does not affect the prognosis of melanoma, although gestation is associated with an increased level of melanocyte-stimulating hormone (Walker *et al.*, 2018). No difference was found in survival of 58 pregnant women with melanoma compared to non-pregnant controls with melanoma (Reintgen *et al.*, 1985). Treatment is usually comprised of surgical resection, with or without lymph node dissection. A variety of chemotherapeutic agents is used, but their success rate is poor, with little success whether chemotherapy is given as neoadjuvant or primary therapy in metastatic disease. In seven studies that included 1836 pregnant women with melanoma, pregnancy was not associated with a poor outcome. In seven studies of 709 women who had melanoma while pregnant, outcome was worse than expected (Walker *et al.*, 2018). Unfortunately, these studies did not report fetal outcomes (birth defects, prematurity, etc.). Among 60 pregnant women who were treated for melanoma during pregnancy, one congenital anomaly was diagnosed before birth and terminated (1/60 = 1.7 percent). Two other pregnancies were terminated for maternal well-being. A maternal-fetal death also occurred (de Haan *et al.*, 2017, 2018).

## OTHER NON-GENITAL CANCERS

Other non-genital types of cancer, such as colorectal carcinoma, gastric carcinoma, pancreatic or hepatic cancer, and sarcoma, are rare during pregnancy. Colorectal cancer is rare, and occurs in 0.8 per 100,000 pregnancies (Kocian *et al.*, 2019). The course of disease seems unaffected by pregnancy, and behaves the same as in the non-pregnant adult patient. Surgery in the first trimester was associated with a 14.3 percent miscarriage rate, but this is not appreciably greater than would be expected in normal pregnancy (Kocian *et al.*, 2019).

Gastric carcinoma is also rare, and occurs in an estimated 0.026 percent to 0.01 percent of pregnancies. Of 137 cases of gastric cancer in pregnancy, the prognosis was poor. One- and two-year survival rates were 18 percent and 15.1 percent, respectively (Sakamoto *et al.*, 2009). The prevalence of pancreatic cancer during pregnancy has not been reported, except to state that is extremely rare, but rates have not been published. Hepatic cancer is also very rare, and its estimated prevalence is one per 100,000 women, with a one year survival rate of approximately 23 percent (Norouzi *et al.*, 2012). Similarly, the prevalence of sarcoma during pregnancy has not been published, and its experience is limited to only a few published cases.

Treatment of these rare neoplasms during pregnancy is similar to that of non-pregnant women, but with the chemotherapeutic and irradiation precautions as described earlier. Diagnoses in the first trimester do not mandate a therapeutic abortion, but it should be discussed as one option. Discovery of these rare cancers in the latter two thirds of pregnancy provide other options such as early delivery (after 28 weeks gestation) followed by antineoplastic treatment. Chemotherapy outside the first trimester is associated with **no increased risk of birth defects** based on biological plausibility, although actual evidence is lacking for antineoplastics. The known **risk of exposure outside the first trimester is fetal growth retardation** (i.e., exposure in the second and third trimesters only). If chemotherapy must be administered in the first trimester, folic acid antagonists should be avoided.

## Pregnancy Following Non-Genital Cancer

No data support the misconception that women with breast cancer should not become pregnant following initial therapy. Similarly, no scientific data support the misconception that pregnancy after mastectomy for breast cancer adversely affects survival of the mother. A meta-analysis of 1244 pregnancies to breast cancer survivors, the rates of birth defects was not greater than would be expected at random (2–3%) in the general population (Azim *et al.*, 2011).

It is suggested subsequent pregnancies be delayed for two to three years following successful treatment of any cancer, and allow an appropriate period for observation for recurrence and retreatment, if necessary. Importantly, more than 90 percent of recurrences happen during the three years following remission of non-genital cancer (Koren and Lishner, 2011).

## Fertility and Outcome in Subsequent Pregnancies

The likelihood of a live birth is significantly decreased in cancer survivors compared to age-matched reproductive age women. Pregnancy rates are an estimated 35–40 percent lower among female cancer survivors compared to women who never had cancer. These rates vary by cancer type and treatment.

Women who were diagnosed with melanomas or thyroid cancers have fertility rates similar to the general population. In contrast, breast cancer survivors have the lowest probability of conceiving and carrying a subsequent pregnancy. The reduction is approximately 70 percent lower than the general population. Reduced fertility among breast cancer survivors may be due to gonadotoxic chemotherapy, or may also be related the widely held misconception that pregnancy may cause cancer recurrence because it is a hormone-driven disease.

A large compilation of childhood cancer survivors (n = 2283 patients) of reproductive age showed that they were less likely to become pregnant than their siblings. Importantly, radiation below the diaphragm was associated with a 25-percent decrease in fertility for both sexes (Byrne *et al.*, 1987).

Of interest, alkylating agent therapy was associated with approximately a 66-percent reduction in male fertility. Interestingly, alkylating agent therapy had no effect on female fertility. In another study, Pregnancy outcome was not adversely affected by childhood or adolescent treatment for acute lymphoblastic leukemia' (Green *et al.*, 1989). In another study of a small group (n = 34) of women treated with polydrug chemotherapy (vincristine, vinblastine, thiotepa, and procarbazine) for stage II and III Hodgkin's disease, fertility was apparently not impaired (Lacher and Toner, 1986).

## Genital Cancers

Cervical and ovarian cancers occur during pregnancy, but cervical cancer occurs more often than ovarian neoplasms.

## Cervical Cancer

Cervical carcinoma is the fourth most frequent cancer in women (Bray *et al.*, 2018), and is usually diagnosed early in pregnancy (Halaska *et al.*, 2019). Between 2001 and 2013, the incidence of cervical and uterine cancer was 9.5 per 100,000 (Cottreau *et al.*, 2019). Previously, it was reported that the incidence of cervical cancer in pregnancy was approximately 1.3 per 1,000 pregnancies (Hacker *et al.*, 1982; Halaska *et al.*, 2019), ranging from 1:1,000 to 1:10,000.

The major difficulties working with this neoplasm is lesion stage determination and treatment plan formulation. The extent of the tumor in the pregnant patient tends to be underestimated (Pentheroudakis and Pavlidis, 2006).

The treatment depends upon the stage of the cancer and gestational age of the pregnancy. In the first half of pregnancy, treatment consists of radical hysterectomy and lymphadenectomy for small lesions and radiotherapy for more extensive lesions (Han *et al.*, 2013). Frequently, radiotherapy results in spontaneous abortion, and therapeutic abortion should be offered as an option (PDQ Editorial Board, 2020).

It is appropriate to follow these patients conservatively and to deliver them when fetal pulmonary maturity is reached when diagnosis of cervical cancer is made in pregnancies close to viability (i.e., 24 weeks gestation and beyond) (PDQ Editorial Board, 2020). Chemotherapy is usually used for advanced or metastatic disease. The best pregnancy outcome prognosis is treatment after the first trimester, if possible. Further, if diagnosis is made close to viability, best outcomes are associated with initiation of chemotherapy after delivery (PDQ Editorial Board, 2020). Microinvasion or pre-invasive lesions can usually be treated with cone biopsy or conservative therapy until after pregnancy (Pentheroudakis and Pavlidis, 2006). Cervical cancer prognosis is not affected by pregnancy. Patients with cervical cancer should be referred to specialized centers with a multidisciplinary team that includes a specialty perinatology center (Halaska *et al.*, 2019).

## OVARIAN CANCER

Ovarian cancer in pregnancy is extremely rare, approximately one in 18 000–25 000 deliveries (Beischer *et al.*, 1971; Chung and Birnbaum, 1973; Jubb, 1963; Munnell, 1963; Mukhopadhyay *et al.*, 2016). Approximately 6 percent of adnexal masses in pregnancy are malignant compared to 15–20 percent in the non-pregnant patient. The most recent incidence estimate for ovarian cancer during pregnancy is 1:10,000 to 1:100,000 (Mukhopadhyay *et al.*, 2016).

Studies of epithelial cell, germ cell, gonadal stromal cell, and endodermal sinus tumors during pregnancy were published, but there are limited epidemiological data. Stage of the disease and gestational age of the pregnancy determine the therapy plan. Stage IA disease may be treated with unilateral oophorectomy and may be satisfactory (Muto *et al.*, 2020).

Advanced disease may indicate hysterectomy or radical surgery depending on the stage of pregnancy and degree of advanced disease. As with other cancers (except acute leukemia), chemotherapy may be indicated as adjuvant therapy, but should be started after the first trimester (Muto *et al.*, 2020).

Diagnosis of ovarian cancer during the first trimester occurred in 44–59.1 percent of cases, and 6.8 percent to 17 percent of cases were diagnosed in the second trimester (Table 7.6). Zero to

---

**TABLE 7.6**

**Type and Trimester of Occurrence in 23[1] and 44[2] Cases of Ovarian Cancer during Pregnancy**

| Stage of pregnancy | Percent[1] | Percent[2] |
|---|---|---|
| First trimester | 44% | 59.1% |
| Second trimester | 17% | 6.8% |
| Third trimester | 9% | 0% |
| Delivery or postpartum | 30% | 67.8% |
| | | |
| **Type of cancer** | | |
| Borderline | 35% | |
| Epithelial | 30% | |
| Dysgerminoma | 17% | |
| Granulosa cell | 13% | |
| Undifferentiated | 5% | |

[1] Dgani *et al.*, 1989.
[2] Cottreau *et al.*, 2019.

9 percent were diagnosed in the third trimester (Cottreau *et al.*, 2019). A review of ovarian carcinoma during pregnancy, 23 cases, found 35 percent were borderline grade; overall survival of those diagnosed in pregnancy was better than expected for ovarian cancer because more early stage cases were studied (Dgani *et al.*, 1989). Fourteen of the 23 women gave birth to normal live-born infants with an overall five-year survival of 61 percent, and 92 percent for stage I lesions (Dgani *et al.*, 1989; Cottreau *et al.*, 2019).

Notably, the purported association between talc powder use and ovarian cancer is very likely false. A recent study reported no association between talc powder and ovarian cancer in 252,745 women of reproductive age (O'Brien *et al.*, 2020).

## OCCUPATIONAL EXPOSURE

There may be an increased frequency of fetal loss from occupational exposure to various chemotherapeutic agents (Selevan *et al.*, 1985).

## SUMMARY

All antineoplastic agents are devoted to the purpose of suppressing cell replication. The conflict arises because the predominant cellular event that occurs during *in utero* development is replication. Cell differentiation and replication dominate embryonic development; increases in cell number (hyperplastic growth) are the major occurrences during fetal growth and development. Hence, the greatest risk of antineoplastic agents during the first trimester is for birth defects, and the greatest risk during the fetal period is for intrauterine/fetal growth retardation.

# 8 Analgesics during Pregnancy

A large proportion of pregnant women take analgesics during gestation, and the frequency is usually higher during the first trimester. The wide variation in survey results indicate rates of medication use during pregnancy, ranging from 30 percent to over 90 percent probably reflect study design differences, targeted intent of the surveys, and analytic approach. Analgesics were taken by an estimated 15.6 percent of women during the first trimester, and 23.7 percent anytime during pregnancy (Haas *et al.*, 2018). Some aches and pains may not require analgesic therapy, but a substantial proportion have chronic conditions. For example, an estimated 20 percent of pregnant women have migraine headaches. Non-migraine headaches and pain secondary after dental procedures are common indications for analgesia use during pregnancy. Many nonnarcotic analgesics are commercially available, a number of which are available over-the-counter medications. With few exceptions that will be highlighted here, most OTC pain relievers can be safely used during pregnancy for treatment of minor pain during pregnancy.

Limited data are available on the pharmacokinetics of analgesics during pregnancy, and the findings are not entirely consistent. For example, acetaminophen has a decreased half-life and increased clearance in one study, but it is unchanged in another at about the same gestational age (Table 8.1). The pharmacokinetics of meperidine in pregnancy are unchanged compared to non-pregnant controls, and the same is true of the kinetics of meptazinol. In contrast, morphine has a decreased half-life and increased clearance, implying the need for increased frequency or dose regimen to maintain adequate analgesia. Indomethacin has a decreased half-life, and $C_{max}$, which also implies dose or frequency regimen adjustment. In contrast, sodium salicylate has an increased half-life during late pregnancy. Low-dose aspirin apparently does not significantly affect umbilical artery circulation (Owen *et al.*, 1993; Veille *et al.*, 1993). Notably, the half-life for aspirin increases during pregnancy, implying that a dose decrease in amount and/or frequency may be needed (Table 8.1).

## TABLE 8.1
## Pharmacokinetics Analgesic Agents during Pregnancy: Pregnant Compared with Non-Pregnant

| Agent | n | EGA (weeks) | Route | AUC | $V_d$ | $C_{max}$ | $C_{ss}$ | $t_{1/2}$ | Cl | PPB | Control group[a] | Authors |
|---|---|---|---|---|---|---|---|---|---|---|---|---|
| Acetaminophen | 8 | 3rd trimester | PO | | | | | ↓ | ↑ | | Yes (1) | Miners *et al.* (1986) |
| Acetaminophen | 6 | 36 | PO | ↑ | | = | = | = | = | | Yes (2) | Rayburn *et al.* (1986) |
| Indomethacin | 5 | 36–38 | IV | | | ↓ | ↓ | ↓ | | | Yes (1) | Traeger *et al.* (1973) |
| Meperidine | 18 | Term | IV | | = | = | = | = | | | Yes (1) | Kuhnert *et al.* (1980) |
| Meptazinol | 5 | 36–38 | IV | = | | = | = | = | = | | Yes (1) | Murray *et al.* (1989) |
| Morphine | 13 | Term | IM, IV | ↑ | = | | | ↓ | ↑ | | Yes (1) | Gerdin *et al.* (1990) |
| *Sodium salicylate* | *20* | *40* | *IV* | | | | | | | | *No* | *Noeschel et al. (1972)* |

*Source:* Little BB. *Obstet Gynecol*, 1999; 93: 858.

*Abbreviations:* EGA, estimated gestational age; AUC, area under the curve; $V_d$, volume of distribution; $C_{ss}$, peak plasma concentration; $C_{ss}$, steady-state concentration; $t_{1/2}$, half life; PPB, plasma protein binding; PO, by mouth; ↓ denotes a decrease during pregnancy compared to nonpregnant values; ↑ denotes an increase during pregnancy compared to nonpregnant values; = denotes no difference between pregnant and nonpregnant values; IV, intravenous; IM, intramuscular.

DOI: 10.1201/9780429160929-8

# NONSTEROIDAL ANTI-INFLAMMATORY AGENTS

Most of the agents in this group are relatively new analgesics and all are prostaglandin synthetase inhibitors. Some of the commonly used agents in this class are listed in Box 8.1.

---

**BOX 8.1 NONSTEROIDAL ANTI-INFLAMMATORY AGENTS**

**Cox-2 Non-Selective**

- Aspirin
- Diclofenac
- Diflunisal
- Etodolac
- Fenoprofen
- Ibuprofen
- Indomethacin
- Ketorulac
- Meclofenamate
- Naproxen
- Phenylbutazone
- Piroxicam
- Rofecoxib
- Sulindac
- Tolmentin

**Cox-2 Selective**

- Celecoxib
- Etodolac
- Rofecoxib

---

## NONNARCOTIC ANALGESICS

### Salicylates (Aspirin)

The main use of aspirin has been as an analgesic, antipyretic, or anti-inflammatory agent. Salicylates were used clinically for over 120 years and are one of the most commonly used nonnarcotic analgesics. Aspirin has been widely used in pregnancy in the past, but acetaminophen has supplanted ASA as the most frequently used analgesic in pregnancy. Prospective study of 1529 pregnant women in 1974 and 1975, reported an estimated 50 percent of the women took aspirin sometime during pregnancy, but less than 5 percent took the drug daily. Salicylates are prostaglandin synthetase inhibitors, and non-selectively inhibit cyclooxygenase (COX) enzymes 1 and 2. COX-1 inhibition blocks normal production of protective esophageal and gastric mucosa, increasing the risk for gastrointestinal bleeds and associated complications. COX-1 suppression blocks synthesis of prostacyclin and thromboxane A (vasoactive prostaglandins). Prostacyclin is a strong vasodilator that is a platelet aggregation inhibitor. Thromboxane A is a potent vasoconstrictor that stimulates platelet aggregation (Bhagwat *et al.*, 1985; Ellis *et al.*, 1976). Prostaglandin E and prostaglandins are also inhibited. COX-2 suppression possesses analgesic activity associated with blocking prostaglandins linked with inflammation.

Therapeutic doses (>325 mg) block production of prostacyclin and thromboxane, and low-dose aspirin (60–83 mg) results in selective block of thromboxane production, favoring the prostacyclin (vasodilation) pathway (Schiff *et al.*, 1989; Sibai *et al.*, 1989; Wallenberg, 1995; Wallenberg *et al.*,

1986). Review of 46 studies of aspirin during pregnancy for preeclampsia found a dose response effect that had either mild or no beneficial effects (Roberge *et al.*, 2017). Low-dose aspirin only partially inhibits thromboxane, but does have an inhibitory effect on prostacyclin.

Salicylates cross the placenta to attain physiologically active fetal levels (Levy *et al.*, 1975; Palminsano and Cassudy, 1969; Turner and Collins, 1975). An increased frequency of birth defects was reported in several species of laboratory animals (rats, animals, when given at several times the human adult dose (Wilson *et al.*, 1977)

Aspirin is probably better studied more than other medications used during pregnancy. Overall, the frequency of birth defects does not appear to be increased among infants whose mothers took aspirin during the first trimester.

## Cohort Studies

Congenital anomalies were not increased in frequency among infants whose mothers took aspirin during the first 16 weeks after the last menstrual period, compared to unexposed infants (Slone *et al.*, 1976). In a large study of 50,282 women who used medications during pregnancy, the frequency of birth defects among 14,864 infants who were born after first trimester exposure to aspirin was not increased (Heinonen *et al.*, 1977). In the US, the major birth defect rate estimated from national study was 6.7 percent among those exposed to chronic aspirin use, 6.8 percent for occasional use, and 6.3 percent among infants whose mothers did not use aspirin during gestation (Heinonen *et al.*, 1977). Analysis of 144 gravidas with "heavy" aspirin use (>325 mg more than twice daily) major congenital anomalies occurred among 4.2 percent, which was not significantly different from the 3.5 percent to 5 percent background rate (Turner and Collins, 1975). In a small cohort analysis, birth defects were not increased in frequency among 62 infants born to women who used aspirin during the first trimester (Aselton *et al.*, 1985). The frequency of congenital anomalies was not increased among 2,069 infants whose mothers used aspirin during the first trimester. Height and weight at 12 and 18 months was normal (CLASP, 1995). Unpublished data indicate no increased frequency of congenital anomalies among 1,709 infants exposed to aspirin during organogenesis (Rosa personal communication, Briggs *et al.*, 2017). Among 3,173 infants whose mothers used aspirin during the first trimester, the frequency of four types of congenital anomalies was increased in frequency: anencephaly/craniofacial, cleft palate, gastroschisis, and anophthalmia/microphthalmia (Hernandez *et al.*, 2012). The authors acknowledged that these findings needed to be replicated in other studies. These patterns are not apparent in other large databases.

## Case-Control Studies

Several early studies from the 1960s and 70s found associations between birth defects and aspirin exposure during the first trimester. The frequency of exposure to aspirin in the first trimester was significantly increased among 833 infants with CNS, alimentary tract, talipes, and miscellaneous birth defects (Richards, 1969). Exposure to aspirin was more frequent among 458 infants with major congenital anomalies (Nelson *et al.*, 1971). Aspirin exposure during the first trimester was significantly more frequent in infants born with cleft palate/cleft lip (Saxen, 1975).

Among 390 infants with congenital heart disease, aspirin use in the first trimester was significantly increased (Rothman *et al.*, 1979). Congenital heart disease was not significantly associated with first trimester exposure to aspirin in case-control analyses among 1381, 5015 and 36 infants born with heart defects (Werler *et al.*, 1989; Kallen, 2003; Zierler *et al.*, 1985).

Chronic high-dose aspirin taken late in the third trimester has been associated with (1) premature closure of the ductus arteriosus, (2) persistent pulmonary hypertension (Levin *et al.*, 1978; Sibai and Amon, 1988), (3) decreased fetal renal function, and (4) oligohydramnios (Witter and Niebyl, 1986). Some investigators (Streissguth *et al.*, 1987), but not others (Klebanoff and Berendes, 1988) have reported lower IQs in offspring of mothers who took aspirin in the first trimester of pregnancy. Chronic high-dose aspirin use is associated with increased frequency of post-term pregnancies (Collins and Turner, 1975), low birth weight (Lewis and Schulman, 1973), neonatal bleeding disorders, and intracranial hemorrhage in premature infants (Rumack *et al.*, 1981; Stuart *et al.*, 1982), and premature closure of the ductus arteriosus in the fetus (Levin *et al.*, 1978). However, these complications are not associated with aspirin use when pharmacologically controlled doses of salicylates were used (Sibai and Amon, 1988). This implies that gravidas may be self-adjusting their doses and/or frequency regimens upward, increasing the risk of untoward outcomes.

The ACOG recommendations (ACOG Committee Opinion, 2018a) for Low-Dose Aspirin (81 mg/day) Use in Pregnancy are:

1. Recommended for women at high risk of preeclampsia; therapy should be initiated 12 to 28 weeks of gestation and continued until delivery.
2. Should be considered for women with moderate risks for preeclampsia.
3. Not recommended for unexplained stillbirth in the absence of risk for preeclampsia.
4. Not recommended for prevention of fetal growth restriction.
5. Not recommended for prevention of preterm birth in the absence of risk for preeclampsia.
6. Not recommended for prevention of early pregnancy loss.

Meta-analysis of 11 clinical trials found no significant difference in the incidence of placental abruption among women taking aspirin compared to controls (Hauth *et al.*, 1995b), but one study found a significantly increased frequency of placental abruption among women who took low-dose aspirin therapy compared to controls (Sibai *et al.*, 1993).

In summary, at therapeutic or low doses, aspirin is not associated with a significant risk of birth defects, although in very large, chronic doses close to the time of delivery, aspirin may be associated with an increase in bleeding disorders in the mother and fetus. Mega-doses as may be used in suicide gestures are discussed in Chapter 14.

## Acetaminophen

In the recent decade, acetaminophen is the most commonly used analgesic in pregnancy (Liew *et al.*, 2014), surpassing aspirin. It has antipyretic action., Forty-one percent of pregnant women reported acetaminophen use during pregnancy in a large longitudinal study (Streissguth *et al.*, 1987). Recent research reported 11.7 percent of pregnant women took acetaminophen during the first trimester, and 15.6 percent took any analgesic during organogenesis (Haas *et al.*, 2018). Birth defects were not increased in frequency above background rate among more than 1200 offspring whose mothers used acetaminophen during the first trimester (Aselton *et al.*, 1985; Heinonen *et al.*, 1977; Jick *et al.*, 1981). Among 26,424 infants born to women who used acetaminophen during the first trimester, the frequency of birth defects was not increased in a Danish registry (Rebordosa *et al.*, 2008). In the National Birth Defects Surveillance program, first-trimester acetaminophen use in 11,610 infants whose used acetaminophen during the first trimester, the frequency of birth defects was not increased (Feldkamp *et al.*, 2010). Offspring average IQ at 4 years old whose mothers used acetaminophen during pregnancy was not different from controls (Streissguth *et al.*, 1987).

It seems unlikely that the putative association of maternal acetaminophen use and polyhydramnios because this is based upon one case report of one infant (Char *et al.*, 1975), and no other reports were published in the ensuing 45 years. Ingestion of large doses of acetaminophen as in a suicide gesture or the protracted use of this drug may result in renal and hepatic failure in the adult and could result in the same complications in the fetus (see **Chapter 14**).

In summary of available data, the data suggest that acetaminophen is one of the safest non-narcotic analgesics available for use in the pregnant woman with doses in the therapeutic range.

## Phenacetin

Phenacetin is one of the major metabolites of acetaminophen. It has analgesic and antipyretic actions with poor anti-inflammatory effects. Phenacetin is often used in combination with other analgesics, and. The frequency of malformations was not increased among more than 18,000 offspring of mothers who used this analgesic either alone or in combination with other agents (Heinonen *et al.*, 1977; Jick *et al.*, 1981). In addition, findings for acetaminophen also are relevant to this drug because a large proportion of acetaminophen is metabolized to phenacetin. No association between birth defects and phenacetin was found in experimental animals according to manufacturer's package insert.

### Phenylbutazone

Phenylbutazone is an NSAID with analgesic, antipyretic, and anti-inflammatory actions commonly used to treat women with arthritic conditions (rheumatoid arthritis, degenerative joint disease). No scientific studies are published regarding the safety or efficacy of this medication in pregnant women. Unpublished data had 27 infants who were exposed to phenylbutazone during the first trimester, and two major birth defects were found (Rosa, personal communication, cited in Briggs *et al.*, 2017). Some prostaglandin synthetase inhibitors are associated with premature closure of the ductus arteriosus in the newborn (Csaba *et al.*, 1978; Levin *et al.*, 1978). Theoretically, phenylbutazone may be associated with premature closure of ductus arteriosus because of known pharmacologic activity of the drug, and known effects of that pharmacologic effect. No reports of this association have been published to date.

### Indomethacin

Indomethacin is used for analgesic, and anti-inflammatory effects in the treatment of rheumatoid arthritis, osteoarthritis, bursitis, and tendonitis. Because of it prostaglandin inhibition, has been used to treat premature labor in the second and third trimesters of pregnancy (Niebyl *et al.*, 1980; Sibony *et al.*, 1994; Zuckerman *et al.*, 1974, 1984). Intravenous indomethacin was used to close a hemodynamically significant patent ductus arteriosus in premature infants. It was also used treat symptomatic leiomyomata during pregnancy (Dildy *et al.*, 1992).

Among more than 400 infants exposed to indomethacin during the first trimester, the frequency of major birth defects was not different from the population background rate (Aselton *et al.*, 1985; Kallen, 1998). The frequency of was not increased in several reports in which animals received several times the usual human dose of congenital malformations indomethacin (Kalter, 1973; Klein *et al.*, 1981; Randall *et al.*, 1987).

Premature closure of the ductus arteriosus and pulmonary hypertension in the fetus and newborn has been reported in several reports (DeWit *et al.*, 1988; Levin *et al.*, 1978; Manchester *et al.*, 1976; Moise *et al.*, 1988). Seven of 14 fetuses in 13 pregnant women who received indomethacin for premature labor at 25–31 weeks gestation had ductal constriction (by echocardiography) (Moise *et al.*, 1988). Ductal constriction was transient and resolved within 24 hours after discontinuation of the indomethacin. Fetal ductus arteriosus closure in the fetus was also associated with indomethacin exposure in several animal models (Harker *et al.*, 1981; Harris, 1980; Levin *et al.*, 1979). No evidence was reported of either premature closure of the ductus arteriosus or pulmonary hypertension in 15 fetuses whose mothers had received indomethacin in a randomized trial (Niebyl *et al.*, 1980). A review of 167 newborns [<35 weeks estimated gestational age (EGA)] whose mothers received indomethacin for tocolysis found no cases of premature closure of the ductus arteriosus or persistent fetal circulation (Dudley *et al.*, 1985).

Among 818 women who received indomethacin during pregnancy close to delivery, 13 percent compared to 1.8 percent for controls had perinatal complications (Marpeau *et al.*, 1994). Among 57 infants born at 30 weeks Necrotizing enterocolitis, intracranial hemorrhage, and patent ductus arteriosus were increased in frequency among 57 infants exposed to indomethacin compared to 57 control infants (Norton *et al.*, 1993), similar to prior reports of adverse neonatal outcomes (Eronen *et al.*, 1994; Major *et al.*, 1994; Rasenen and Jouppila, 1995; van der Heijden *et al.*, 1994). Among 15 infants exposed to indomethacin chronically during gestation, no instances of patent ductus occurred (Al-Alaiyan *et al.*, 1996).

### Ibuprofen

Ibuprofen is another commonly used NSAID analgesic. The frequency of congenital anomalies was no greater than expected among 51 infants whose mothers took ibuprofen during the first trimester of pregnancy (Aselton *et al.*, 1985).

Among 1117 infants whose mothers took ibuprofen during the first trimester the frequency of birth defects was not increased compared to 2229 non-exposed women (Dathe *et al.*, 2018).

In the Danish National Birth Cohort during 1996–2002, 980 boys with cryptorchidism were identified among whom maternal use of ibuprofen at least 4 weeks during the first trimester was increased in frequency (Jensen *et al.*, 2010). Cryptorchidism was increased with increased maternal use. It is important to keep in mind that the reasons for taking ibuprofen in consecutive weeks may be a confounding factor (e.g., fever over a protracted period, the disease with which the fever is associated such as influenza), or perhaps a causative factor. Analyses of analgesics, antibiotics, and other drugs must be tempered with these cautionary guidelines. In a case series, five infants were reported with abnormalities at birth, but no distinct anomaly syndrome (Barry *et al.*, 1984). Ibuprofen was associated with decreased amniotic fluid volume in one report (Hickok *et al.*, 1989), but subsequent studies have not confirmed this finding.

## Meclofenamate

The frequency of congenital anomalies (3.6 percent) was not increased compared the expected rate in the general population (3.5–5 percent) in 166 infants exposed to meclofenamate during the first trimester (Rosa, unpublished data, Briggs *et al.*, 2017).

## Naproxen

In a series of children born to 23 women who took naproxen throughout pregnancy for rheumatic disease, no congenital anomalies were found (Ostensen and Ostensen, 1996). The frequency of certain birth defects (orofacial clefts, gastroschisis, hypospadias) was slightly increased above baseline among 7,299 infants exposed to naproxen during the first trimester (Iterrante *et al.*, 2017). The same caution applies to interpretation of data for naproxen as for ibuprofen. Drugs with analgesic AND antipyretic properties are likely to be used in instances of hyperthermia, such as influenza or other viral syndromes associated with fever. The birth defects may be associated with the disease being treated and not the drug per se. For example, gastroschisis has been associated with hyperthermia (Little *et al.*, 1991).

## Sulindac

Sulindac is an NSAID used to treat rheumatoid arthritis, osteoarthritis, ankylosing spondylitis, and acute shoulder pain. Major congenital anomalies were not increased in frequency (4.3 percent) among 69 infants born to women who used sulindac during the first trimester, which is not different from the general population (Rosa, unpublished data, Briggs *et al.*, 2005). Sulindac is another of several NSAIDs that has been used as a tocolytic. Sulindac was superior to indomethacin for tocolysis in two studies sulindac had equivalent efficacy but fewer side effects than indomethacin (Carlan *et al.*, 1992; Rasenen and Jouppila, 1995).

## Miscellaneous NSAIDs

NSAIDs used infrequently during pregnancy (<5 percent) include fenoprofen, tolmentin, rofecoxib, celecoxib, and etodolac. Importantly, each of these drugs are prostaglandin synthetase inhibitors, and may theoretically cause premature closure of the ductus arteriosus and/or oligohydramnios based upon experience with better studied NSAIDs that have highly similar modes of action.

## COX-2 Inhibitors

Cox inhibitors are indicated for the relief of the signs and symptoms of osteoarthritis and rheumatoid arthritis. The Cox-selective drugs are a class of analgesics that target only Cox-2, and does not inhibit Cox-1, which is the protective enzyme that produces protective gastric mucosa. This class of drugs is gastric protective compared to non-specific Cox inhibitors such as aspirin, naproxen, sulindac, etc. Among 174 infants born to women who took coxibs in the first trimester, the frequency of congenital anomalies was not increased compared to 521 randomly selected controls (Dathe *et al.*, 2018). In another study of 114 infants whose mothers took one of several coxibs (celecoxib, etoricoxib, rofecoxib) in the first trimester exposures, the frequency of birth defects was not increased (Daniel *et al.*, 2012). Cox selective agents apparently have the same prostaglandin inhibition as non-selective Cox analgesics as they have been effective in management of ductus arteriosus in preterm infants (Lainwala and Hussain, 2016).

### Rofecoxib

Rofecoxib is a cyclooxygenase-2 (COX-2) selective analgesic. No studies of congenital anomalies in offspring exposed to rofecoxib during embryogenesis have been published. Premature closure of the ductus arteriosus is a theoretical risk of maternal therapy with rofecoxib because of the pharmacologic action of the drug. Rofecoxib (Vioxx) was withdrawn from the market in September 2004 because an increased risk of myocardial infarction or stroke was found. Among 109 infants exposed to rofecoxib during pregnancy the frequency of major congenital anomalies was not increased (Kallen, 2019).

### Celecoxib

Celecoxib is a COX-2 selective analgesic. Among 109 infants exposed to celecoxib during the first trimester, the frequency of congenital anomalies (n = 6, 5.5 percent) was not significantly increased above control rates (Kallen, 2019). Premature closure of the ductus arteriosus is a theoretical risk because of the pharmacologic action of celecoxib. Ductus closure has been demonstrated in animal models, but not reported in humans. In 24 pregnancies exposed to celecoxib, the rate of prematurity (n = 6) was increased (Bérard *et al.*, 2018). The clinical significance of this finding is unclear.

### Etoricoxib

Data on etoricoxib exposure in the first trimester is limited to 36 infants, in the Swedish registry, and no birth defects were reported (Kallen, 2019).

### Etodolac

Etodolac is a COX-2 selective analgesic. No studies of congenital anomalies in offspring exposed to etodolac during the first trimester have been published. Premature closure of the ductus arteriosus is a theoretical risk because of the pharmacologic action of etodolac. Etodolac was found to be safer for the gastrointestinal tract (i.e., fewer bleeding ulcers than naproxen) with chronic therapy (Weideman *et al.*, 2004). The frequency of congenital anomalies was increased among rats or rabbits exposed to etodolac during embryogenesis (Ninomiya *et al.*, 1990a, 1990b). Among 265 infants whose mother took etodolac during the first trimester, the frequency of birth defects was not increased (Daniel *et al.*, 2012).

### Narcotic Analgesics

Commonly used analgesics are listed in Box 8.2. All opioid narcotic analgesics cross the placenta, and all opioids can cause dependence and withdrawal symptoms in the fetus, newborn and mother if there is abuse, ***even if regularly used*** as prescribed (see Chapter 16 regarding substance abuse). A number of opiates are frequently used for pain management during labor. Use for acute pain in appropriate doses, opiates are associated with few, if any, adverse fetal effects. At high doses with fetal exposure intrapartum, fetal respiratory depression may occur, and maternal respiratory depression may occur with opioids used in sufficiently large doses close to delivery. A 2.2-fold increase in the risk for neural tube defects was among 20,630 infants born following periconceptional opioid use in a case-control study (Yazdy *et al.*, 2013). Meta-analysis of 68 studies was not definitive, but 17 of 30 studies found a statistically significant increased frequency of birth defects among infants exposed opioid during organogenesis (Lind *et al.*, 2017).

---

### BOX 8.2 NARCOTIC ANALGESICS

- Alphaprodine
- Butorphanol
- Codeine
- Fentanyl
- Hydrocodone
- Hydromorphone
- Meperidine

- Morphine
- Nalbuphine
- Oxycodone
- Oxymorphone
- Pentazocine
- Propoxyphene
- Sufentanil

---

## Meperidine

Meperidine is one of the most commonly used analgesics during labor. Within 7 min of maternal injection, fetal levels are about equal to maternal levels (Fishburne, 1982; Spielman, 1987). The half-life in the newborn may be up to 23 hours (Spielman, 1987). Meperidine is metabolized predominantly in the liver, and its major metabolite, normeperidine, is more potent and potentially more toxic than the parent compound itself.

Birth defects were not increased in frequency among more than 300 infants born to women who took meperidine in the first trimester (Heinonen *et al.*, 1977; Jick *et al.*, 1981). Among 62 newborns exposed to meperidine during the 1st trimester, the frequency of birth defects was not increased (F. Rosa, Unpublished data, Briggs *et al.*, 2017).

Among 30 infants with birth defects, exposure to meperidine was not increased in frequency (Broussard *et al.*, 2011).

Neonatal respiratory depression and behavioral changes have been reported, and attributed to the relatively long half-life of this drug in the fetus and newborn whose enzymatic activity is naturally immature (Belsey *et al.*, 1981; Busacca *et al.*, 1982; Koch and Wendel, 1968; Morrison *et al.*, 1973; Schnider and Moya, 1964). Neonatal behavioral changes are transient, and at 5- to 10-year follow-up of 70 children born to mothers who received meperidine during labor, behavior did not differ from controls.

No significant persisting physical or psychological effects were found in the meperidine-exposed children compared to unexposed controls (Buck, 1975). Among the offspring of hamsters given meperidine at doses several times the usual human dose during organogenesis, an increased frequency of birth defects was produced (Geber and Schramm, 1975).

Meperidine is apparently a safe drug for use during pregnancy *when taken within the therapeutic dose range, especially during labor*. Dose management requires close attention because of the long half-life of this drug in the neonate.

## Morphine

Morphine is no longer commonly used as an analgesic during labor because neonatal respiratory depression occurred with a significantly greater frequency than with meperidine (Spielman, 1987). In some cases, pregnant women may be exposed to this narcotic analgesic for other indications (e.g., postoperative pain), and will need to be managed carefully.

Among the offspring of 70 women who took morphine during the first trimester, the frequency of birth defects was not increased in frequency (Heinonen *et al.*, 1977). In the Swedish registry, the frequency of birth defects was not increased in 297 infants born to women who used morphine during the first trimester (Kallen, 2019).

Two animal studies found that morphine exposure during embryogenesis did not increase the frequency of congenital anomalies (Fujinaga and Mazze, 1988; Yamamoto *et al.*, 1972). Three other experimental animal studies did find an increase in the central nervous system and other structural anomalies in the offspring of animals treated with morphine in doses several times larger than those used in humans (Geber, 1977; Geber and Schramm, 1975; Harpel and Gautierie, 1968).

Newborns of addicted mothers may experience withdrawal symptoms, and more detail is given in the chapter on substance abuse (Chapter 16).

### Pentazocine

Pentazocine is a narcotic analgesic used for relief of moderate to severe pain. Similar to other narcotics, it is associated with a risk of respiratory depression at high doses. Pentazocine crosses the placenta, but evidently not to the same extent as meperidine (Spielman, 1987).

Congenital anomalies were not increased in frequency in two studies including a total of 63 infants born to mothers who used pentazocine in association with tripelennamine (an antihistamine, blue pill) in a street drug combination, i.e., Ts and blues (see Chapter 16) (Chasnoff et al., 1983; Senay, 1985). The frequency of birth defects was increased but concomitant heavy alcohol use during pregnancy was likely the true cause of the observed birth defects (Little et al., 1990). It was concluded that it was very unlikely the birth defects observed were associated with the abuse of pentazocine. Only five infants (with no birth defects) were exposed to pentazocine in the Swedish registry (Kallen, 2019).

An increased frequency of low birth weight infants was associated with the use of pentazocine and tripelennamine during pregnancy (Chasnoff et al., 1983; Dunn and Reynolds, 1982; Little et al., 1990; von Almen and Miller, 1986). No epidemiologic studies are published regarding the possible association of congenital anomalies with the therapeutic use of pentazocine.

An increased frequency of central nervous system defects were observed in the offspring of hamsters that had received large doses of pentazocine, but not with smaller doses (Geber and Schramm, 1975).

As with all narcotics, fetal addiction and severe neonatal withdrawal symptoms occur with habitual maternal use of pentazocine (Goetz and Bain, 1974; Kopelman, 1975; Little et al., 1990; Scanlon, 1974).

### Butorphanol

Another narcotic analgesic, butorphanol is parenterally administered for labor analgesia. The drug has agonist and antagonist actions (Spielman, 1987). Butorphanol is more efficacious than other narcotic analgesics. However, the risk of respiratory depressive effects is greater with butorphanol than with other narcotics. The butorphanol metabolite is biologically inactive (i.e., has no analgesic or toxic effect) unlike meperidine, which produces active metabolites. This is a distinct advantage over other labor analgesics in the management of maternal dose and potential untoward neonatal effects (Spielman, 1987). Importantly, this agent readily crosses the placenta and affects fetal respiration (Pittman et al., 1980), possibly causing fetal and neonatal cardiorespiratory depression with frequent and high dose regimens. If butorphanol is used chronically or abused during pregnancy, fetal dependence and severe neonatal withdrawal symptoms may develop.

No studies are published on butorphanol use during pregnancy and the frequency of congenital anomalies, but the drug likely does not substantially increase the risk of birth defects. Birth defects were not increased in frequency among offspring exposed to butorphanol during embryogenesis compared to controls (Takahashi et al., 1982). Butorphanol is compatible with breastfeeding (American Academy of Pediatrics, 1994).

### Hydrocodone

A synthetic narcotic, hydrocodone, is used to treat moderate pain but is infrequently used during labor and delivery. Hydrocodone is a component of cough suppressant formulations. Congenital anomalies were slightly increased in frequency (7.2 percent) compared to the background rate in the general population (5 percent) in an unpublished study of 332 infants born to women who used this drug during the first trimester (Rosa, unpublished data, Briggs *et al.*, 2017). Congenital anomalies in a clinical case series of 40 infants whose mothers used hydrocodone during the first trimester were heterogeneous, and did not seem to comprise a constellation or pattern, as would be expected in a syndrome. (Schick *et al.*, 1996). Analysis of the association of birth defects with hydrocodone use in the first trimester in the National Birth Defects Prevention Study found several associations. Spina bifida, five types of heart defects (atrioventricular septal defect, tetralogy of Fallot, left ventricular outflow tract obstruction defect, hypoplastic left heart syndrome, pulmonary valve stenosis, ventricular septal defect plus atrial septal defect) and cleft palate were significantly increased in frequency among infants whose mothers used hydrocodone during pregnancy (Broussard *et al.*, 2011). Birth defects were increased in frequency in the offspring of hamsters injected with extremely large doses of this agent (Geber and Schramm, 1975).

## Oxymorphone

Oxymorphone is narcotic analgesic that has been in use for more than 50 years, but no studies are published of its use during pregnancy. Several early studies regarding the use of this analgesic during labor associate it with newborn respiratory depression (Sentnor *et al.*, 1962; Simeckova *et al.*, 1960), which is a known risk with all opioids.

An increased frequency of malformations was observed in offspring of animals given oxymorphone during embryogenesis at a dose >1000 times the usual human dose, which was associated with a 25 percent maternal mortality (Geber and Schramm, 1975).

## Oxycodone

Among 78 infants exposed to oxycodone during the first trimester, the frequency of birth defects was not increased above population background levels (3.5–5 percent) (Schick *et al.*, 1996). In an unpublished study, the frequency of birth defects among 281 infants born to women who were prescribed oxycodone during the first trimester was not increased (Briggs *et al.*, 2021). The frequency of birth defects among infants whose mothers used oxycodone in the first trimester was increased in The National Birth Defects Prevention Study, specifically for pulmonary valve stenosis (Broussard *et al.*, 2011).

Pharmacologically, oxycodone is pharmacologically expected to produce neonatal respiratory depression, and possibly withdrawal symptoms. Although there is a paucity of information regarding the last three drugs (hydrocodone, oxymorphone, and oxycodone), they are listed as FDA category B drugs under the old system.

## Alphaprodine

Alphaprodine is an early narcotic analgesic and has been in use since the 1940s (Hapke and Barnes, 1949). No studies of the use of alphaprodine are published that could be located. Alphaprodine crosses the placenta readily and may result in newborn respiratory depression. This agent is no longer commonly used during pregnancy because of the potential for causing a sinusoidal heart rate pattern in the fetus (Gray *et al.*, 1978).

## Fentanyl

Fentanyl, a synthetic narcotic, is 1000 times more potent than meperidine (Spielman, 1987). No studies have been published on the use of fentanyl during the first trimester. However, fentanyl can cause respiratory depression with chronic maternal use in the third trimester (Regan *et al.*, 2000). Birth defects were not increased in frequency among offspring of rats born to mothers given high doses of fentanyl throughout gestation (Fujinaga *et al.*, 1986).

Alfentanil and sufentanil are discussed in Chapter 6.

## Propoxyphene

Propoxyphene is no longer available, but it was a commonly used analgesic agent similar in structure to methadone. It was an analgesic only, and had no antipyretic or anti-inflammatory actions. The frequency of congenital anomalies was not increased among the offspring of almost 800 women who used this agent during early pregnancy (Heinonen et al., 1977; Jick et al., 1981). Several case reports of malformations in the offspring of mothers who used propoxyphene during pregnancy were published (Golden et al., 1982; Williams et al., 1983), but no causal links can be established. Propoxyphene was not teratogenic in rabbit, hamster, rat, or mouse animal models at doses 40-fold greater than the usual human dose (Buttar and Moffatt, 1983; Emmerson et al., 1971).

Neonatal withdrawal syndrome (irritability, hyperactivity, tremors, high-pitched cry) was reported among neonates born to mothers who used propoxyphene chronically during late pregnancy (Ente and Mehra, 1978; Klein et al., 1975; Quillian and Dunn, 1976; Tyson, 1974). Propoxyphene was opined to be safe for breastfeeding mothers (American Academy of Pediatrics, 1994).

## Nalbuphine

An opiate analgesic given parenterally for moderate to severe pain, nalbuphine may also be used an adjunct to balanced general anesthesia or regional techniques. Nalbuphine crosses the placenta readily. As with other narcotics, nalbuphine may result in neonatal respiratory depression, fetal and neonatal addiction, fetal cardiac function alterations, and withdrawal symptoms in the newborn. This drug was associated with a sinusoidal fetal heart rate pattern, similar to that produced by alphaprodine (Feinstein et al., 1986).

No studies were published on the use of nalbuphine during the first trimester. According to the manufacturer, this agent was not teratogenic in animal studies.

## Narcotic Antagonists

Narcotic antagonists are agents used primarily for the treatment of central nervous system and cardiorespiratory depression secondary to narcotic agonists. They are also used in some opioid addiction treatment programs.

## Naloxone

Naloxone (Narcan) is a synthetic congener of oxymorphone, and its most common use is as an antagonist agent to revere narcotic respiratory depression in the newborn. No studies have been published regarding congenital anomalies among the offspring of women who took this drug in the first trimester. In a polydrug therapy, buprenorphine-naloxone combination was given to 30 women during the first trimester, and the frequency of birth defects was not increased (Dooley et al., 2016).

The frequency of congenital anomalies was not increased among offspring of hamsters and mice exposed to naloxone at many times the usual human dose during organogenesis (Geber and Schramm, 1975; Jurand, 1985). Naloxone is known to precipitate withdrawal symptoms in newborns whose mothers are habitual users/addicted to narcotics, and used very high doses of opiates near the time of delivery.

## Naltrexone

Another narcotic antagonist, naltrexone (Trexan), is also a congener of oxymorphone. Naltrexone is also used in the treatment of opioid dependence, and for weight loss in combination with another drug. The frequency of birth defects after exposure to naltrexone during pregnancy was not increased among 68 infants, but it was unclear exactly when the exposure occurred (Kelty and Hulse, 2017). Importantly, these gravidas were given naltrexone as part of a treatment regimen for heroin addiction. Three case series comprising reportedly unduplicated patients contained 31 infants whose mothers used naltrexone during the first trimester, and there were no congenital anomalies present (Hulse and O'Neil, 2002; Hulse et al., 2001, 2004). According to its manufacturer, this agent was shown to be embryocidal in animal studies. The frequency of birth defects was not increased among rats or rabbits exposed during embryogenesis (McLaughlin *et al.*, 1997).

## OTHER ANALGESICS

### BUTALBITAL

Butalbital is a short-acting barbiturate that is contained in a variety (over 40) of available prescription analgesic compounds. Butalbital is usually combined with aspirin or acetaminophen (with or without caffeine). The most common indication for butalbital-containing analgesic compounds is tension headaches. All barbiturates cross the placenta, as do acetaminophen and aspirin. Barbiturate use in the first trimester was not associated with an increase in the frequency of congenital anomalies in exposed offspring. However, barbiturates have been associated with fetal dependence and newborn withdrawal symptoms when used chronically by the mother in the third trimester. Butalbital use during the first trimester in 73 women resulted in increased frequency of congenital heart defects during pregnancy (Browne *et al.*, 2014). In a large birth defects study, a case-control analysis that contained only 8 exposed cases found a significant increase in the frequency of hypospadias (Lind *et al.*, 2013).

### NON-BARBITURATE HEADACHE TREATMENTS

Medical compounds comprised of isometheptene, dichloralphenazone and acetaminophen (Midrin, Amidrin, Migratine) are used to treat vascular headaches or migraines. The combination of isometheptene, a sympathomimetic drug that causes vasoconstriction and dichloralphenazone, a mild sedative, is commonly used during pregnancy. However, no studies of the risk of congenital anomalies are published for either of the two components (isometheptene, dichloralphenazone).

### SUMATRIPTAN AND OTHER TRIPTANS

Sumatriptan (Imitrex) is a selective 5-hydroxytryptamine receptor agonist. It is used primarily as acute therapy for migraine headaches. The frequency of birth defects was not increased among 658 infants born to women who used sumatriptan during the first trimester (Kallen and Lynger, 2001). Among 479 first-trimester exposures to sumatriptan, the frequency of major birth defects was not increased (Cunnington *et al.*, 2009). According to the manufacturer's registry, 52 infants born after first trimester exposure did not have an increased frequency of birth defects (Sumatriptan Registry, 2009). Sumatriptan has been shown to cause birth defects in rabbits, but it was not teratogenic in rats. Sumatriptan was shown to cross the placenta by passive transport in the *ex vivo* isolated perfused cotyledon technique (Schenker *et al.*, 1995). Under the old FDA classification system, it is a category C agent. However, available data suggest the drug is safe for use during pregnancy (Table 8.2). Other triptans include naratriptan, almotriptan, rizatriptan, zolmitriptan. None of these migraine drugs has been adequately studied during pregnancy.

### NARATRIPTAN

The frequency of major birth defects was not increased among 52 infants whose mothers took naratriptan during the first-trimester exposures to naratriptan (Eprhoss and Sinclair, 2014).

### TREXIMET

Treximet is a combination of naproxen and sumatriptan. The individual components have been studied (see earlier), but no studies of this combination preparation have been published.

**TABLE 8.2**

**Comparison of Teratogen Information System (TERIS) Risk and Food and Drug Administration (FDA) Pregnancy Risk Ratings**

| Drug | Risk | Risk Rating |
|------|------|-------------|
| Acetaminophen | None | B |
| Butalbital | Unlikely | C* |
| Butorphanol | Undetermined | C* |
| Fenoprofen | Undetermined | B* |
| Fentanyl | Undetermined | C* |
| Hydrocodone | Unlikely, small risk cannot be excluded | C* |
| Hydromorphone | Unlikely, small risk cannot be excluded | B* |
| Ibuprofen | Minimal | B* |
| Indomethacin | None to minimal | B* |
| Isometheptene | Undetermined | C |
| Meclofenamate | Undetermined | B* |
| Meperidine | Unlikely | B* |
| Methadone | Unlikely | B* |
| Morphine | Congenital anomalies: unlikely neonatal neurobehavioral Effects: moderate | C* |
| Nalbuphine | Undetermined | B* |
| Naloxone | Undetermined | B |
| Naltrexone | Undetermined | C |
| Naproxen | Undetermined | B* |
| Oxycodone | Undetermined, small risk cannot be excluded | B* |
| Oxymorphone | Undetermined, small risk cannot be excluded | B* |
| Pentazocine | Unlikely | C* |
| Phenacetin | None | B |
| Phenylbutazone | Undetermined | C* |
| Promethazine | None | C |
| Propoxyphene | None | C* |
| Propranolol | Undetermined | C* |
| Sulindac | Undetermined | B* |
| Sumatriptan | Unlikely | C |

*Sources:* Compiled from: Friedman *et al.*, 1990; Briggs *et al.*, 2005; Friedman and Polifka, 2006.

## ZOLMITRIPTAN

Zolmitriptan is another triptan used to treat migraine headaches. No studies of its use in human pregnancy are published. In rats, mice and rabbits given up to several thousand times the usual human dose, the frequency of birth defects was not increased. At the usual human dose, no adverse effects were observed, but at high doses, embryolethality was increased in frequency (Manufacturer's information).

## SPECIAL CONSIDERATIONS

### LABOR ANALGESICS

#### Meperidine

Meperidine provides effective pain relief for two to four hours in most patients who need systemic labor analgesics. It is important to keep in mind that fetal clearance of meperidine may be slow

**TABLE 8.3**

**Suggested Dosage Regimens for Some Commonly Used Parenteral Narcotic Analgesic Agents for Postoperative Pain[a]**

| Agent | Dosage |
|---|---|
| Butorphanol | 2–4 mg IM q 3–4 h, or 0.5–1 mg IV q 3–4 h |
| Hydromorphone | 1–2 mg IM q 3–4 h, or 0.5–1 mg IV q 3 h |
| Meperidine | 50–100 mg IM q 3–4 h |
| Morphine | 10 mg (5–20 mg) IM q 4 h |
| Nalbuphine | 10 mg IM or IV q 3–6 h |
| Pentazocine | 30 mg IM or IV q 3–4 h |

[a] Refer to manufacturer's recommendations.

because of the immature hepatic enzyme complement. The usual dose is 25–50 mg IV or 50–75 mg IM. Promethazine, in a dose of 25 mg, is also given as an adjunct to prevent nausea (Table 8.3).

## Butorphanol

Butorphanol is effective narcotic for systemic analgesia and is usually given in a dose of 1–2 mg either IV or IM. This agent provides pain relief for up to 4 h.

### ANALGESIA FOLLOWING MINOR PROCEDURES

Several oral narcotic agents (hydrocodone, oxycodone) provide satisfactory relief for moderate pain associated with minor surgical procedures, such as dental procedures. Narcotic agents should not be used over a protracted period (more than seven days) late in pregnancy because of the potential for neonatal dependence or withdrawal symptoms. Recent findings also suggest that use during the first trimester is associated with an increased risk of certain congenital anomalies (spina bifida, heart defects, cleft palate), but the increased risk is small.

### HEADACHE

Frequency of migraines apparently increases in frequency in the first trimester, usually improves during the second and third trimester. However, among 4 to 8 percent of pregnant women, migraines may worsen during the latter trimesters. Migraine headache frequency usually returns to pre-pregnancy rates post-delivery. Pregnancy outcomes in women who have migraine headaches during pregnancy are at increased risk of low birth infants, preterm birth, cesarean section, and preeclampsia (Chen *et al.*, 2010)

Non-migraine headaches are common during pregnancy, and may increase in frequency during gestation. In all headache syndromes, potential identifiable causes of headaches should be ruled out before a long-term treatment plan is implemented. Etiology of headaches in most patients is unknown.

Two major categories of headache are recognized, namely, (1) tension and (2) vascular (migraine). For mild to moderate headaches, aspirin, acetaminophen, ibuprofen, or naproxen usually provide satisfactory acute relief. Acetaminophen is the preferred analgesic for use during pregnancy. Aspirin in frequent and large doses should be avoided during pregnancy to maintain hemostasis, especially when headaches occur close to term. Aspirin increases the potential for bleeding because of decreased platelet activity. NSAIDs should not be used after 34 weeks gestational age because of the theoretical potential for premature closure of the ductus arteriosus and other potential adverse effects. If non-NSAID agents have failed, ibuprofen seems associated with the smallest risk for increased bleeding and premature ductus closure.

Migraine (vascular) headaches are difficult to treat during pregnancy. Ergotamine agents used to treat migraine headaches in non-pregnant patients are vasoconstrictive. Ergotamines are not recommended for use during pregnancy because they have (1) vasoconstrictive and (2) oxytocin-like actions. Propranolol at a dose of 40 mg or higher per day (several divided doses) has been effective for the treatment of migraines in some pregnant patients, and seem to pose negligible risk to the unborn child.

Amitriptyline, a tricyclic antidepressant, has been used to treat migraine headaches in pregnant women. However, this agent should be used as a third line of medical treatment for migraine headaches among pregnant women with vascular headaches who have not responded to triptans, analgesics or propranolol.

The combination of isometheptene, dichloralphenazone, and acetaminophen is also used for treatment of migraine headaches during pregnancy. Unfortunately, the effects of isometheptene and dichloralphenazone are unknown. It is known that this combination of drugs should be avoided in women with hypertension because of isometheptene's associated vasoconstrictive effects. The usual dose is two capsules orally at the beginning of an attack and then one capsule every hour; up to five capsules in any one 12-h period (see manufacturer's prescribing recommendations).

Sumatriptan (Imitrex) has been studied among 1,137 infants born to mothers who took the drug during the first trimester to state that the risk of congenital anomalies following first trimester exposure is not greater than that in the general population (Kallen and Lygner, 2001; Cunnington *et al.*, 2009).

Serious emphasis must be placed on the cautionary statement that *narcotic analgesics should not be used chronically for headaches because of the potential for addiction in the mother and withdrawal symptoms in the fetus, and birth defects following first trimester exposure*. However, narcotic analgesics may be efficacious for the treatment of an acute migraine episode with little to no risk to the fetus.

### ANALGESIA FOLLOWING OPERATIVE PROCEDURES

Acute narcotic analgesic therapy is most commonly indicated for postoperative pain relief. Women who require surgery during pregnancy can be safely treated **for acute pain relief** with a variety of analgesic agents for postoperative pain with relative safety for the fetus. Two commonly used regimens are meperidine (Demerol), 50–100 mg IM every three to four hours, or hydromorphone (Dilaudid), 1–2 mg every three to four hours. Caution should be exercised with large doses during breastfeeding. Dosage regimens for various parenteral preparations are summarized in Table 8.3.

## SUMMARY

In general, analgesics are not a high-risk drug class for use during pregnancy (Table 8.2). The major change that has occurred is the recognition and validation that opioid analgesics are associated with an increased risk for certain birth defects (Broussard *et al.*, 2011). Other than opioid analgesics, analgesics are not associated with an increased risk of congenital anomalies, where the risk is known (Table 8.2). Importantly, dose and dose frequency must be managed carefully during pregnancy, especially in the third trimester for all analgesics. For example, meperidine probably requires no adjustment in dose or frequency because its pharmacokinetics do not change appreciably from the non-pregnant to pregnant states. Slow fetal clearance of meperidine must be considered when this drug is used near term. Depressed perinatal respiration may occur with large doses prior to delivery.

Morphine, on the other hand, has a decreased half-life and increased clearance, indicating likely need for increasing dose and/or frequency (Table 8.3). Neonates exposed to analgesics during gestation need to be monitored for possible complications, including (1) bleeding disorders (salicylates), (2) neonatal dependence (narcotics and barbiturates), and (3) withdrawal (narcotics and barbiturates). High doses of narcotic analgesics may be associated with maternal and/or neonatal respiratory depression. Large doses of analgesic are often an attempt to compensate for more increased volume of distribution, more rapid metabolism, and clearance of opiates, and other analgesics during pregnancy (Table 8.2).

# 9 Anticonvulsant Drugs during Pregnancy

Seizure disorders occur among 0.5–1 percent of all pregnancies (Royal College Ob Gyn, 2016). An estimated 1.1 million women of childbearing age have a seizure disorder (Patel and Pinnell, 2016), and an estimated three to 10 of 1,000 gravidas are epileptic (Razaz *et al.*, 2017). Available AEDs to treat seizures are classed into three groups: first, second and third generation drugs. Medical treatment with antiseizure medications date to at least 1857 (Table 9.1).

## PREGNANCY COMPLICATIONS

Epilepsy is associated with an increased frequency in pregnancy, with complications occurring in both the mother and the fetus (Razaz *et al.*, 2017). Maternal complications include an increased risk of pregnancy-induced hypertension, preterm delivery, and low birth weight (Table 9.2). Major congenital anomalies are the predominant risk to the fetus, and occur among infants exposed to antiepileptic drugs that is two- to threefold higher than the general population (Jazayeri *et al.*, 2018; Yerby, 1994). Specifically, clusters of anomalies seem present with some drugs. For example, neural tubes defects (i.e., spina bifida) are associated with valproic acid and carbamazepine (Tomson *et al.*, 2019; **Yerby, 2000, 2003**).

Antiepileptic medications (AEDs) during pregnancy and the occurrence of syndromes (fetal hydantoin syndrome, fetal valproate syndrome) are an emerging area of pharmacogenomics which has made some progress, but research in pregnancy is limited. The genetic enzyme complement of the gravida and her fetus are intermediate in the effects of these AEDs because metabolism varies between women. Limited data suggest that some poor metabolizers may be at a higher risk of having a baby with a

**TABLE 9.1**
**First-, Second-, and Third-Generation AEDs**

### Antiepileptic Drugs

| First Generation | | Second Generation | | Second Generation | |
|---|---|---|---|---|---|
| **Drug** | **Year** | **Drug** | **Year** | **Drug** | **Year** |
| Potassium br. | 1857 | Vigabatrin | 1989 | Fosphenytoin | 2007 |
| Phenobarbital | 1912 | Oxcarbazepine | 1990 | Rufinamide | 2008 |
| Phenytoin | 1939 | Lamotrigine | 1991 | Lacosamide | 2008 |
| Ethosuximide | 1960 | Felbamate | 1994 | Stiripemtol | 2008 |
| Primidone | 1960 | Gabapentin | 1994 | Piracetam | 2010 |
| Sultiame | 1960 | Topiramate | 1995 | Retigabine/Ezogabone | 2011 |
| Diazepam | 1963 | Tiagabine | 1996 | Clobazam | 2011 |
| Clonazepam | 1965 | Levetiracetam | 2000 | Pregabalin | 2012 |
| Carbamazepine | 1965 | Zoisamide | 2007 | Perampanel | 2012 |
| Valproic acid | 1970 | | | Eslicarbazepine | 2013 |
| Clorazepate | 1976 | | | Brivaracetam | 2016 |
| | | | | Safinamide | 2017 |
| | | | | Ganaxolone | 2017 |

*Source:* Adapted from Singh and Verma, 2019.

DOI: 10.1201/9780429160929-9

**TABLE 9.2**

**Complications of Epilepsy and Pregnancy Reported**

| Maternal | Fetal or Neonatal |
|---|---|
| Abortion (elective or spontaneous) | |
| Abruptio placentae | Congenital anomalies |
| Cesarean delivery | Drug withdrawal |
| Eclampsia | Feeding difficulties |
| Hyperemesis gravidarum | Hypoxemia |
| Hypotonic labor | Low birth weight |
| Increased seizure activity | Malnutrition |
| Preeclampsia | Neonatal hemorrhage |
| Pregnancy-induced hypertension | Perinatal deaths |
| Preterm delivery | Prematurity |
| Vaginal bleeding | Stillbirths |
| Seizures | |

*Source:* Adapted from Razaz *et al.*, 2017.

**TABLE 9.3**

**Overview of Recommended Management of AED Use in Pregnancy**

| Stage of Pregnancy | AED Level Management during Pregnancy | | |
| | Clearance | Drug Level | Dose Change |
|---|---|---|---|
| First Trimester | Possible ↑ | Begin monitoring | Possible ↑ |
| Second Trimester | ↑ | Monitor | ↑—titrate |
| Third Trimester | ↑ | Monitor | ↑—titrate |
| Postpartum | ↓ | Monitor | ↓—taper down, titrate |

*Source:* Compiled from Thomson *et al.*, 2019.

birth defect. Pharmacokinetics are important in the management of pregnancy complicated by epilepsy. Piecemeal information is available regarding pharmacokinetics of AEDs during pregnancy (Table 9.3).

## EFFECT OF PREGNANCY ON ANTICONVULSANT LEVELS

Pharmacokinetics of several anticonvulsants showed that the levels of phenytoin and phenobarbital decreased during pregnancy associated with physiologic changes of pregnancy affect metabolism, plasma protein binding, maternal serum level, and clearance of anticonvulsants. Clearance of phenytoin, phenobarbital, carbamazepine, and valproate increase during pregnancy (Deligiannidis *et al.*, 2014; Levy and Yerby, 1985; Tomson *et al.*, 2013). Anticonvulsant levels vary during pregnancy for a given dose and cannot be predicted. Insufficient data exist to allow adequate modeling for more than a few drugs such as acetaminophen (Little, 1999). Anticonvulsant levels should be monitored throughout pregnancy in order to control seizure activity which may increase in some pregnant women (Levy and Yerby, 1985). The published literature on anticonvulsant pharmacokinetics indicates that dose and frequency of anticonvulsants given during pregnancy to control seizures very likely require adjustment to maintain therapeutic levels (Table 9.4).

The frequency of birth defects associated with epilepsy during pregnancy over the past two decades is attributed in part to management of epilepsy with lower risk AEDs and dose management (Tomson *et al.*, 2019). Management included regimen adjustment while maintaining seizure control. The frequency of birth defects from five international birth defect registries that include polytherapy

**TABLE 9.4**

**Summary of Pharmacokinetics of AED Medications during Pregnancy**

| Agent | N | $C_{ss}$ | Cl | 3rd Trimester Concentration |
|---|---|---|---|---|
| Carbamazepine | 100 | ↓ 5/5 | ↑ 4/5 | ↓ 42% |
| Gabapentin | 3 | = | = | No change |
| Lamotrigine | 17 | ↓ 2/2 | ↑ 2/2 | ↓ 250% |
| Levetiracetam | 45 | ↓ 1/1 | ↑ 1/1 | ↓ 60% |
| Oxcarbazine | 27 | ↓ 1/1 | ↑ 1/1 | ↓ 40% |
| Phenobarbital | 48 | ↓ 2/2 | ↑ 2/2 | ↓ 55% |
| Phenobarbitone | 31 | — | ↑ 1 /2 | ↓ 55% |
| Phenytoin | 185 | ↓ 3/3 | ↑ 4/8 | ↓ 55% |
| Primidone | 15 | = 1 /2 | = 1 /2 | ↓ 70% |
| Topiramate | 34 | ↓ 1/1 | ↑ 1/1 | ↓ 40% |
| Valproic acid | 28 | ↓ | ↑= 1/1 | ↓ 50%* |
| Zonisamide | 2 | ↓ 1/1 | ↑ 1/1 | ↓ 50% |

* Dose not adjusted in 24/38 pregnancies, increased in 7/38.

*Abbreviations:* EGA, estimated gestational age; AUC, area under the curve; $V_d$, volume of distribution; $C_{ss}$, peak plasma concentration; $C_{ss}$, steady-state concentration; $t_{1/2}$- half life; PPB, plasma protein binding; PO, by mouth; ↓ denotes a decrease during pregnancy compared to nonpregnant values; ↑ denotes an increase during pregnancy compared to nonpregnant values; = denotes no difference between pregnant and nonpregnant values; IV, intravenous; IM, intramuscular.

*Sources:* Little BB. *Obstet Gynecol*, 1999; **93**: 858; Tomson *et al.*, 2013, Tomson and Hiilesmaa 2007; Ohman *et al.*, 2008a, 2008b; Deligiannidis *et al.*, 2014; Landmark *et al.*, 2018; Reimers *et al.*, 2018.

**TABLE 9.5**

**Comparison of Prevalence of Major Congenital Anomalies in National and International Birth Defect Registries**

| Drug | Prevalence Range | Number of Studies | Number of Infants |
|---|---|---|---|
| Carbamazepine | 2.6%–5.5% | 4 | 7,327 |
| Gabapentin | 1.7% | 1 | 59 |
| Lamotrigine | 1.9%–6.5% | 5 | 233,999 |
| Levetiracetam | 0%–2.8% | 5 | 228,217 |
| Oxcarbazepine | 2.2%–3.0% | 3 | 908 |
| Phenobarbital | 5.5%–6.5% | 2 | 493 |
| Phenytoin | 1.2%–10.2% | 4 | 227,429 |
| Topiramate | 1.5%–11.9% | 5 | 227,495 |
| Valproate | 5.4%–10.3% | 4 | 229,730 |

*Sources:* Compiled from Tomson *et al.*, 2019. The primary data come from the International Registry of Antiepileptic Drugs and Pregnancy (EURAP), North American AED Pregnancy Registry, UK Epilepsy and Pregnancy Register.

indicate that valproate is associated with the highest incidence of birth defects (Table 9.5). The estimated risks for birth defects associated with each monotherapy indicates valproate is the highest risk ranked treatment (Table 9.6).

Dose may be increased, or the frequency increased to optimize AED therapy management during pregnancy. Published data on pharmacokinetics of anticonvulsant during pregnancy, observed that

**TABLE 9.6**
**AED Monotherapy: Comparison of Rates of Major Congenital Anomalies**

First Trimester
Exposure:

| Monotherapy | n/N% | Associated Malformation(s) |
|---|---|---|
| Carbamazepine | 74/4647 = 1.59% | Neural tube defects |
| Lamotrigine | 154/6174 = 2.49% | Club foot |
| Levetiracetam | 30/1353 = 2.22% | No increase |
| Oxcarbazepine | 14/515 = 2.72% | No increase |
| Phenobarbital | 30/493 = 6.09% | No increase |
| Phenytoin | 23/623 = 3.69% | Congenital heart defects, syndrome |
| Topiramate | 24/581 = 4.13% | Oral clefts |
| Valproate | 254/2924 = 8.69% | Neural tube defects; syndrome |

*Source:* Compiled from Tomson *et al.*, 2019.

(1) clearance is increased, (2) steady state concentration is decreased, and (3) plasma protein binding is decreased. These changes indicate that ***dose adjustment and monitoring levels should be considered because of the expanded volume of distribution associated with pregnancy, the decreased steady state concentrations, and the increased clearance of the drug*** (Tomson *et al.*, 2019).

## FORMULATING A TREATMENT PLAN: CONGENITAL ANOMALIES AND MATERNAL ANTICONVULSANT THERAPY

AED use in pregnancy is an example of how the frequency of birth defects can be reduced through careful management of individual patients (Figure 9.1).

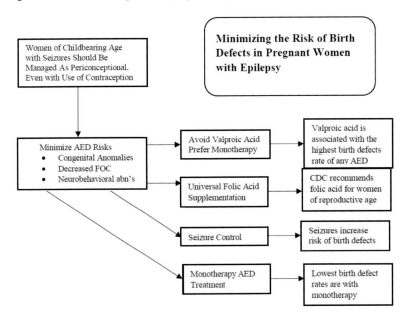

**FIGURE 9.1**    AED use in pregnancy.

(Compiled from data in Tomson *et al.*, 2019.)

Women with epilepsy requiring anticonvulsant therapy have a two- to threefold increased risk of having an infant with a congenital anomaly (Hill, 1973; Janz, 1975, 1982; Kelly, 1984). An aggregated analysis of approximately 750,000 pregnancies (13 separate cohort studies) indicated that the birth defect rate for newborns of epileptic mothers was 7 percent compared to 3 percent for controls (Kelly, 1984) in the absence of known or suspected teratogens used to treat the disease (i.e., AEDs).

Personalized medicine needs to be practiced to maintain seizure control and avoid toxicity. AED levels must be adjusted during pregnancy to maintain seizure control, and drug levels need to be adjusted specific to the medication used and the specific patient.

$C_s$ decreases for all the drugs listed in Table 9.4, except for gabapentin and valproic acid. Data are limited for gabapentin (n = 3), while protein binding seemed more influential than the increased volume of distribution in late pregnancy. Therefore, drug level monitoring needs to include the protein bound and unbound fractions. By late third trimester, maternal doses usually are increased approximately 50 percent over non-pregnant states to maintain seizure control, with the exception of lamotrigine which may require much larger doses.

## ETIOLOGY OF MALFORMATIONS

Why epilepsy is associated with an increased frequency of birth defects remains unknown because the etiologic pathophysiology mechanisms remain unknown for epilepsy-associated congenital anomalies. Even in the absence of AEDs during pregnancy, epilepsy is associated with an increased frequency of birth defects, debate continues whether or not the disease is associated with birth defects, or whether the treatment for the disease is mainly responsible (Tomson et al., 2015). One report stated that among women who took AEDs for indications other than epilepsy the frequency of birth defects was similar to that of epileptics (Jazayeri et al., 2018).

Available evidence suggests that a combination of AED exposure in an individual with epilepsy who may be "genetically" susceptible to poor metabolism of the AED agents may be responsible. The birth defect risk of certain anticonvulsant drugs may be secondary to a genetic "defect" (lowered or no activity) in the epoxide hydrolase enzyme system. This results in an inability to completely metabolize "toxic" intermediary oxidative metabolites (Bielec et al., 1995; Buehler et al., 1990; Finnell et al., 1992; Jones et al., 1989; Stickler et al., 1985; Van Dyke et al., 2000; Zhang et al., 2019).

Cytochrome P450 (CYP) metabolism is better studied in pregnancy than other pathways. Several CYP and/or non-CYP pathways metabolize AEDs. Other metabolic pathways include uridine diphosphate glucuronosyltransferase (UGT) and N-acetyltransferase. Pregnancy associated increase in sex steroids affect CYP-450 and UGT metabolism in a clinically important way through several CYP-450 pathways by inhibition (e.g., CYP1A2, CYP2C19, CYP2B6, CYP3A429), induction (CYP2A630), or increased glucuronidation (UGT1A4, UGT2B7). Cytochrome P450 and UGT alter drug levels through metabolism. These changes in maternal drug pharmacokinetics affect placental transfer and fetal drug metabolism. Cytochrome P1A2 is inhibited by sex steroids, and is less active in women than men. Compared with the non-pregnant state, CYP1A2 is reduced by 65–70 percent. Increased CYP3A4 activity is induced in pregnant women by progesterone, and increases metabolism and decreases drug plasma levels of carbamazepine, for example. CYP2C19 activity during pregnancy is reduced by almost 50 percent. During pregnancy, cytochrome P2D6 is induced, causing pharmacokinetic changes, usually increasing drug metabolism and clearance compared to non-gravid women. Maternal CYP metabolic phenotype is a major determinant of metabolism and drug clearance. Maternal polymorphisms of CYP2D6 can result in different therapeutic dosing requirements because phenotypes can vary from no/very slow metabolism to normal to very rapid. Non-pregnant women may require dose adjustments because of differences in CYP2D6 phenotype, and during pregnancy, differences in metabolism may require dose adjustment to maintain seizure control (Singh and Verma, 2019; Tomson et al., 2011; Zhang et al., 2019).

Certain anticonvulsants, especially the hydantoins (e.g., phenytoin), may be associated with folic acid anemia and may depress vitamin D (Lane and Hathaway, 1985). Therefore, vitamin (D and K) and folic acid supplements have been recommended for the pregnant woman with epilepsy who is taking anticonvulsant medications (Stephen *et al.*, 2019). Phenytoin and other AEDs that depress Vitamin K levels may be associated with hemorrhagic disease in the neonate, and may progress to severe or fatal with an event in the first 24 hours following delivery (Allen *et al.*, 1980; Lane and Hathaway, 1985). Other than avoiding salicylates during pregnancy, vitamin K supplementation during the last 2 months of pregnancy (10 mg PO) or in the last 2 weeks (20 mg PO) was recommended (Lane and Hathaway, 1985). If seizure control is maintained, tapering the AED level down within 2 weeks of expected delivery date is recommended to avoid perinatal AED toxicity.

## SYNDROMES AND ISOLATED CONGENITAL ANOMALIES ASSOCIATED WITH ANTICONVULSANTS

Anticonvulsant syndromes are constellations or clusters of congenital anomalies that recur as a pattern in infants exposed to AEDs during the first trimester. Dysmorphic features (facies, hypoplastic distal phalanges, other minor anomalies) and other birth defects associated with exposure to anticonvulsants during embryogenesis varies considerably (Table 9.7). Syndrome specialists who are "splitters" tend to assign a new syndrome name to each drug's collection of defects. Others who study syndromes are "lumpers" and use the label "fetal anticonvulsant syndrome" as an umbrella for the spectrum of defects that occur with anticonvulsants. Each AED is associated with birth

**TABLE 9.7**

**Syndromic and Isolated Congenital Anomalies Associated with Exposure to AEDs during Embryogenesis**

| Drug | Minor Anomalies | | Clefting | | Major Birth Defects | | | Growth | |
| | Distinctive Facies | Hypoplastic Phalanges | Facial | Lip/Palate | NTDs | CHD | UGD | Delay | Microcephaly |
|---|---|---|---|---|---|---|---|---|---|
| Carbamazepine | + | – | – | – | + | – | – | – | – |
| Clonazepam | + | + | – | – | – | – | – | – | – |
| Diones* | + | – | – | + | – | + | + | + | + |
| Felbamate** | ? | ? | ? | ? | ? | ? | ? | ? | ? |
| Gabapentin | +/– | – | – | – | + | – | – | – | – |
| Lamotrigene | – | – | – | – | +/– | – | – | – | – |
| Levetiracetam | – | – | – | – | – | – | – | – | – |
| Oxcarbazine | – | – | – | – | +/– | – | – | – | – |
| Phenobarbital | + | + | + | + | – | + | – | + | + |
| Phenytoin | + | – | – | + | – | + | – | + | + |
| Pregabalin | ? | ? | ? | ? | ? | + | ? | ? | ? |
| Primidone | + | + | – | – | – | + | – | + | – |
| Topiramate | + | – | – | + | – | – | – | – | – |
| Valproic acid | + | + | – | – | + | – | + | + | + |

* Paramethadione, trimethadione.

** Not in general use because of liver failure and aplastic anemia associations.

*Sources:* Compiled from published reports (Dansky and Finnell, 1991; Dieterich *et al.*, 1980; Eller *et al.*, 1997; Hanson, 1986; Iqbal *et al.*, 2001; Jager-Roman *et al.*, 1986; Koch *et al.*, 1996; Lajeunie *et al.*, 2001; McMahon and Braddock, 2001; Nulman *et al.*, 1997; Ornoy *et al.*, 1998; Rodriguez-Pinilla, 2000; Samren *et al.*, 1997, 1999; Waters *et al.*, 1994; Williams *et al.*, 2001; Yerby and Devinsky, 1994; Winterfield *et al.*, 2016).

defects seems to have a signature constellation of anomalies, ranging from minor craniofacial dysmorphia to spina bifida (Table 9.7). Dysmorphic features and congenital anomalies associated with first generation anticonvulsants are well characterized, although less information was available regarding birth defects of syndromes associated with newer AEDs.

Four large studies registries are available to inform on epilepsy, AEDs use in pregnancy, and birth defects.

The overall frequency of major congenital anomalies was reported from four major data sources. Across five registries, the rates of birth defects ranged from 0 percent (zero) to 10.3 percent (Table 9.5). Compared to an estimated 3.5 percent background rate for birth defects, valproic acid was associated with a higher frequency of congenital anomalies (10.3 percent), higher than any other anticonvulsants in the registries.

Notably, high doses (>200 mg) of lamotrigine were associated with an increased frequency of congenital anomalies (5.4 percent). Similarly, high doses of valproic acid (>800 mg) were associated with a 9.1 percent congenital anomaly rate. When valproic acid was a component of polytherapy, the frequency of congenital anomalies was significantly increased (Morrow *et al.*, 2006)

## ANTICONVULSANT POLYTHERAPY

AED polytherapy during pregnancy increases the frequency of congenital anomalies above than monotherapy. For example, four (7 percent) of 55 newborns with *in utero* exposure to two epileptic drugs had congenital anomalies, compared to six (17 percent) of 36 exposed to three agents and four (25 percent) of 16 exposed to four anticonvulsant agents (Lindhout *et al.*, 1984). Some combinations carry a greater risk than others do. Carbamazepine, phenobarbital, and valproic acid (with or without phenytoin) polytherapy were reported to be associated with congenital anomalies in seven (58 percent) of 12 infants compared to only three (7.5 percent) of 40 infants with birth defects who were exposed to other combinations of three or four anticonvulsants (Lindhout *et al.*, 1984). The authors argue that combinations of certain anticonvulsants may result in accumulation of toxic epoxide intermediates. The frequency of congenital anomalies was reported to be 1.6 to 4.2 times higher among fetuses of women taking four anticonvulsants compared to those taking only two (Hauser and Hesdorffer, 1990). Polytherapy for epilepsy during the first trimester is uniformly associated with an increased risk for congenital anomalies (Perucca, 2005). In addition, higher doses during polytherapy increase the frequency of birth defects (Tomson *et al.*, 2011). Composite estimates indicate that the highest prevalence of birth defects, 15.5 percent, was observed with valproic acid plus carbamazepine polytherapy (Table 9.8).

**TABLE 9.8**

**Composite Estimates of Major Birth Defect Frequency by AED Polytherapy**

| Drug | n | N |
|---|---|---|
| Lamotrigine + CBZ | 3/ 99 | 3.0% |
| Lamotrigine + Non-VPA AEDS | 10/ 450 | 2.2% |
| Lamotrigine + VPA | 5/ 55 | 9.1% |
| Lamotrigine+Phenobarbital | 20 / 355 | 5.7% |
| VPA + CBZ | 56 / 365 | 15.5% |

*Source:* Holmes *et al.*, 2011.

## BIRTH DEFECTS, EPILEPSY, AND ANTICONVULSANTS

Cardiac defects are the most frequent birth defects in infants born to women who used AEDs during early pregnancy (Tomson *et al.*, 2015). Among AED exposed infants the frequency of congenital heart defects was 0.5 percent compared to the expected rate of 0.3 percent. Cleft lip/palate was the second most frequent congenital anomaly in AED-exposed pregnancies (Table 9.7). In one review, the estimated rate of cleft lip/palate was 13.8 per 1000 compared to the background rate of 1.5 per 1,000 (Kelly, 1984), which agrees with more recent reviews (Tomson *et al.*, 2015). (Kelly, 1984). Other birth defects are associated with AED exposure during the first trimester, and vary by the specific drug (Table 9.6).

## ANTICONVULSANT AGENTS

A number of AEDs approved by the FDA for treatment of seizure disorders in the USA. AEDs cross the placenta; it is not medically safe for women with epilepsy to discontinue medication except under close supervision of her neurologist. Ideally, in a planned pregnancy, AEDs would be discontinued preconceptually, but this is usually not possible. A two- to threefold increase in the frequency of birth defects was observed in infants exposed to AEDs in the first trimester, but no specific birth defect was associated with a given drug (Speidel and Meadow, 1972). A recognizable cluster of anomalies among infants exposed during early pregnancy is called a syndrome. Since 1975, a number of syndromes were described in association with AED exposure include (1) phenytoin (Hanson and Smith, 1975), (2) phenobarbitone (Seip, 1976), (3) carbamazepine (Jones *et al.*, 1989), (4) primidone (Rudd and Freedom, 1979), (5) trimethadione (Zackai *et al.*, 1975), and (6) valproic acid (DiLiberti *et al.*, 1984). Authorities have advocated "lumping" these drug specific observations into a loose grouping of major and minor anomalies called 'the fetal anticonvulsant drug syndrome' (Zackai *et al.*, 1975). A two- to threefold increase in birth defects is reported from the most recent information published (Veroniki *et al.*, 2017).

### PHENYTOIN

Phenytoin is a hydantoin (Dilantin, Diphenylan, Mesantoin, Peganone), and has been used as an anticonvulsant for over 100 years. It is chemically related to barbiturates, is also used to treat arrhythmias, trigeminal neuralgia, and myotonic muscular dystrophy.

"Fetal hydantoin syndrome" is characterized by a pattern of multiple minor and major craniofacial and limb anomalies (Hanson and Smith, 1975) (Box 9.1).

---

**BOX 9.1   CHARACTERISTICS OF FETAL HYDANTOIN SYNDROME**

- Craniofacial anomalies
- Cleft lip/palate
- Broad nasal bridge
- Hypertelorism
- Epicanthal folds
- Growth deficiency
- Limb defects
- Hypoplasia of distal phalanges, nails
- Mental deficiency

*Source:* Hanson and Smith, 1975.

Phenytoin is among the 200 frequently prescribed drugs, and the most commonly prescribed anticonvulsant drug. Hemorrhagic complications in the neonate have occurred in neonates of mothers who received phenytoin (Gimovsky and Petrie, 1986; Solomon *et al.*, 1972). In three prospective studies, IQ was 10 points lower among preschool- and school-aged children exposed *in utero* to phenytoin compared to controls (Gladstone *et al.*, 1992; Scolnick *et al.*, 1994; Vanoverloop *et al.*, 1992). Importantly, none of the children was diagnosed intellectually deficient. Among 142 infants whose mothers took phenytoin during embryogenesis did not have an increased frequency of birth defects in the Swedish Birth Defects Registry (Kallen, 2019).

Cleft palate, cardiac anomalies, and skeletal defects were increased in the offspring of experimental animals that received phenytoin (Finnell, 1981; Finnell and Chernof, 1984; McClain and Langhoff, 1980).

A large meta-analysis (Veroniki *et al.*, 2018) assembled the largest collection of information on phenytoin exposure during organogenesis shows a similar pattern. The information indicates major congenital anomalies are increased, specifically cleft lip/palate (Box 9.2).

## BOX 9.2   PHENYTOIN EXPOSURE AND BIRTH DEFECTS

| Anomaly | N | Increased | Investigator |
|---|---|---|---|
| Major birth defects | 140/79,049 | Yes | Kallen, 2019 |
| Major congenital anomalies | 2237 | Yes | Veroniki *et al.*, 2018 |
| Congenital heart defects | 1697 | No | Veroniki *et al.*, 2018 |
| Cleft lip/palate | 1172 | Yes | Veroniki *et al.*, 2018 |
| Club foot | 932 | No | Veroniki *et al.*, 2018 |
| Hypospadias | 1350 | No | Veroniki *et al.*, 2018 |
| IUGR | 519 | No | Veroniki *et al.*, 2018 |

*Source:* Veroniki *et al.*, 2018.

## CARBAMAZEPINE

Carbamazepine (Tegretol) is a widely prescribed anticonvulsant, also used as an analgesic for trigeminal neuralgia and in psychiatry as a mood stabilizer. Previously, this agent was considered ideal for use during pregnancy, and in one review of 94 exposed infants, the rate of congenital anomalies was not increased over the expected rate (Niebyl *et al.*, 1979). More data became available later that indicated carbamazepine (Jones *et al.*, 1989) is associated with a pattern of congenital anomalies similar to that of phenytoin. These findings possibly indicate a syndrome associated with carbamazepine exposure during early pregnancy (Box 9.3). Two large studies indicate an increased

## BOX 9.3   CHARACTERISTICS OF FETAL CARBAMAZEPINE SYNDROME

- Craniofacial abnormalities
- Upslanting palpebral fissures
- Short nose
- Epicanthal folds
- Growth deficiency
- Limb defects
- Hypoplasia of distal phalanges, nails
- Mental deficiency
- Neural tube defects

*Sources:* Jones *et al.*, 1989; Rosa, 1991.

frequency of a variety of congenital anomalies (Box 9.4). Similarities in malformations may be related to the similarity in toxic arene epoxide intermediates when epoxide hydrolase activity is lowered, or absent.

## BOX 9.4   CARBAMAZEPINE

| | | | |
|---|---|---|---|
| All malformations | 97/79,049 | Yes | Kallen, 2019 |
| Other CNS malformations | 4/830 | Yes | Kallen, 2019 |
| Major congenital anomalies | 8237 | Yes | Veroniki *et al.*, 2017 |
| Congenital heart defects | 6336 | No | Veroniki *et al.*, 2017 |
| Cleft lip/palate | 5577 | No | Veroniki *et al.*, 2018 |
| Club foot | 450 | No | Veroniki *et al.*, 2017 |
| Hypospadias | 3540 | No | Veroniki *et al.*, 2017 |
| IUGR | 2897 | No | Veroniki *et al.*, 2017 |

As with phenytoin, it remains uncertain whether birth defects are caused by the disease process itself, the medication, a metabolite, an enzyme deficiency, or a combination of these effects (Scialli and Lione, 1989; Holmes *et al.*, 2011; Veroniki *et al.*, 2017).

In 1991 a report was published that carbamazepine may be associated with neural tube defects among 1 percent of offspring whose mothers took carbamazepine during the first trimester, similar to valproic acid (Rosa, 1991). IQ was not different between carbamazepine-exposed and controls in preschool- and school-aged children (Scolnick *et al.*, 1994). A large lumbar meningomyelocele was reported in a patient who took a megadose carbamazepine (~4.8 grams) during the period of neural tube closure (Little *et al.*, 1993). Twenty-three carbamazepine-exposed infants (n = 23) included one infant with a similar neural tube defect (myeloschisis) and multiple other major congenital anomalies (Gladstone *et al.*, 1992). Among 3,625 infants from Sweden, whose mothers took carbamazepine during pregnancy the frequency of spina bifida was increased (Kallen, 1994). In the EUROCAT birth defects monitoring system, the frequency of spina bifida was increased among 2680 carbamazepine exposed infants (Jetnik *et al.*, 2010). Among 1605 infants born to women who took carbamazepine during organogenesis, the frequency of congenital malformations was not increased in the Swedish Birth Defects Registry (Kallen, 2019), but the result approached significance (OR = 1.22, 95 percent CI: 0.95–1.58).

Birth defects were increased in frequency in offspring of pregnant animals given carbamazepine during organogenesis, including central nervous system anomalies (Finnell *et al.*, 1986; Paulson *et al.*, 1979).

## PARAMETHADIONE AND TRIMETHADIONE

The dione anticonvulsants, paramethadione (Paradione) and trimethadione (Tridione) were used primarily for the treatment of petit mal seizures, and is indicated for the of petit mal seizure control that are refractory to other drug treatments. The association between trimethadione and malformed newborns was published in 1970 (German *et al.*, 1970). Following this 1970 report, numerous reports of fetal malformations associated with maternal dione use were published. A review of 65 *in utero* exposures to either trimethadione or paramethadione was summarized in the statement: "a normal child resulting from such a pregnancy is the exception" (Kelly, 1984). No controlled studies have been published of birth defects following exposure during embryogenesis with either of these agents. However, a distinct syndrome has been described for trimethadione (Zackai *et al.*, 1975), termed the "trimethadione syndrome" (Box 9.5). Note that this syndrome differs from the hydantoin and carbamazepine syndromes only in the absence of distal digital hypoplasia (Kelly, 1984). Dione anticonvulsants are contraindicated for use during pregnancy.

---

**BOX 9.5  CHARACTERISTICS OF FETAL TRIMETHADIONE SYNDROME**

**Craniofacial Abnormalities**

- Cleft palate
- V-shaped eyebrows
- Irregular teeth
- Epicanthal folds
- Backward-sloped ears

**Other Anomalies**

- Cardiac anomalies
- Growth deficiency
- Hearing loss
- Mental deficiency
- Microcephaly
- Simian creases
- Speech difficulty

*Sources:* Kelly, 1984; Zackai *et al.*, 1975.

---

CAUTION: The diones are still available but should not be prescribed to women of reproductive age if at all possible. If diones are the only effective treatment, patients should be counseled of the risks, and directed to use effective contraception because pregnancy outcomes are very frequently complicated by multiple congenital anomalies and intellectual deficits.

## VALPROIC ACID

Valproic acid (Depakane, Myproic Acid, Depakote) is used to treat petit mal seizures. It is also used to treat myoclonic and tonic-clonic (grand mal) seizures. With the use of valproic acid an increased risk of neural tube defects and microcephaly was reported in 1980 (Dalens *et al.*, 1980; Gomez, 1981). Valproic acid during the first trimester increases the risk for neural tube defects to approximately 2 percent, compared to about 0.1 percent (one per 1,000) in the general population (CDC, 1983; Jager-Roman *et al.*, 1986; Jeavons, 1982; Koch *et al.*, 1983; Lindhout and Schmidt, 1986; Lindhout *et al.*, 1992; Omtzigt *et al.*, 1992; Padmanabhan and Hameed, 1994; Yerby *et al.*, 1992). Major and minor anomalies comprise the constellation malformations called "fetal valproate syndrome" (Box 9.6). Valproic acid in the first trimester was associated with an increased frequency of major congenital anomalies (Box 9.7). The Swedish Birth Defects Registry reported an increased frequency of birth defects among 731 infants exposed to valproic acid during embryogenesis (Kallen, 2019).

**BOX 9.6   MALFORMATIONS REPORTED TO BE ASSOCIATED
WITH VALPROIC ACID: FETAL VALPROATE SYNDROME**

| | |
|---|---|
| Brachycephaly | Hypospadias |
| Cleft palate | Low-set ears |
| Congenital heart defects | Neural tube defects |
| Hypertelorism | Small nose and mouth |

*Sources:* Compiled from Dalens *et al.*, 1980; DLiberti *et al.*, 1984; Jager-Roman *et al.*, 1986; Jeavons, 1982; Koch *et al.*, 1983; Lindhout and Meinardi, 1984; Lindhout and Schmidt, 1986; Mastroiacovo *et al.*, 1983; Tein and MacGregor, 1985; Thomas and Buchanan, 1981.

---

**BOX 9.7   VALPROIC ACID**

| Birth Defect | N | Increased Risk |
|---|---|---|
| Major congenital anomalies | 4,455 | Yes |
| Congenital heart defects | 3,194 | No |
| Cleft lip/palate | 2,721 | Yes |
| Club foot | 802 | Yes |
| Hypospadias | 802 | Yes |
| IUGR | 1,622 | No |

*Source:* Compiled from Tomson *et al.*, 2016, 2018, 2019.

---

Increased frequency of congenital anomalies was reported in offspring of pregnant animals who received valproic acid (Mast *et al.*, 1986; Moffa *et al.*, 1984).

### SUCCINIMIDES

Ethosuximide (Zarontin), methsuximide (Celontin), and phensuximide (Milontin) are succinimide anticonvulsants utilized primarily for petit mal seizures. Among more than 90 (42 and 57) infants exposed to ethosuximide during the first trimester, the frequency of congenital anomalies was not increased among the population background risk for epileptics (9–11 percent) (Samren *et al.*, 1997, 1999). Importantly, these drugs are anticonvulsant medications and are probably associated with a higher risk of congenital anomalies than these two small series indicate. The frequency of major malformations associated with ethosuximide during the first trimester is given in (Box 9.8).

**BOX 9.8   ETHOSUXIMIDE**

| Birth Defect | N | Increased Risk |
|---|---|---|
| Major congenital anomalies | 61 | Yes |
| Congenital heart defects | 31 | Yes |
| Cleft lip/palate | 29 | Yes |
| Club foot | -- | -- |
| Hypospadias | 31 | No |
| IUGR | -- | -- |

*Source:* Compiled from Tomson *et al.*, 2016, 2018, 2019.

Skeletal and central nervous system and other congenital anomalies have been observed in the offspring of pregnant animals that received ethosuximide (el-Sayed *et al.*, 1983; Sullivan and McElhatton, 1977) or methsuximide (Kao *et al.*, 1979). Ethosuximide use in late pregnancy has been reported to be associated with neonatal hemorrhage (Bleyer and Skinner, 1976).

## PHENOBARBITAL

Phenobarbital is often used in combination with other anticonvulsants. It has also been used for many years in pregnant women for a variety of other indications. There is no firm scientific evidence that phenobarbital is teratogenic, although it is often implicated because of its frequent use with other anticonvulsants. Specifically, facial clefts and heart defects seem to be increased in frequency among infants whose mothers took phenobarbital during the first trimester (Box 9.9). Detailed dysmorphic examinations indicated that phenobarbital monotherapy during pregnancy was associated with minor congenital anomalies previously associated with the fetal anticonvulsant syndrome (Holmes *et al.*, 2001). A mild reduction in the IQs of adult males exposed to phenobarbital prenatally was found in two studies (Reinisch *et al.*, 1995; Dessens *et al.*, 2000).

---

### BOX 9.9   PHENOBARBITAL

| Birth Defect | N | Increased Risk |
|---|---|---|
| Major congenital anomalies | 1709 | Yes |
| Congenital heart defects | 1255 | No |
| Cleft lip/palate | 894 | Yes |
| Club foot | 1057 | No |
| Hypospadias | 1024 | No |
| IUGR | 400 | Yes |

*Source:* Compiled from Tomson *et al.*, 2016, 2018, 2019.

---

## FELBAMATE

No studies of human neonates born after exposure to felbamate during the first trimester have been published. Two experimental animal studies were published that found no increased frequency of congenital anomalies in rats or rabbits that were exposed during embryogenesis.

## LAMOTRIGINE

The FDA warning label for use of lamotrigine during pregnancy indicates a 20- to 30-fold increase in the incidence of non-syndromic (i.e., isolated) cleft palate with the use of this drug during the first trimester. Congenital anomalies were increased in frequency ($n = 6$, 12 percent) among 51 infants whose mothers took lamotrigine during the first trimester (Lamotrigine Pregnancy Registry, 2004; Mackay *et al.*, 1997; Wilton *et al.*, 1998). Among 414 infants exposed to lamotrigine monotherapy in a registry-based study only 12 (2.9 percent) had congenital anomalies (Lamotrigine Pregnancy Registry, 2004; Tennis and Eldridge, 2002). The frequency of congenital anomalies appeared to be increased among 270 infants whose mothers took lamotrigine polytherapy (combined with one or more other anticonvulsants) during embryogenesis, 16 (5.9 percent). Frequency of major congenital anomalies was greatest among infants whose mothers took lamotrigine with valproic acid during the first trimester (11 of 88, 12.5 percent).

The frequency of congenital anomalies (2.1 percent) was not increased among 390 infants born to women who took lamotrigine monotherapy during the first trimester of pregnancy in another registry-based study (Morrow *et al.*, 2003). No birth defects were reported in 61 infants whose mothers were treated with lamotrigine monotherapy during pregnancy. Four major congenital anomalies (5.9 percent) were found in 68 infants born to women treated with an anticonvulsant polytherapy that contained lamotrigine (Vajda *et al.*, 2003). The frequency of birth defects (*n* = 1, or 2 percent) was not increased among 51 infants born following lamotrigine monotherapy during the first trimester (Sabers *et al.*, 2004). Importantly, at least 16 fetuses or infants with neural tube defects have been reported when the mother took lamotrigine, often in polytherapy with valproic acid or carbamazepine, during the first trimester (Lamotrigine Pregnancy Registry, 2004). Among 1,330 infants whose mothers used lamotrigine during organogenesis, the frequency of birth defects was not increased in the Swedish Birth Defects Registry (Kallen, 2019), but the result was almost significant (OR = 1.26, 95 percent CI: 0.94–1.69). See Box 9.10 for a summary of lamotrigine in pregnancy.

## BOX 9.10   LAMOTRIGINE

| Birth Defect | N | Increased Risk |
|---|---|---|
| Major congenital anomalies | 6290 | No |
| Congenital heart defects | 4788 | No |
| Cleft lip/palate | 4664 | No |
| Club foot | 1621 | No |
| Hypospadias | 95 | No |
| IUGR | 2882 | No |

*Source:* Compiled from Tomson *et al.*, 2016, 2018, 2019.

Experimental animal studies of lamotrigine during embryogenesis are equivocal, with a report of no increased frequency of congenital anomalies, and another reporting an increased frequency of birth defects.

### LEVETIRACETAM

The frequency of birth defects was not increased in 1,015 infants born after exposure to levetiracetam during the first (Box 9.11). Nonetheless, the nature of the disease being treated (seizure disorder) and the drug (anticonvulsive agent) have raised concerns that infants exposed to levetiracetam during gestation may be at an increased risk of birth defects. However, there was no increased frequency of birth defects in more than 1,000 infants exposed during the first trimester (Box 9.11). Among 87 infants whose mothers took levetiracetam during the first trimester in the Swedish Birth Defects Registry, no birth defects were observed (Kallen, 2019)

### BOX 9.11 LEVETIRACETAM

| Birth Defect | N | Increased Risk |
|---|---|---|
| Major congenital anomalies | 1015 | No |
| Congenital heart defects | 754 | No |
| Cleft lip/palate | 872 | No |
| Club foot | 450 | No |
| Hypospadias | 754 | No |
| IUGR | 81 | No |

*Source:* Compiled from Tomson *et al.*, 2016, 2018, 2019.

## GABAPENTIN

Congenital anomalies have been reported among 44 women who used gabapentin during pregnancy (Montouris, 2003), but (1) the anomalies (hypospadias, renal agenesis) are not consistent with the fetal anticonvulsant syndrome and (2) it is not clear from the published report precisely when during pregnancy the women were exposed. A case report of an infant with holoprosencephaly and cyclopia whose mother took carbamazepine and gabapentin during pregnancy has been published (Rosa, 1995), but it is unclear what, if any, association this has with prenatal drug exposure. Other isolated case reports have also been published (Bruni, 1998; Morrell, 1996), but their relationship to risks associated with gabapentin use during pregnancy is unknown. A case report described a child whose features resembled the 'fetal anticonvulsant syndrome' and whose mother took gabapentin and valproic acid during pregnancy (Moore *et al.*, 2000). Among 133 infants whose mothers used gabapentin during organogenesis, the frequency of birth defects was not increased in the Swedish Birth Defects Registry (Kallen, 2019). In 329 infants whose mothers used gabapentin during the first trimester, the frequency of major birth defects was not increased (Box 9.12).

### BOX 9.12 GABAPENTIN

| Birth Defect | N | Increased Risk |
|---|---|---|
| Major congenital anomalies | 329 | No |
| Congenital heart defects | 35 | Yes |
| Cleft lip/palate | 33 | No |
| Club foot | -- | -- |
| Hypospadias | 33 | Yes |
| IUGR | 70 | No |

*Source:* Compiled from Tomson *et al.*, 2016, 2018, 2019.

Experimental animal studies with mice, rats, and rabbits have not found an increased frequency of congenital anomalies among offspring exposed to gabapentin during embryogenesis.

## OXCARBAZEPINE

***Important note:*** oxcarbazepine is an anticonvulsant drug closely related to a known human teratogen, carbamazepine. This drug has been part of a polytherapy regimen in most published reports of its use during pregnancy, confounding its possible causal role. Among 248 pregnancies exposed to oxcarbazepine monotherapy during pregnancy, there were six congenital anomalies (2.4 percent), which is similar to that expected in the general population. Among 61 infants whose mothers were given polytherapy that included oxcarbazepine, four birth defects (6.6 percent) occurred (Montouris, 2005), which is greater than that in the general population. Among 372 infants exposed to oxcarbazepine during the first trimester, the frequency of birth defects was not increased (Box 9.13)

---

**BOX 9.13   OXCARBAZEPINE**

| Birth Defect | N | Increased Risk |
|---|---|---|
| Major congenital anomalies | 372 | No |
| Congenital heart defects | 346 | No |
| Cleft lip/palate | 372 | No |
| Club foot | 198 | No |
| Hypospadias | 200 | No |
| IUGR | 1002 | No |

*Source:* Compiled from Tomson *et al.*, 2016, 2018, 2019.

---

Among 35 infants born to epileptic women treated with oxcarbazepine monotherapy in one series, no congenital anomalies were found (Meischenguiser *et al.*, 2004). Among 20 infants born to women who took polytherapy anticonvulsant regimen that included oxcarbazepine, one baby was born with a major cardiac congenital anomaly. One of nine infants born to epileptic women treated in the first trimester with oxcarbazepine monotherapy had multiple major birth defects involving the genitourinary tract (Kaaja *et al.*, 2003). Isolated case reports involving polytherapy (including oxcarbazepine) of single infants with spina bifida, short spine, hypospadias, or limb reduction defects have been published (Lindhout *et al.*, 1992; Lindhout and Omtzigt, 1994). Among 51 infants exposed to oxcarbazepine during the first trimester, there were three birth defects observed in the Swedish Birth Defects Registry (Kallen, 2019), which was judged not significant.

Mølgaard-Nielsen and Hviid (2011) found 11 birth defects among infants of 393 women using oxcarbazepine, which gave an OR = 0.86 (95 percent CI: 0.46–1.59). Veroniki *et al.* (2017) in their review and meta-analysis identified 372 monotherapies with an OR of 1.32 (95 percent CI: 0.72–2.29). Among 375 infants whose mother used clonazepam during the first trimester, the frequency of congenital anomalies was not increased (Box 9.14). The causal meaning of case reports is not

---

**BOX 9.14   CLONAZEPAM**

| Birth Defect | N | Increased Risk |
|---|---|---|
| Major congenital anomalies | 375 | No |
| Congenital heart defects | 47 | No |
| Cleft lip/palate | 375 | No |
| Club foot | 34 | Yes |
| Hypospadias | 42 | No |
| IUGR | 411 | No |

*Source:* Compiled from Tomson *et al.*, 2016, 2018, 2019.

possible to ascertain. Animal teratology studies (one published, Bennett *et al.*, 1996, one unpublished) of oxcarbazepine were negative. Among 114 infants exposed to clonazepam during the first trimester, the frequency of birth defects was not increased (Kallen, 2019).

## PREGABALIN

Pregabalin is similar to gabapentin and is used to treat epilepsy, usually as an adjuvant agent. Among 164 pregnancies exposed to pregabalin during pregnancy, the frequency of birth defects was increased to 6 percent compared to 2.1 percent in 656 controls (Winterfield *et al.*, 2016). Rodents born to mothers treated with pregabalin during organogenesis had an increased frequency of skeletal malformations, neural tube defects, and pregnancy losses according to manufacturer's information. Among 184 infants whose mothers took pregabalin during embryogenesis, the frequency of birth defects was not increased in the Swedish Birth Defects Registry (Kallen, 2019).

## TIAGABINE

Among nine infants whose mothers took tiagabine during pregnancy, one infant had a congenital anomaly, but this was not similar to any of the anomalies in "fetal anticonvulsant syndrome" (Morrell, 1996).

In unpublished experimental animal studies (rats, rabbits) employing doses much higher than the human dose, and at doses toxic to the mother, there were increased frequencies of congenital anomalies in rats but not rabbits. None of this information is relevant to the assessment of human risk of birth defects following exposure to tiagabine during embryogenesis.

## TOPIRAMATE

In a case series three normal infants were reported whose mothers were treated with topiramate sometime during gestation (Morrell, 1996). In another case report, a pattern of minor anomalies similar to the 'fetal anticonvulsant syndrome' was observed in an infant whose mother took topiramate monotherapy throughout pregnancy (Hoyme *et al.*, 1998). The relevance of these anecdotal reports, if any, to human risks following exposure to topiramate during embryogenesis is unknown. Among 58 infants whose mothers took topiramate during organogenesis, the frequency of birth defects was significantly increased 4.38 fold (Kallen, 2019).

The results of studies of rats, mice, and rabbits exposed to topiramate during embryogenesis are conflicting. Rats had limb defects at the highest doses, mice had craniofacial defects, and rabbits had vertebral anomalies. The inconsistent findings and the lack of peer review of these unpublished studies confound any possible interpretation of these data.

## VIGABATRIN

Among 47 infants born to women who took vigabatrin during the first trimester two (4.3 percent) had congenital anomalies (Wilton *et al.*, 1998).

In several studies, major anomalies were increased among mice exposed to vigabatrin during embryogenesis, and cleft palate occurred among rabbits exposed to maternally and fetotoxic doses. No increased frequency of congenital anomalies was found among rats exposed to vigabatrin during embryogenesis.

## ZONISAMIDE

Zonisamide is an anticonvulsant used either in monotherapy or in polytherapy to treat a broad spectrum of epileptic conditions (Oguni *et al.*, 1988; Schmidt *et al.*, 1993). In a small prospective case series of 26 infants born to women treated throughout pregnancy with zonisamide as part of a polytherapy anticonvulsant regimen, two infants (7.7 percent) were reported with major congenital anomalies (anencephaly, atrial septal defect) (Kondo *et al.*, 1996). A child whose mother took zonisamide, carbamazepine, phenytoin, sodium valproate, and a barbiturate during pregnancy was reported with features of anticonvulsant embryopathy (Noda *et al.*, 1996).

Increased frequencies of congenital anomalies were found in animal studies of teratogenicity of zonisamide in rats (cardiac), mice (visceral, skeletal), dogs (cardiac), and monkeys (pregnancy wastage) (Terada *et al.*, 1987a, 1987b, 1987c).

## SPECIAL CONSIDERATIONS

In general, women with epilepsy should be given preconception counseling, and a management plan developed (Box 9.5). If a pregnant woman presents on anticonvulsant therapy, she should be given counseling regarding the two- to threefold increased risk of malformations. She should also be offered high-resolution ultrasound and alpha-fetoprotein screening at appropriate gestational intervals. It should be emphasized that these techniques, although helpful, may not rule out anticonvulsant embryopathy. Anticonvulsant therapy should be continued if necessary. It may be possible to discontinue medications in certain patients who have been seizure-free for protracted periods, especially in patients who have had petit mal seizures. Trimethadione and paramethadione are generally contraindicated during pregnancy, and valproic acid should be avoided if possible. One of the succinimides, ethosuximide, would appear to be a better choice for petit mal seizures in the rare pregnant patient where it is indicated. Monitoring of serum levels of anticonvulsants may be indicated in some pregnant women, especially those with increased seizure activity. A suggested management protocol for pregnant patients with epilepsy is summarized in Box 9.15.

---

### BOX 9.15   SUGGESTED PROTOCOL FOR COUNSELING MANAGEMENT OF PREGNANT WOMEN WITH EPILEPSY

Preconceptional or gravid epileptics counseling regarding a possible epilepsy-associated two- to threefold increased risk of malformations above population background rate (3.5–5 percent)

Explain that risk for neural tube defects (NTDs) is increased (see Table 9.4), as indicated
Continue anticonvulsants if necessary to control seizures

The disease itself—seizure disorder—may cause congenital anomalies and threaten maternal health; therefore, controlling seizures is a high priority

During embryogenesis [2–10 weeks estimated gestation age (EGA) by menstrual dates, or first 8 weeks of gestation by conception dates] avoid certain anticonvulsants if possible:

- Avoid trimethadione and paramethadione if seizure control can is possible with other agents.
- Avoid valproic acid, if possible.
- Avoid carbamazepine, if possible.
- Avoid polytherapy of any sort, if possible.
- Lower doses to minimum dose for seizure control.
- Avoid large anticonvulsant doses, use minimal necessary to control seizures.

- Discontinue anticonvulsants in only select patients and with neurological medical consultation serial high-resolution ultrasound examinations at appropriate intervals.
- Maternal alpha-fetoprotein screening at appropriate intervals.
- Serum anticonvulsant level monitoring.

- Dose titration to achieve therapeutic levels.
- Bear in mind that pregnancy changes the pharmacokinetics of anticonvulsants, which may indicate the need to adjust dose and/or frequency to prevent maternal seizures.
- Clearance (Cl) is uniformly increased during pregnancy (steady state concentration) is lowered.
- Plasma protein binding (PPB) is decreased during pregnancy for anticonvulsants that have been studied.

Patients should be counseled that anticonvulsant therapy during pregnancy is associated with risks of serious birth defects. For example, with valproic acid and carbamazepine, the risk for neural tube defects, spina bifida in particular, is increased with exposure during the first trimester (Table 9.6). Risks for other congenital anomalies are increased when associated with exposure to other anticonvulsants during embryogenesis (Table 9.8). Risk for valproic acid-associated neural tube defects is increased at (1) high doses (>800 mg/day) and (2) polytherapy. Interestingly, recent analyses indicate that the risk for neural tube defects with exposure to oxcarbazepine or to lamotrigine is not different from the risk with carbamazepine (Perucca, 2005).

Ratings by the FDA Pregnancy Risk Categories and Teratogen Information System (TERIS) Risk for Congenital Anomalies (Table 9.5) provide informative support for clinical decisions.

## PHARMACOGENETICS/PHARMACOGENOMICS

Many anticonvulsant drugs inhibit the metabolism of folic acid. This alteration in folate metabolism is presumed to be provoked by hepatic enzyme induction and folate malabsorption (Janz, 1982; Maxwell *et al.*, 1972). Phenobarbitone, phenytoin, carbamazepine, valproic acid, and primidone have been implicated in these metabolic alterations (Donaldson, 1991). Human and animal studies support the finding that folic acid supplementation decreases the rate of congenital malformations in infants of epileptic mothers who are receiving anticonvulsants during pregnancy (Biale and Lewenthal, 1984; Dansky *et al.*, 1987; Zhu and Zhou, 1989). Therefore, it is recommended that all women of childbearing age receive 0.4–0.5 mg per day of folic acid preconceptually and at least through the first trimester of pregnancy. Epileptic mothers with a positive history of neural tube defects or orofacial clefts in previous children, or paternal or maternal family history should be supplemented preconceptually and through the first trimester with 4–5 mg per day of folic acid, especially women taking valproic acid or carbamazepine (Perucca, 2005).

In addition, mothers receiving these anticonvulsants should be given 20 mg of vitamin K in the final month of pregnancy (Delblay *et al.*, 1982). The newborn should receive 1 mg of vitamin K at birth and again in 12 hours. Umbilical cord prothrombin, partial thromboplastin values, and vitamin-K-dependent clotting factors should be evaluated shortly after delivery (Bleyer and Skinner, 1976; Srinivasan *et al.*, 1982). Folic acid and vitamin D supplements should be considered for pregnant women on phenytoin and other similar anticonvulsants, in addition to vitamin K supplementation in the third trimester (Yerby, 2003).

Unfortunately, no anticonvulsant is known to be free from risk. Further, it is not possible to unravel the relationship of the disease being treated, the treatment for the disease, and the genetic complement of the mother and fetus in assessing the risk for birth defects in epileptic pregnancies.

The management of pregnancy in women with epilepsy requires the coordinated efforts of the patient's primary treating physician and her neurologist. With proper management, 90 percent of women with epilepsy can anticipate uneventful pregnancies and normal children.

# 10 Psychotropic Use during Pregnancy

The frequency of psychiatric disorders is relatively low during pregnancy. Bipolar disorders (0.5–1.5 percent) or schizophrenia (1–1.5 percent) are relatively infrequent during pregnancy, although 5 to 10 percent of pregnant women take psychoactive agents during pregnancy. In one survey, the frequency of depression in one large survey exceeded 25 percent. Obstetrical physicians may regularly treat patients who have used psychotropic drugs during pregnancy. In most cases, management of psychiatric disorders during pregnancy differs little from the non-pregnant state, with notable exceptions. *Pharmacokinetics of psychotropics is the major exception, and vary considerably from the non-pregnant state.* The pharmacokinetics of most drugs change with the physiological alterations of pregnancy that affect volume of distribution, clearance rate and steady-state concentration. These key parameters change during pregnancy and usually require dose adjustment to maintain therapeutic levels.

The psychotropics class that includes mood stabilizers contains drugs known to increase the risk for birth defects (valproic acid, carbamazepine, lithium). These agents are generally viewed as teratogenic) and should be avoided during embryogenesis. Newer antidepressants, serotonin selective reuptake inhibitors (SSRIs) are not associated with significant birth defect risks (Einarson and Einarson, 2005), but may be associated with complications in neonatal adaptation (Kallen, 2004; Oberlander *et al.*, 2004) or prematurity (Chambers *et al.*, 1996).

Severity of mental illness usually remains stable, does not worsen during pregnancy given that doses are adjusted properly to maintain therapeutic drug levels. The prognosis for pregnant women with a psychiatric disorder remains similar to the non-gravid state. Notably, second and third generation antidepressants (e.g., SSRIs/SNRIs) are more effective in women than the older agents (e.g., first generation or tricyclics) (Yonkers, 2003). However, the risk of depression relapse after delivery is high. *In the postpartum period, medication dose management is a key criterion for avoiding relapse because the three key parameters ($V_d$, $C_b$, $C_{ss}$) that determine drug levels decrease after delivery.*

Major diagnostic criteria for depression include anhedonia (lack of pleasure) and a chronically depressed mood. Depression is an affective disorder, and is unipolar or bipolar Depressed patients are also characterized by physical symptoms (too much or too little sleep, altered appetite, altered activity, decreased motion, or agitated pacing, low energy) and cognitive symptoms (ruminative guilty thoughts, suicidal ideation, poor concentration, indecision). Bipolar disorders have periods of mania and depression (American Psychiatric Association, 1993). Medical treatment of depression is based on the hypothesis that depression, in some cases, may be caused by an insufficient amount of serotonin and/or norepinephrine in certain areas of the brain. Similarly, the molecular basis of psychosis is thought to be secondary to abnormally elevated dopamine concentration in certain brain regions.

Pregnant women take a variety of psychotropic agents. All psychotropic drugs that have been studied cross the placenta and the embryo/fetuses will be exposed. The psychotropics used during pregnancy include antidepressants, antipsychotics, sedatives, hypnotics, and tranquilizers.

Pregnancy-associated physiological changes affect pharmacokinetics of most drugs, and psychotropics are not an exception.

## PHARMACOKINETICS

The limited data on pharmacokinetics of psychotropics during pregnancy are not consistent. While diazepam has no change in the clearance and increased half-life in gravidas compared to non-pregnant women, oxazepam has a decreased half-life and increased clearance (Table 10.1). Notably,

 DOI: 10.1201/9780429160929-10

**TABLE 10.1**

**Pharmacokinetics during Pregnancy of Some Psychotropic Drugs**

| Agent | n | EGA (weeks) | Route | AUC | $V_d$ | $C_{max}$ | $C_{ss}$ | $t_{1/2}$ | Cl | PPB | Control Group[a] | Source |
|---|---|---|---|---|---|---|---|---|---|---|---|---|
| Clorazepate | 7 | 37–42 | IM | | = | ↓ | | ↓ | ↑ | | Yes (1) | Rey *et al.* (1979) |
| Diazepam | 14 | 37–39 | IV | | ↑ | | | ↑ | = | | Yes (1) | Moore and McBride (1978) |
| Nortriptyline | 6 | 12–40 | PO | | | | ↓ | | | | Yes (2) | Wisner *et al.* (1993) |
| Oxazepam | 8 | 40 | PO | | ↑ | | | ↓ | ↑ | | Yes (3) | Tomson *et al.* (1979) |

*Abbreviations:* EGA, estimated gestational age; AUC, area under the curve; $V_d$, volume of distribution; $C_{ss}$, peak plasma concentration; $C_{ss}$, steady-state concentration; $t_{1/2}$- half life; PPB, plasma protein binding; PO, by mouth; ↓ denotes a decrease during pregnancy compared to nonpregnant values; ↑ denotes an increase during pregnancy compared to nonpregnant values; = denotes no difference between pregnant and nonpregnant values; IV, intravenous; IM, intramuscular.
*Source:* From Little, 1999.

nortriptyline levels are lower in the pregnant state compared to non-pregnant, suggesting that an increase in dose or frequency may be needed to maintain therapeutic levels.

## ANTIDEPRESSANTS

Antidepressants can generally be classified into three major groups, namely, (1) tricyclics, (2) selective serotonin reuptake inhibitors (SSRIs), and (3) monoamine oxidase inhibitors (MOAs) (Box 10.1).

---

### BOX 10.1    COMMONLY USED ANTIDEPRESSANT AGENTS

**Tricyclics**

- Amitriptyline (Amitril, Elavil, Endep, Emitrip, Enovil)
- Amoxapine (Asendin)
- Clomipramine (Anafranil)
- Desipramine (Norpramin, Pertofrane)
- Doxepin (Adapin, Sinequan)
- Imipramine (Janimine, Tofranil, Tipramine)
- Nortriptyline (Aventyl, Pamelor)
- Protriptyline (Vivactil)

**Tetracyclics**

- Isocarboxazid (Marplan)
- Maprotiline (Ludiomil)
- Monoamine oxidase inhibitors (MAOIs)
- Phenelzine (Nardil)
- Selegeline (MAO A and MAO B activity)
- Tranylcypromine (Parnate)

**Selective serotonin reuptake inhibitors (SSRIs)**

- Citalopram (Celexa)
- Escitalopram (Lexapro)

- Fluoxetine (Prozac)
- Fluvoxamine (Luvox)
- Paroxetine (Paxil)
- Sertraline (Zoloft)

**Serotonin norepinephrine reuptake inhibitors (SNRIs)**

- Duloxetine (Cymbalta)
- Venlafaxine (Effexor)

**Other**

- Bupropion (Wellbutrin)
- Mirtazapine (Avanza, Norset, Remergil, Remeron, Zispin)
- Nefazodone
- Serzone
- Trazodone (Desyrel)

## Tricyclics

Women of reproductive age are frequently prescribed tricyclic antidepressants, and with no apparent decline in their use over time.

Reviews of antidepressant use during the first trimester have associated several antidepressants with an increased risk of birth defects, including (1) citalopram (heart defects), (2) paroxetine (heart defects, anencephaly, gastroschisis), (3) venlafaxine (heart defects, neural tube defects, gastroschisis) (Table 10.2).

**TABLE 10.2**
**Birth Defects and Antidepressant Use in the First Trimester**

| Drug | Exposed Cases | Odds Ratio (95% CI) | Specific Birth Defect(s) |
|------|---------------|---------------------|--------------------------|
| Bupropion | 57 | **None significant** | None |
| Citalopram | 50 | 4.59 (0.90–23.52) | AVSD |
| Escitalopram | 43 | **None significant** | |
| Fluoxetine | 125 | **None significant** | |
| Paroxetine | 6 | 4.29 (1.13–16.32) | APVR |
| | 4 | 4.13 (0.86–19.85) | TAVPR |
| | 6 | 3.76 (1.06–13.33) | Anencephaly/ Cranioschisis |
| | 15 | 2.30(1.03–5.14) | Gastroschisis |
| Sertraline | 17 | 2.60 (0.80–8.49) | Diaphragmatic hernia |
| Venlafaxine | 15 | 2.58 (1.13–5.88) | LVOTO |
| | 8 | 4.77 (1.58–14.36) | Coarctation of aorta |
| | 18 | 2.28 (1.08–4.84) | Septal defects |
| | 9 | 2.50 (0.97–6.45) | ASD-secundum |
| | 9 | 2.47 (0.95–6.40) | Any NTD |
| | 5 | 9.82 (1.88–51.20) | Anencephaly/ Cranioschisis |
| | 22 | 2.83 (1.35–5.93) | Any oral cleft |
| | 11 | 3.11 (1.21–8.00) | Cleft palate only |
| | 7 | 4.09 (1.25–13.46) | Gastroschisis |

Tricyclic antidepressants have been reported to be associated with fetal and neonatal effects (e.g., tachycardia, cyanosis, and other withdrawal symptoms), and may cause adverse maternal effects, such as hypotension, constipation, sedation, tachycardia, and light-headedness (Miller, 1996; Prentice and Brown, 1989). However, the putative association of tricyclics (amitriptyline) with limb reduction defects has not been borne out, and may be a chance finding because of small sample size.

A recent epidemiological analysis found a higher than expected frequency of birth defects among infants, but the sample sizes for drug-specific analyses were small in several instances. Nonetheless, the study was published in a *JAMA* journal. The most conservative analysis was women who were using a specific antidepressant compared to women who used a specific antidepressant during pregnancy. Using this type of control group has the strength of comparing women with prior use of drugs in this category, but not using during the first trimester (Anderson *et al.*, 2020). The authors state that this controls for the effect of "underlying conditions" such as having a depressive disorder (Table 10.2).

## IMIPRAMINE

The prototype of tricyclic compounds is imipramine. It has efficacy in treatment of endogenous depression, and potent anticholinergic activity. Small numbers of first-trimester imipramine exposures are reported, but no sufficiently large study of imipramine is published that associated the drug with birth defects (Banister *et al.*, 1972; Crombie *et al.*, 1972; Heinonen *et al.*, 1977; Idanpaan-Heikkila and Saxen, 1973; Kuenssberg and Knox, 1972; Miller, 1994a; Rachelefsky *et al.*, 1972; Scanlon, 1969). There were 30 cases of first-trimester imipramine exposure recently reported, and the frequency of anomalies was not increased (McElhatton *et al.*, 1996) (Table 10.3). Small series have been published with 10 and 20 infants exposed in the first trimester (McElhatton *et al.*, 1996; Kallen, 2019), and these provide no signal of an increased risk for congenital anomalies.

Purported associations of limb reduction birth defects with imipramine in the first trimester raised early suspicions of teratogenicity (McBride, 1972; Morrow, 1972). **Of interest, McBride was one of the early human teratologists who correctly attributed phocomelia (limb reduction defect) to thalidomide** (McBride, 1961). McBride described other limb reductions possibly associated with drug exposure during pregnancy.

Most authorities believe chance occurrence and not causal association were related to the early reports of limb reduction birth defects with imipramine in the first trimester. Birth defects surveillance groups in North America examined drug exposure histories of hundreds of women who delivered children with limb reduction defects, and concluded evidence was insufficient to support a cause-and-effect relationship with imipramine (Banister *et al.*, 1972; Rachelefsky *et al.*, 1972) or other tricyclic antidepressants.

Three neonates whose mothers used imipramine during late third trimester exhibited symptoms consistent with withdrawal (transient respiratory, circulatory, and neurological adaptation abnormalities) (Eggermont *et al.*, 1972).

Animal studies indicate an increased frequency of congenital anomalies among the offspring of mice, rabbits, and hamsters whose mothers were given imipramine at doses several times greater than in the usual human dose (Guram *et al.*, 1980; Harper *et al.*, 1965; Jurand, 1980), but not at lower doses (Harper *et al.*, 1965; Hendrickx, 1975; Larsen, 1963; Wilson, 1974).

## AMITRIPTYLINE

Another tricyclic antidepressant, amitriptyline has marked anticholinergic and sedative activity, but has been effective in treating depression. The frequency of birth defects was not increased among 427 infants whose mothers took amitriptyline during the first trimester, 25 birth defects (5.9 percent) occurred, a rate not increased above background (Rosa, personal communication, Briggs *et al.*, 2017). One of 89 infants in another study was malformed, a rate not greater than the general population (McElhatton *et al.*, 1996).

**TABLE 10.3**

**Meta-Analyses of Psychotropic Exposure during the First Trimester**

| | Total | Elective Abortions | Miscarriages | Live Births | Anomalies n (%) | | Source |
|---|---|---|---|---|---|---|---|
| *European Network*[a] | | | | | | | McElhatton *et al.*, 1996 |
| *Tricyclics* | | | | | | | |
| Amitriptyline | 118 | 18 | 10 | 85 | 1 | 1.2 | |
| Clomipramine | 134 | 20 | 22 | 87 | 2c | 2.3 | |
| Imipramine | 30 | 1 | 3 | 27 | 2 | 7.4 | |
| *Nontricyclics* | | | | | | | |
| Amineptine | 40 | 7 | 7 | 25 | 1 | 4.0 | |
| Fluoxetine | 96 | 15 | 13 | 65 | 2 | 3.1 | |
| Fluvoxamine | 66 | 9 | 6 | 50 | 1 | 2.0 | |
| Maprotiline | 107 | 17 | 11 | 77 | 2 | 2.6 | |
| Mianserin | 48 | 5 | 7 | 37 | 1 | 2.7 | |
| Viloxazine | 23 | 4 | 2 | 17 | 0 | 0 | |
| *Meta-analysis*[b] | | | | | | | |
| Amitriptyline | 467 | - | - | 467 | 25 | 5.4 | Rosa, unpublished, 1993 |
| Amitriptyline | 742 | | | 742 | 8 | 1.1 | Kallen, 2019 |
| Clomipramine | 838 | - | - | 838 | 15 | 1.8 | Kallen and Olausson, 2003 |
| Clomipramine | 1425 | | | 1425 | 28 | 2.0 | Kallen, 2019 |
| Imipramine | 75 | - | - | 75 | 6 | 8 | Rosa, unpublished, 1993 |
| Nortriptyline | 61 | - | - | 61 | 2 | 3.3 | Rosa unpublished, 1993 |
| Nortriptyline | 108 | | | 108 | 0 | 0 | Kallen, 2019 |
| Bupropion | — | — | — | 72 | 0 | 0 | Chan *et al.*, 2005 |
| Fluoxetine | — | — | — | 300 | 9 | 3.0 | Chambers *et al.*, 1996; Goldstein, 1995; Patsuzak *et al.*, 1993 |
| Fluoxetine | 109 | - | - | 109 | 2 | 1.8 | Rosa, unpublished, 1993 |
| Fluoxetine | 453 | | 72 | 379 | 40 | 4.4 | Goldstein and Marvel, 1993 |
| Fluoxetine | 3310 | | | 3310 | 104 | 3.1 | Kallen, 2019 |
| *Meta-analysis, 21 studies* | | | | | | | |
| Fluoxetine | 11,914 | | | 11,914 | 613 | 5.1 | Gao *et al.*, 2017 |
| *Other studies* | | | | | | | |
| Paroxetine | — | — | — | 222 | 9 | 4.1 | Kulin *et al.*, 1998 |
| Paroxetine | 63 | 12 | 9 | 44 | 0 | 0 | Inman *et al.*, 1993 |
| Trazodone/Nefazodone | — | — | — | 121 | 2 | 1.7 | Einarson *et al.*, 2003 |
| Venlafaxine | — | — | — | 125 | 2 | 1.6 | Einarson *et al.*, 2001 |
| Venlafaxine | | | | 154 | 2 | 1.3 | Einarson *et al.*, 2009 |

[a] European Network of Teratology Services Surveillance of Psychotropics in Pregnancy, Adapted from McElhatton *et al.*, 1996.

[b] Einarson and Einarson, 2005.

—: not analyzed; background risk is 3.5–5%.

[c] Excludes one case of Down syndrome.

A national study, Collaborative Perinatal Project, included 21 infants whose mothers were treated with amitriptyline during the first trimester. The rate of birth defects was not increased in the exposed offspring (Heinonen *et al.*, 1977). Another large multinational study included 118 first-trimester exposures to amitriptyline among whom there was no increased frequency of congenital anomalies (McElhatton *et al.*, 1996). Transient central nervous system depression was reported in a newborn whose mother was exposed to amitriptyline throughout gestation (Vree and Zwart,

1985). However, maternal levels were high, with serum levels in the moderately toxic range; and the infant's levels were in the severely toxic range.

Animal teratology studies are not consistent, and any relevance of these findings to therapeutic use in humans is unknown.

## DESIPRAMINE

An active metabolite of imipramine, desipramine, is used to treat depression. It has sedative and anticholinergic effects, but they are much less severe than are those of imipramine. One in 31 infants whose mothers were treated with desipramine during the first trimester was malformed (Briggs *et al.*, 2021), a rate which is not increased. Similar to imipramine, neonatal symptoms consistent with withdrawal were observed when the drug was used taken throughout gestation (Webster, 1973).

## NORTRIPTYLINE

Nortriptyline is an active metabolite of amitriptyline. Two (3.3 percent) of 61 infants whose mothers had prescriptions for nortriptyline had birth defects (Rosa, personal communication, 1993, not peer reviewed). The frequency of birth defects was not increased among 108 infants whose mothers took nortriptyline during the first trimester (Kallen, 2019). A single newborn was reported with limb reduction anomalies and a dermoid cyst was born to a mother who took 30 mg nortriptyline daily in the early first trimester (Bourke, 1974). It is highly probable this is not a causal relationship, but the 'urban legend' of limb reduction with the tricyclics (amitriptyline, imipramine, nortriptyline). Transient newborn urinary retention was associated with maternal use of nortriptyline during late pregnancy (Shearer *et al.*, 1972).

## DOXEPIN

Doxepin is another tricyclic antidepressant with efficacy equivalent to imipramine, nortriptyline, and amitriptyline in treating depression, but has a stronger sedative effect than the other tricyclics. No reports have been published on studies of congenital anomalies among the infants born to women treated with doxepin during the first trimester. The frequency of congenital anomalies was not increased among rats and rabbits exposed to doxepin during embryogenesis (Owaki *et al.*, 1971a, 1971b). However, at doses 40 to 100 times those used in humans, an increase in fetal loss and neonatal death was found.

## PROTRIPTYLINE AND AMOXAPINE

No teratologic studies in animals or epidemiological studies of malformations among the newborns of pregnant women treated with protriptyline or amoxapine are published. The manufacturer reported that no birth defects were increased in frequency among the offspring of rats, mice, and rabbits given up to 10 times the usual human dose of protriptyline during organogenesis. Amoxapine was not associated with birth defects in mice, rats, and rabbits given 3 to 10 times the usual human dose of amoxapine during embryogenesis, but embryotoxicity, stillbirths, and intrauterine deaths were increased in frequency.

A metabolite of loxapine, amoxapine is an antipsychotic and antidepressant. Data on its use in pregnancy are very limited. Among 19 infants, there were three (15.8 percent) with congenital anomalies (Rosa, unpublished), high compared to the expected rate of 5.3 percent but is based on a very small number of exposed infants. This is not a sufficiently large number of exposed infants on which to base any risk assessment.

## CLOMIPRAMINE

Congenital anomalies were not increased in 134 infants exposed to clomipramine during the first trimester (McElhatton *et al.*, 1996). In a large Swedish registry analysis of 1,425 infants exposed to clomipramine during the first trimester, infants (n = 28) had an increased frequency of heart defects. In newborns exposed to clomipramine during late pregnancy, seizures and abnormalities of perinatal adaptation were observed (Cowe *et al.*, 1982; Ostergaard and Pedersen, 1982). Symptoms observed in one infant whose mother took clomipramine in late pregnancy were similar to withdrawal symptoms (increased irritability, alternating hypertonia and hypotonia, hyperreflexia, cyanosis, and hypothermia) (Boringa *et al.*, 1992). An increased frequency of central nervous system and other anomalies was found among the offspring of pregnant mice exposed to clomipramine in doses 36 times those used in humans (Jurand, 1980). Persistent behavior changes were observed in offspring of pregnant rats treated with clomipramine at doses several fold the usual human dose (de Ceballos *et al.*, 1985; Drago *et al.*, 1985; File and Tucker, 1983).

## MAPROTILINE

Maprotiline is a tetracyclic antidepressant. The frequency of congenital anomalies was not increased among 107 pregnancies exposed to maprotiline during the first trimester (McElhatton *et al.*, 1996; see Table 10.3). The frequency of birth defects was not increased among experimental animals (Esaki *et al.*, 1976; Hirooka *et al.*, 1978).

### Newer Antidepressants or Selective Serotonin Reuptake Inhibitors

Selective serotonin uptake inhibitors (SSRIs) are a relatively new class of antidepressants including citalopram, escitalopram, fluoxetine, paroxetine, and sertraline. Fluoxetine (Prozac) is probably the most commonly used and best-known agent in this group.

However, the neonatal behavioral alterations noted earlier may comprise a withdrawal syndrome.

Some authorities have anecdotally noted similar symptoms of abstinence among adults who abruptly discontinue SSRI use. Furthermore, it is suggested by some psychiatrists that infants antenatally exposed to SSRIs, and perhaps other antidepressants, remain at risk for depression as teenagers and adults.

### Citalopram

Citalopram is an SSRI used to treat depression. Among 125 pregnancies with 114 live-born infants whose mothers took citalopram during the first trimester, there was one (0.9 percent) congenital anomaly (Sivojelezova *et al.*, 2005). The authors concluded that the drug was not associated with congenital anomalies with exposure during early pregnancy, but that use of citalopram in late pregnancy was associated with increased frequency of poor neonatal adaptation, recently reported with other SSRIs (Chambers *et al.*, 1996; Costei *et al.*, 2002; Kallen, 2004; Nordeng *et al.*, 2001; Oberlander *et al.*, 2004). Analysis of the Swedish registry of 8015 pregnancies exposed to citalopram during the first trimester found no increased frequency of birth defects with first trimester exposure (Kallen, 2019). The frequency of diaphragmatic hernia was increased among 126 infants exposed to citalopram during organogenesis (Anderson *et al.*, 2020).

## ESCITALOPRAM

Among 196 infants born to women who used escitalopram in the first trimester the frequency of birth defects was not increased (5/196 = 2.6 percent) (Hoog *et al.*, 2013). In addition, the Swedish birth defects registry 1,214 infants were exposed to escitalopram during the first trimester, and the frequency of congenital anomalies was not increased (Kallen, 2019). In a recent study from the CDC (Anderson *et al.*, 2020) of 102 infants exposed to escitalopram in the first trimester in a case-control study, the frequency of birth defects was not increased.

## FLUOXETINE

Fluoxetine (Prozac) inhibits serotonin reuptake at neuronal cleft (Goldstein *et al.*, 1991). The manufacturer's registry has collected outcome information on 184 pregnancies exposed to this agent (Goldstein *et al.*, 1991). Of these, 35 resulted in spontaneous abortions and 41 pregnancies were electively terminated. Of the 114 live-born infants, 93 were normal, nine were premature, nine had perinatal complications, and three had malformations of a nonspecific type. One of these infants had major cardiac malformations and was born to a mother who took fluoxetine in the second trimester, beyond the period of embryonic cardiac development. The spontaneous abortion rate of 19 percent and malformation rate of 2–3 percent is similar to the rate of these complications in the general population.

Review of pregnancy outcomes following first-trimester exposure to fluoxetine showed no increase in congenital anomalies (Pastuszak *et al.*, 1993). In a European study, no increased frequency of birth defects among 96 first-trimester exposed pregnancies was reported (McElhatton *et al.*, 1996; see Table 10.3). The frequency of congenital anomalies was not increased above background in 493 infants exposed to fluoxetine during the first trimester (Goldstein and Marvel, 1993). Meta-analysis indicated no increased risk of congenital anomalies among 300 infants exposed to fluoxetine during the first trimester (Einarson and Einarson, 2005). Another meta-analysis of 11,914 infants exposed to fluoxetine during the first trimester, the frequency of birth defects was not increased (Gao *et al.*, 2017). In an unpublished study (Briggs *et al.*, 2021), the frequency of birth defects was not increased among 109 infants whose mothers took fluoxetine in the first trimester. Among 3,310 infants exposed to fluoxetine during the first trimester, the frequency of birth defects was not increased (Kallen, 2019). Recently, among 125 infants exposed to fluoxetine during organogenesis, birth defects were not increased (Anderson *et al.*, 2020) Congenital anomalies were not increased in frequency among 174 infants whose mothers used fluoxetine throughout pregnancy (including first trimester) (Chambers *et al.*, 1996). The rate of preterm delivery was significantly increased in the fluoxetine-exposed group. No differences in IQ or neurodevelopment were found compared to matched controls at 1.5–3 years of age among 43 children whose mothers took fluoxetine during pregnancy (Nulman and Koren, 1996).

Problems in neonatal adaptation have been reported with SSRI use in late pregnancy.

## PAROXETINE

Paroxetine and sertraline are listed under the old FDA category B drugs, but recent research calls the safety of paroxetine use during pregnancy into question. The frequency of congenital anomalies was not increased above background among 394 infants exposed to paroxetine during the first trimester (Diav-Citrin *et al.*, 2002; Ericson *et al.*, 1999; Inman *et al.*, 1993; Kulin *et al.*, 2002; McElhatton *et al.*, 1996; Wilton *et al.*, 1998). However, as recently as July 2006, the manufacturer of Paxil (paroxetine) reported that first trimester use increased the risk of birth defects by between two and three times, with the risk of congenital heart defects being doubled. This contradicts prior studies of the drug's use during the first trimester.

Further research has shown that in 1,786 infants first trimester paroxetine exposure was associated with an increased frequency of congenital heart defects (Kallen, 2019), and among 166 case infants the frequency of heart defects, anencephaly, and gastroschisis were increased (Anderson *et al.*, 2020).

## SERTRALINE

Another SSRI, sertraline is also a category B under the old FDA system. The frequency of birth defects was not increased among infants born to 326 women who took sertraline during the first trimester (Chambers *et al.*, 1999; Hendrick *et al.*, 2003; Kulin *et al.*, 2002; Wilton *et al.*, 1998).

Similarly, the frequency of congenital anomalies was not increased among 390 infants whose mothers used sertraline (Anderson *et al.*, 2020). The Swedish registry contained 8,162 infants whose mothers took sertraline during the first trimester among whom the frequency of birth defects was not increased (Kallen, 2019).

Transient problems in neonatal adaptation termed the 'neonatal adaptation syndrome' was described in infants exposed to paroxetine in late pregnancy (Costei *et al.*, 2002).

### OTHER NON-TRICYCLIC ANTIDEPRESSANTS

Data have been published for other non-tricyclic antidepressants that are not discussed earlier. No increased frequency of congenital anomalies was found among 40, 66, 48, and 23 infants exposed during the first trimester to amineptine, fluvoxamine, mianserin, and viloxazine, respectively (McElhatton *et al.*, 1996; see Table 10.3).

## BUPROPION

Bupropion is used as an antidepressant and also in tobacco smoking cessation treatment. Bupropion use in the first trimester was not associated with an increased risk of congenital anomalies among 354 infants whose mothers used the drug during the first trimester (12 birth defects, or 3.4 percent) (Bupropion Registry, 2004). One study reported no birth defects in 105 infants after first trimester exposure to bupropion (Chun-Fai-Chan *et al.*, 2005), another study reported no increased frequency in 1213 (Cole *et al.*, 2007), and among 675 infants exposed to the drug during organogenesis the rate of congenital anomalies was not increased (2.7 percent) (GlaxoSmithKline, 2008). Among 8856 infants exposed to bupropion during organogenesis, the frequency of congenital heart defects was not increased (Huybrechts *et al.*, 2014). Bupropion is an FDA category B drug under the old classification. In a recent analysis of 229 infants whose mothers used bupropion during the first trimester, the frequency of diaphragmatic hernia and intestinal atresia were increased in frequency (Anderson *et al.*, 2020).

## TRAZODONE

Trazodone is an antidepressant that is also given for its sedative activity. First-trimester exposure to trazodone in 100 infants was not associated with an increased frequency of congenital anomalies (Rosa, personal communication, cited in Briggs *et al.*, 2021), although this study is not peer reviewed. In another investigation that was peer reviewed, 121 women took trazodone or nefazodone during the first trimester. The frequency of congenital anomalies was not increased above that expected in the general population (3.5 percent) (Einarson *et al.*, 2003). Trazodone is a category C drug.

### MONOAMINE OXIDASE INHIBITORS

Monoamine oxidase inhibitors (MAOIs) are another medication class to treat depression. No epidemiological studies are published that analyzed the safety of MAO agents during pregnancy. Only 21 pregnancies with first trimester exposure to the monoamine oxidase inhibitors are published, with an apparent increase in birth defects (Heinonen *et al.*, 1977). It is impossible to make clinically useful recommendations because the sample size is too small.

Animal teratology studies of monoamine oxidase inhibitors are not consistent. Some investigations have reported no increased frequency of birth defects with tranylcypromine (Poulson and Robson, 1963), but others studies reported an increase in mortality and stillbirth rates in the isocarboxazid group (Werboff *et al.*, 1961). Placental infarcts were more frequent in pregnant rats treated with iproniazid during gestation (Poulson *et al.*, 1960). No animal teratology studies are published regarding phenelzine.

MAOIs are not commonly used during pregnancy because of potential adverse maternal side effects, and are FDA category C drugs under the old system. Women who use this class of drugs must follow a diet low in tyramine. Hypertensive crises may occur if patients on monoamine oxidase inhibitors consume foods high in tyramine Importantly, monoamine oxidase inhibitors given with meperidine, or other similar agents, may cause hyperthermia (Happe, 2007).

## ANTIPSYCHOTICS

Antipsychotics are used to treat psychosis of any cause (e.g., psychotic depression, bipolar disorder, substance-induced hallucinations, delirium-induced psychosis). These medications are used "Off-label" to augment antidepressant and anti-anxiolytic therapy. Antipsychotic drugs are usually continued only as long as the underlying cause of psychosis is present because tardive dyskinesia occurs in association with these medications, and is not always transient. Antipsychotic drugs were formerly called neuroleptics or major tranquilizers.

Antipsychotics, with the exception of clozapine (Box 10.2), are dopamine antagonists. Antipsychotics have numerous side effects including anticholinergic effects such as constipation, dryness, marked sedation and orthostatic hypotension, and extrapyramidal side effects such as akathisia (Miller, 1996). Transient neonatal side effects including withdrawal symptoms and extrapyramidal dysfunction (hand posturing, tremors, and irritability) are associated with antipsychotic use in late pregnancy (Auerbach *et al.*, 1992; Miller, 1994a, 1996; Sexson and Barak, 1989).

There are two major problems confounding the possible associations of antipsychotics and congenital anomalies. A number of antipsychotics are used for indications other than psychosis (hyperemesis, anxiety), but lower doses may be used. In addition, the psychiatric disease itself may be associated with an increased frequency of malformations (Elia *et al.*, 1987; Anderson *et al.*, 2020).

---

**BOX 10.2   COMMONLY USED ANTIPSYCHOTIC AGENTS**

- Chlorpromazine (Thorazine)
- Fluphenazine (Prolixin, Permitil)
- Haloperidol (Haldol, Decanoate)
- Loxapine (Loxitane, Daxolin)
- Mesoridazine (Serentil)
- Molindone (Moban, Lidone)
- Perphenazine (Etrafon, Trilafon)
- Thioridazine (Mellaril)
- Thiothixene (Navane)
- Trifluoperazine (Stelazine)
- Aripiprazole (Abilify)
- Clozapine (Clozaril)

**Newer Antipsychotics**

- Amisulpride (Solian)
- Aripiprazole (Abilify)
- Amisulpride (Solian)
- Clozapine (Clozaril)
- Olanzapine (Zyprexa)
- Risperidone (Risperdal)
- Sertindole (Serdolect)
- Ziprasidone (Geodon)

## Butyrophenones

### Haloperidol

Haloperidol, a butyrophenone derivative, is a major tranquilizer that has actions similar to the piperazine phenothiazines, but is chemically related to this drug group. It is used to treat psychosis, Tourette's syndrome, mania, and severe hyperactivity. At lower doses, it is used to treat nausea or anxiety. In a cohort study of 90 pregnant women who received haloperidol for hyperemesis gravidarum during the first trimester at lower doses than for psychosis (1.2 mg b.i.d.), no birth defects or adverse fetal effects were reported (van Waes and van de Velde, 1969). In an unpublished study, 56 infants exposed to haloperidol during the first trimester (for unknown indications and at unknown doses), congenital anomalies were not increased in frequency (n = 3, or 5.4 percent) (Rosa, personal communication, 1993) It is unknown how this finding relates to treatment of psychosis. In the Swedish registry, 124 infants were exposed to haloperidol in the first trimester, and the frequency of congenital anomalies (4.0 percent) was not increased (Kallen, 2019). Three cases of newborns with limb reduction malformations after haloperidol exposure during the first trimester have been published (Dieulangard et al., 1966; Kopelman et al., 1975; Diav-Citrin et al., 2005), but anecdotal observations cannot address cause-effect relations.

Large doses of haloperidol in pregnant animals and adverse fetal effects and pregnancy losses have been reported (Druga et al., 1980; Gill et al., 1982; Szabo and Brent, 1974), but not at lower doses (Bertelli et al., 1968; Hamada and Hashiguchi, 1978). As noted throughout this volume, the relevance of animal studies to safety of drugs in human pregnancy is inconsistent and not reliably predictive.

### Loxapine

Loxapine, a dibenzoxazepine derivative, is used to treat schizophrenia. No information on the use of this tricyclic antipsychotic during pregnancy in humans has been published as of 2020. In mice and rats whose mothers were treated with loxapine during embryogenesis, a low incidence of exencephaly and an increase in fetal loss was observed in only one mouse litter out of 20 studied (Mineshita et al., 1970).

## Phenothiazines

Phenothiazines have potent adrenergic-blocking action that depress the central nervous system and prolongs effects of narcotic or hypnotic drugs. They are also associated with hypotensive, antiemetic, and antispasmodic activity. Severe side effects include extrapyramidal symptoms (including akathisia and tardive dyskinesia), hyperprolactinemia, and weight gain.

### Chlorpromazine

Another phenothiazine derivative, chlorpromazine, is used to treat psychoses. It has tranquilizing and sedative effects. Chlorpromazine is used at low doses as an antiemetic during pregnancy. Hypotension and extrapyramidal tract symptoms are well-described side effects of this drug that need special attention. Birth defects were not increased in frequency among 142 infants born to women exposed to chlorpromazine during the first trimester (Heinonen et al., 1977). The frequency of congenital anomalies was not increased in 264 infants whose mothers took chlorpromazine for hyperemesis gravidarum in the first trimester (Farkas and Farkas, 1971). Among 57 infants whose mothers used chlorpromazine during the first trimester, the frequency of birth defects (n = 4, microcephaly/clubfoot, syndactyly, endocardial fibroelastosis, microcephaly, or 7 percent) was elevated compared to controls (Rumeau-Rouquette et al., 1977). These findings are confounded by multiple drug exposure in three of the four infants with birth defects, and microcephaly was delivered of a woman who had a prior child with microcephaly. The frequency of congenital anomalies or pregnancy loss in 52 pregnancies was not increased among those exposed to chlorpromazine. However, three infants were reported with respiratory distress delivered from mothers treated with 500–600 mg per day (Sobel, 1960). In an unpublished study, 36 infants were exposed to chlorpromazine, none of whom had a birth defects (Rosa personal communication, Briggs *et al.*, 2021). A case of congenital defects involving the heart in association of phenothiazine use during gestation was reported (Vince, 1969), but this is anecdotal and its significance is unknown. Chlorpromazine use during late pregnancy was associated with transient newborn neurological dysfunction (Hammond and Toseland, 1970; Hill *et al.*, 1966; Levy and Wisniewski, 1974; Tamer *et al.*, 1969). Extrapyramidal signs in exposed infants included muscle rigidity, hypertonia, and tremor.

Experimental teratology studies are inconsistent, with several finding an increased frequency of congenital anomalies in animals exposed to chlorpromazine during embryogenesis (Brock and von Kreybig, 1964; Jones-Price *et al.*, 1983b; Singh and Padmanabhan, 1978; Yu *et al.*, 1988). However, four other studies did not find an association between chlorpromazine and exposure during early pregnancy (Beall, 1972; Jelinek *et al.*, 1967; Jones-Price *et al.*, 1983a; Robertson *et al.*, 1980).

## Fluphenazine

Fluphenazine is a piperazine phenothiazine used to treat psychosis. The frequency of congenital anomalies was not increased among 226 infants whose mothers who took fluphenazine as an antiemetic during the first trimester, (King *et al.*, 1963). Transient extrapyramidal signs in the newborn were observed several weeks after delivery of a newborn exposed to fluphenazine *in utero* (Cleary, 1977). The frequency of congenital anomalies was not increased in the offspring of pregnant rats exposed to this phenothiazine during organogenesis compared to unexposed controls (Jahn and Adrian, 1969; Adrian, 1973).

## Mesoridazine

Mesoridazine, a piperidyl phenothiazine, is the major active metabolite of thioridazine and is an effective antipsychotic agent. No published epidemiological studies or case reports are available of mesoridazine use in the first trimester. Phenothiazines that have been studied appear to be safe to use during gestation. It was given to pregnant rats and rabbits at doses 12 times in the usual human dose, of mesoridazine during organogenesis, and the frequency of congenital anomalies was not increased among the offspring of rats and rabbits (Van Ryzin *et al.*, 1971).

## Perphenazine

Perphenazine, another a piperazine phenothiazine tranquilizer, is used to treat psychoses. At lower doses, it is used to treat nausea and vomiting. Birth defects were not increased in 63 infants whose mothers used perphenazine during the first trimester (Heinonen *et al.*, 1977). Unpublished data indicated no increased frequency of birth defects in 140 infants exposed to this drug during the first trimester (Rosa, unpublished data, 1993). According to the Swedish Registry, the frequency of birth defects was not increased among 124 infants whose mothers took perphenazine during the first trimester (Kallen, 2019).

The frequency of somatic chromosomal abnormalities (breaks and rearrangements) in peripheral blood lymphocytes was reported in patients who took perphenazine (Nielen *et al.*, 1969), but the relevance of this to gametic chromosomes is unknown. Typically, somatic chromosomes are not conserved because they have no genetic progeny. Only breaks in gametic chromosomes are relevant to reproduction or genetic toxicity. Offspring of pregnant rats treated with perphenazine at many times the usual human dose had an increased frequency of cleft palate and micromelia (Beall, 1972; Druga, 1976). It is speculated that suppression of the mother's appetite was a proximate cause in cleft palate teratogenesis (Szabo and Brent, 1974, 1975). However, an infant born after megadose perphenazine in a suicide gesture during the first trimester had birth defects similar to the animal models that were exposed to high doses (Wertelecki *et al.*, 1980). The infant had birth defects similar to those observed in animal models, and included microcephaly, cleft palate, micrognathia, ambiguous genitalia, and foot deformities.

## Thioridazine

The prototype piperidine compound, thioridazine is a piperidyl phenothiazine tranquilizer. It used to treat psychoses, emotional disorders, and severe behavioral problems. A small series of 23 newborns exposed to this medication during the first trimester was reported and no congenital defects were found (Scanlon, 1972). Unpublished data (Rosa, 1993) from Michigan reported no increased frequency of birth defects (n = 2, 3.2 percent) among 63 infants who were exposed to thioridazine during the first trimester. The Swedish Birth Defects Registry reported another small cohort of 33 infants exposed during the first trimester, and there was one birth defect (3 percent) (Kallen, 2019). An increased frequency of cleft palate was observed in offspring of mice and rats whose mothers were thioridazine at doses several times the usual humans dose during embryogenesis (Szabo and Brent, 1974). However, the frequency of cleft palate was not increased in frequency when mothers were force fed (Szabo and Brent, 1975).

## Thiothixene

Thiothixene, a phenothiazine derivative, is a tranquilizer used to treat psychosis. Its chemical structure and pharmacological activity are similar to the piperazine phenothiazine compounds. First-trimester exposure to thiothixene was not associated with an increased frequency of congenital anomalies among 38 infants in one study (Rosa, 1993, unpublished). Birth defects were not increased in frequency in offspring of pregnant mice or rabbits given 20–180 times the usual human dose of thiothixene during embryogenesis (Owaki *et al.*, 1969a, b).

## Molindone

Molindone is an indole derivative not related chemically to other antipsychotic drugs. No studies have been published of birth defects in newborns that were exposed to molindone *in utero*, and no studies in animals evaluating its teratogenic effects are available. In pregnant rats or rabbits given 6 and 69 times the usual human dose during organogenesis, no birth defects were reported (Gopalakrishnan *et al.*, 2018).

## Lithium Salts and Bipolar Treatment

Bipolar disorder is treated with mood stabilizers (lithium, anticonvulsants, antipsychotics) with an adjuvant antidepressant, if necessary. Lithium is effective in the prophylaxis and treatment of affective psychiatric disorders.

Of all the psychotropic agents currently available, lithium has received the greatest attention as a possible teratogen, particularly for Ebstein's anomaly, which is induced between two and six weeks post-conception.

Congenital heart defects, particularly Ebstein's anomaly, were increased among the infants of mothers who took lithium carbonate during the first trimester (Nora *et al.*, 1974). However, the magnitude of these risks has been questioned (Cohen *et al.*, 1994), and recent analyses seem to attenuate the risks associated with lithium use during pregnancy to levels lower than previously thought (Table 10.4).

Three congenital anomalies (5 percent) were reported among 60 infants exposed to lithium *in utero*, which is not different from the background rate in the general population (Schou and Amidsen, 1971). Among 50 women who took lithium during gestation, one infant had myelomeningocele, one had unilateral hernia, and none had congenital heart defects (Cunniff *et al.*, 1989). No maternal history of lithium ingestion was found among 40 infants with Ebstein's anomaly and in 44 with tricuspid atresia (Kallen, 1988). The risk of Ebstein's anomaly and other birth defects was reevaluated, and the risk of cardiac anomalies appears to be much less than estimated in previous studies (Cohen *et al.*, 1994; Miller, 1994a, 1996). The early recommendation that women who take lithium salts during early gestation should undergo prenatal diagnosis with fetal echocardiography (Allan *et al.*, 1982) is still valid (Yonkers *et al.*, 2004). The risk of birth defects associated with

**TABLE 10.4**

**Lithium Exposure during First Trimester and Congenital Anomalies: A. Cohort Studies, B. Case-Control Studies, and C. Metanalyses**

| | Exposed N | Non-Heart Anomalies n/N | % | Heart Anomalies n/N | % | Ebstein's Anomaly | n/N% |
|---|---|---|---|---|---|---|---|
| **A. Cohort Studies** | | | | | | | |
| Background | | 35/1000 | 3.5% | 8/1000 | 0.8% | 1/20 000 | 0.005% |
| Weinstein (1980) | 225 | 7/225 | 3.1% | 18/225 | 8.0% | 6/225 | 2.7% |
| Jacobsen *et al.* (1992) | 138 | 3/138 | 2.2% | 0/138 | 0% | 1/138[a] | 0.8% |
| Kallen and Tandberg (1983) | 59 | 11/59 | 1 8.6% | 4/59 | 6.8% | 0/59 | 0% |

| | Ebstein's Anomaly Lithium Exposure | | Unaffected Control Lithium Exposure | |
|---|---|---|---|---|
| **B. Case-Control Studies** | **Yes** | **No** | **Yes** | **No** |
| Kallen (1988) | 69 | 0 | 128 | 0 |
| Edmonds and Oakley (1990) | 34 | 0 | 34 | 0 |
| Zalzstein *et al.*, 1990 (1994) | 59 | 0 | 168 | 0 |
| Correa-Villasenor *et al.* (1994) | 47 | 0 | 3572 | 0 |

**C. Meta-Analysis (Munk-Olsen *et al.*, 2018)**

| | N Anomalies | Pooled | N | Anomalies Pooled | | OR | |
|---|---|---|---|---|---|---|---|
| Major anomalies | 621 | 47 | 7.4% | 20,957 | 856 | 4.3% | 1.71 (1.07–2.72) |
| Major cardiac anomalies | 621 | 16 | 2.1% | 20,957 | 316 | 1.6% | 1.54 (0.64–3.70) |

[a] The case of Ebstein's anomaly was a therapeutic abortion.

lithium was probably overestimated in the past (Yonkers *et al.*, 2004). The risk is "likely to be weak if it exists" and the 'data certainly do not support the 30-fold increased risk of Ebstein's anomaly suggested by the Register of Lithium Babies' (Moore, 1995). Nonetheless, first-trimester exposure to lithium is an indication for a fetal echocardiogram, targeting the competence and function of the tricuspid valve.

Physical and mental anomalies were found in a follow-up study of 60 school-aged children who were exposed to lithium *in utero* (Schou, 1976). Newborns whose mothers took lithium salts near term suffer lithium toxicity, including cardiac, hepatic, and neurological abnormalities, it has been reported (Morrell *et al.*, 1983; Woody *et al.*, 1971). Diabetes insipidus and polyhydramnios are also complications attendant to lithium-exposed pregnancies: "In light of this evidence and our study results, we suggest that lithium exposure is associated with an increased risk of malformations and these findings should guide treatment decisions and future studies" (Munk-Olsen *et al.*, 2018).

Cleft palate, eye and ear defects, and fetal loss were increased in frequency in animal teratology studies among the offspring exposed to lithium carbonate *in utero* (Smithberg and Dixit, 1982; Szabo, 1970; Wright *et al.*, 1971). Animal teratology studies of lithium are inconsistent and it is not possible to interpret these data for use in evaluation of human exposures.

In summary, prenatal screening for possible congenital heart defects remains recommended because cardiac anomalies remain the main known risk, although the most recent data suggests Ebstein's anomaly risk may have been overestimated in prior years.

## SEDATIVES, HYPNOTICS, AND TRANQUILIZERS

### Barbiturates

Barbituric acid salts are the active ingredient in barbiturates, a family of drugs that have analgesic, anticonvulsant, sedative, and hypnotic actions.

### Phenobarbital

Phenobarbital is a barbiturate used to treat seizure disorders. In the past this drug was used for mild anxiety or sedation, but it is now rarely used for that purpose today. Administration of phenobarbital is usually via the oral route, but it may be given parenterally if necessary.

Possible teratogenic effects of phenobarbital and phenytoin were suspected early among 262 infants whose mothers used phenobarbital and phenytoin because three cases of cleft palate occurred in the treatment group (Janz and Fuchs, 1964), but it was later reported that epilepsy may be associated with cleft palate (Meadow, 1968). In another study of 65 infants born to women with epilepsy, 10 infants had major birth defects, and five of those were cleft palate (Elshove and van Eck, 1971).

The risk for the pregnant woman treated with phenobarbital and other seizure medications of having an infant with congenital malformations is two to three times greater than that of the general population. It is not clear whether the increased risk is secondary to the anticonvulsants, genetic factors, the seizure disorder itself, or possibly a combination of these factors (Kelly, 1984).

Evidence implicates anticonvulsants as the etiology (Hanson and Buehler, 1982). An increased frequency of minor and major congenital anomalies was found among offspring of pregnant women who received phenobarbital during gestation for seizure disorders compared to women who received the drug for other reasons (Hanson and Buehler, 1982). The frequency of congenital anomalies was not increased in several studies of children born to women who were treated with phenobarbital for epilepsy when compared to the offspring of women with epilepsy who were not treated (Greenberg *et al.*, 1977; Nakane *et al.*, 1980; Robert *et al.*, 1986; Rothman *et al.*, 1979). In an analysis of phenobarbital monotherapy exposure separately (i.e., no other concomitant anticonvulsants), the frequency of congenital anomalies was not always increased (Nakane *et al.*, 1980). In a multinational European collaborative study of 250 infants born to women with epilepsy, the frequency of congenital malformations was the same among those who received phenobarbital monotherapy and those who received monotherapy with other anticonvulsants (Bertollini *et al.*, 1987). A slight, but significant, reduction in birth weight and head circumference was found among 55 newborns born to epileptic women who used phenobarbital during gestation, compared to newborns of women without epilepsy (Mastroiacovo *et al.*, 1988). Notably, a similar effect on head circumference was observed among the newborns of women with epilepsy who received no treatment, implicating the disease. No increased frequency of congenital malformations was found among the offspring of over 1400 pregnant women who received phenobarbital during the first trimester (Heinonen *et al.*, 1977).

Characteristic dysmorphic features of the fetal hydantoin syndrome are commonly seen in newborns of women with epilepsy treated with both phenytoin and phenobarbital during gestation, and are discussed in Chapter 9 in the section on antiseizure medications during pregnancy. Sporadic reports of similar dysmorphic features among the infants of women with epilepsy who received phenobarbital monotherapy have been published (Robert *et al.*, 1986; Seip, 1976).

The frequency of cleft palate, cardiovascular defects, and other congenital malformations were increased among the offspring of pregnant mice or rats given phenobarbital in doses greater than those used in humans (Finnell *et al.*, 1987; Fritz *et al.*, 1976; Nishimura *et al.*, 1979; Sullivan and McElhatton, 1977; Vorhees, 1983). Malformations observed included facial anomalies similar to those observed in human newborns delivered to women with epilepsy who received anticonvulsants during gestation. A decrease in the number of specific brain cells and changes in neonatal behavior have been observed in animal studies of gestational exposure to the drug (Bergman *et al.*, 1980;

Takagi *et al.*, 1986; Vorhees, 1983, 1985). The relevance of these observations to the clinical use of phenobarbital in humans is unknown.

Transient neonatal sedation or withdrawal symptoms that include hyperactivity, irritability, and tremors have been observed among newborns exposed to phenobarbital during pregnancy (Desmond *et al.*, 1972; Koch *et al.*, 1985). Hemorrhagic disease of the newborn has been associated with phenobarbital use during pregnancy and typically begins within the first 24 hours of life (Gimovsky and Petrie, 1986; Mountain *et al.*, 1970). The exact cause of this hemorrhagic defect is unknown, but is probably related to phenobarbital induction of fetal liver microsomal enzymes that deplete fetal vitamin K and suppress the synthesis of vitamin-K-dependent clotting factors II, VII, IX, and X. In contrast, maternal phenobarbital therapy immediately before delivery has been used to prevent intraventricular hemorrhage in premature newborns (Morales and Koerten, 1986; Shankaran *et al.*, 1986).

A follow-up study of 114 adult males whose mothers used phenobarbital while pregnant showed lowered IQ scores by approximately 7–10 points, and it was concluded that phenobarbital exposure during early development could have long-term deleterious cognitive effects. However, detrimental environmental conditions (i.e., maternal epilepsy) may intensify such negative outcomes (Reinisch *et al.*, 1995).

## Amobarbital

Amobarbital, a barbiturate, is an effective sedative usually administered orally. The frequency of major and minor congenital anomalies was not increased among 298 infants born to women treated with amobarbital exposure during the first trimester (Heinonen *et al.*, 1977). Amobarbital use during the first trimester was possibly associated with cardiovascular defects (seven cases), inguinal hernia (nine cases), clubfoot (four cases), genitourinary anomalies (three cases), and polydactyly in Black infants (two cases). In a survey including over 1,300 women exposed to multiple agents, of whom 175 infants were exposed to amobarbital during the first trimester, the frequency of congenital anomalies was increased (Nelson and Forfar, 1971). Authorities in the field generally believe that this drug is not likely to be a teratogen and that the significant associations may be due to chance and conducting multiple statistical comparisons (Friedman and Polifka, 2006).

## Aprobarbital

Aprobarbital is a barbiturate used as a sedative and hypnotic agent. No information has been published regarding its safety for use during pregnancy. Furthermore, no studies in animals evaluating the teratogenic effects of aprobarbital have been published.

## Butalbital

A number of analgesic compounds contain butalbital, a short-acting barbiturate with hypnotic and sedative properties. Among 112 infants whose mothers took butalbital during the first trimester, no increased frequency of congenital anomalies was found among the offspring (Heinonen *et al.*, 1977). Transient neonatal withdrawal was reported in association with butalbital use late in gestation (Ostrea, 1982). No animal studies of possible teratogenic effects of butalbital have been published.

## Pentobarbital

Pentobarbital is an effective, short-acting barbiturate that is used as a hypnotic and sedative agent, and is typically given orally. Among 250 infants whose mothers took pentobarbital during the first trimester, the frequency of congenital malformations was not increased (Heinonen *et al.*, 1977). Similarly, among more than 50 newborns born to women exposed to pentobarbital during the first trimester of gestation, the frequency of birth defects was no greater than expected (Jick *et al.*, 1981).

Skeletal and craniofacial defects, as well as fetal loss, were increased among the offspring of pregnant mice, golden hamsters, and rabbits given pentobarbital many times the doses that are used in humans (Hilbelink, 1982; Johnson, 1971; Setala and Nyyssonen, 1964). Changes in behavior and decreased brain-body weight ratios were reported among the offspring of pregnant rats administered 20–40 times the human dose of pentobarbital during embryogenesis (Martin *et al.*, 1985). The relevance of these findings in animals to the clinical use of this barbiturate in humans is unknown.

## Mephobarbital

Mephobarbital, which is used as an anticonvulsant and sedative, is metabolized by the liver to phenobarbital and thus has similar properties. Results in a Japanese multi-institutional study found no increased frequency of congenital anomalies in a cohort of 111 infants born to women who used mephobarbital during the first trimester.

One hundred and eleven infants born to pregnant epileptics who used mephobarbital during the first trimester were similar to those for the infants of pregnant epileptics treated with other medications (Nakane *et al.*, 1980). In a small case series, the frequency of congenital malformations was no greater among the newborns of 17 epileptic mothers exposed to mephobarbital during the first trimester of pregnancy than among the newborns of epileptic mothers who received no treatment (Annegers *et al.*, 1974). No animal teratology studies of mephobarbital have been published.

## Secobarbital

Secobarbital is as effective as pentobarbital and is generally administered orally. Among 378 infants born to women who took secobarbital during the first trimester, the frequency of congenital anomalies was not increased (Heinonen *et al.*, 1977). One report of an infant with neonatal withdrawal symptoms of hyperirritability and seizures associated with maternal use of large doses of secobarbital throughout gestation has been published (Bleyer and Marshall, 1972).

## BENZODIAZEPINES

Benzodiazepines are minor tranquilizers with mild anticonvulsant and sedation properties (Box 10.3). These agents differ in potency and duration of effect, and indications for their use are based upon these features. They are commonly used anxiolytic agents. Of these, diazepam is probably the most frequently used drug.

---

### BOX 10.3   COMMONLY USED SEDATIVES, HYPNOTICS, AND TRANQUILIZERS

**Barbiturates**

- Amobarbital (Amytal)
- Aprobarbital (Alurate)
- Butalbital
- Mephobarbital (Mebaral)
- Pentobarbital (Nembutal)
- Phenobarbital
- Secobarbital (Seconal)

**Benzodiazepines**

- Alprazolam (Xanax)
- Chlordiazepoxide (Librium)
- Clonazepam (Klonopin)
- Diazepam (Valium)

- Lorazepam (Ativan)
- Oxazepam (Serex)

**Miscellaneous sedatives and hypnotics**

- Chloral hydrate
- Eszopiclone (Lunesta)
- Ethchlorvynol (Placidyl)
- GHB: Gamma hydroxy butyrate
- Hydroxyzine (Vistaril, Atarax)
- Meprobamate (Equanil, Equagesic, Miltown, Deprol)
- Methaqualone (Quaalude, Sapor, Parest)
- Ramelteon (Rozerem)
- Zaleplon (Sonata)
- Zolpidem (Ambien)

## Diazepam

Diazepam is a benzodiazepine used as a tranquilizer, skeletal muscle relaxant, and preanesthetic medication. Diazepam is also used to treat alcohol withdrawal and as an adjunct to anticonvulsants in the treatment of seizure disorders. It is the most extensively used drug in the benzodiazepine family.

Inconsistencies in the currently available epidemiological data on the risk of congenital anomalies among newborns of women who were exposed to diazepam during gestation confound the issue. Diazepam use during the first trimester was not associated with an increased frequency of malformations among the newborns of more than 150 women in two cohorts, or among 60 newborns of women who used the drug in the first trimester (Aselton *et al.*, 1985; Crombie *et al.*, 1975; Jick *et al.*, 1981).

In contrast, first-trimester diazepam use was increased almost threefold among 1427 infants with congenital malformations compared to controls in one study (Bracken and Holford, 1981), but not in another case-control study that included 417 newborns with multiple congenital malformations (Czeizel, 1988). A hypothesized "benzodiazepine embryofetopathy" (typical facial features, neurological dysfunction, and other anomalies) (Laegreid *et al.*, 1987, 1989) is not widely accepted in the human teratology community. Some early evidence suggested that maternal use of diazepam or other benzodiazepines during the first trimester of gestation was associated with facial clefts in the infants (Aarskog, 1975; Safra and Oakley, 1975; Saxén, 1975; Saxén and Saxén, 1975); more extensive studies have not confirmed this association. Among the infants of women who had first-trimester exposure to antineurotics (mainly diazepam) the frequency of congenital anomalies was not increased (Crombie *et al.*, 1975; Rosenberg *et al.*, 1983; Shiono and Mills, 1984). On balance, the possible risk of cleft lip or palate in the infant of a women exposed to diazepam during the first trimester, if increased at all, is less than 1 percent. Notably, family history of congenital anomalies is a confounder in at least two of these studies.

Maternal use of diazepam or related compounds during the first trimester of pregnancy and an increased risk for cardiovascular anomalies was observed in two case-control studies involving 773 infants (Bracken and Holford, 1981; Rothman *et al.*, 1979). However, in a reanalysis, no significant association was found (Bracken, 1986). In a follow-up study of 298 infants with congenital heart defects, no association with first-trimester diazepam was found (Zierler and Rothman, 1985). The risk for congenital heart disease among the infants of women who have first-trimester exposure to diazepam, is probably not increased, but if it is increased the magnitude is small (<1–2 percent).

Diazepam is readily transferred across the placenta to the human fetus and is concentrated in the fetal compartment with a 2:1 ratio (Erkkola *et al.*, 1974). Apnea, hypotonia, and hypothermia were observed in newborns of women who took diazepam during the third trimester of pregnancy or peripartum (Cree *et al.*, 1973; Gillberg, 1977; Owen *et al.*, 1972; Speight, 1977). Tremors, irritability, and hypertonia similar to neonatal narcotic withdrawal was observed in some infants chronically exposed *in utero* during the third trimester to diazepam (Rementeria and Bhatt, 1977). Loss of beat-to-beat fetal heart rate variability was associated with diazepam exposure during late pregnancy (Scher *et al.*, 1972) and decrease in fetal movement (Birger *et al.*, 1980). The effect of prenatal exposure to this drug and any untoward central nervous system function in later life is unknown. A few reports of normal infants born to women who took toxic doses of diazepam during gestation, with the majority of cases occurring after the first trimester have been published (Cerqueira *et al.*, 1988; Czeizel, 1988).

Animal studies indicate that diazepam is a teratogen in mice and hamsters, but only when doses hundreds of times greater than those used in humans are administered (Kellogg, 1988; Weber, 1985).

## Chlordiazepoxide

Chlordiazepoxide is a benzodiazepine tranquilizer that has less potency than diazepam on a milligram basis. It also has less anticonvulsant, muscle relaxant and sedative properties, but is effective in treating alcohol withdrawal. In several cohort studies, the frequency of congenital defects was not increased among more than 480 newborns whose mothers had first-trimester exposure to chlordiazepoxide (Crombie *et al.*, 1975; Hartz *et al.*, 1975; Heinonen *et al.*, 1977; Kullander and Kallen, 1976a, 1976b). Two case-control studies reported no association between maternal use of this benzodiazepine in the first trimester and congenital defects (Bracken and Holford, 1981; Rothman *et al.*, 1979). In contrast, in a small cohort study an association was reported between congenital malformations in 35 infants and maternal use of chlordiazepoxide in the first 42 days of gestation (Milkovich and van den Berg, 1974). However, there was no pattern to the anomalies observed.

Maternal chlordiazepoxide was associated with neonatal withdrawal beginning on day 26 of life (Athinarayanan *et al.*, 1976), which is an unusually long lag time for such an effect. Withdrawal symptoms included extreme tremulousness and irritability. Chlordiazepoxide given to pregnant hamsters in doses greater than those used in humans during embryogenesis resulted in an increased frequency (dose-dependent) of central nervous system anomalies and maternal toxicity (Guram *et al.*, 1982). The frequency of congenital anomalies was not increased among the offspring of pregnant rats given benzodiazepine, but fetal loss, growth retardation, and skeletal variants were increased in frequency with higher doses (Buttar, 1980; Saito *et al.*, 1984).

## Lorazepam

Lorazepam is a benzodiazepine class minor tranquilizer. The drug is used as an anti-anxiolytic and hypnotic drug. It is also used as a preanesthetic medication because of its amnesic action. In a case-control study, a significant association between first-trimester exposure to lorazepam and anal atresia was published (Bonnot *et al.*, 1999), but the meaning of the association is unclear. Several investigators (de Groot *et al.*, 1975; Kanto *et al.*, 1980; McBride *et al.*, 1979) reported placental transfer of lorazepam.

Transient neonatal hypotonia was observed in newborns of women who took lorazepam late in gestation, either chronically or intrapartum (McAuley *et al.*, 1982; Whitelaw *et al.*, 1981). Intravenously administered maternal lorazepam in hypertensive gravidas was associated with low Apgar scores, hypothermia, poor feeding, and a requirement for assisted ventilation in the infant. No congenital anomalies were reported among the offspring of pregnant rats and mice given up to 4 mg/kg/day lorazepam during organogenesis (Esaki *et al.*, 1975).

## Alprazolam

Alprazolam is a benzodiazepine tranquilizer. The rate of malformations was approximately 5 percent in over 400 births reported to the manufacturer (St Clair and Schirmer, 1992). In a case-control study from Hungary, the association between alprazolam exposure and congenital anomalies was slightly elevated, but not significantly so (Eros *et al.*, 2002). Several series containing more than 300 pregnancies followed through teratogen information services found no apparent increase in congenital anomalies (Friedman and Polifka, 2006) This agent, as other benzodiazepines, may cause hypotonia and hypothermia in the newborn (Yonkers and Cunningham, 1993).

## Other Benzodiazepines

Oxazepam and clonazepam are benzodiazepine tranquilizers. Among 89 infants born to women who used oxazepam during the first trimester, there were no congenital anomalies (Ornoy *et al.*, 1998). Small numbers of first-trimester exposure to clonazepam are published in clinical case series, but they are confounded by concomitant use of other known teratogens (anticonvulsants), as well as small sample sizes and sample selection bias (Friedman and Polifka, 2006).

Congenital anomalies were not increased in frequency among the offspring of pregnant rabbits or rats administered oxazepam in doses greater than those used in humans (Owen *et al.*, 1970; Saito *et al.*, 1984). Changes in behavior were observed among the offspring of pregnant mice given oxazepam in doses four to 42 times those used clinically (Alleva and Bignami, 1986).

## MISCELLANEOUS

### HYDROXYZINE

Hydroxyzine is a piperazine antihistaminic compound that is used to treat anxiety, pruritus, nausea, and vomiting. The frequency of congenital anomalies in a double-blind controlled study was not increased among 74 newborns exposed *in utero* to hydroxyzine (50 mg/day) during the first trimester (Erez *et al.*, 1971). Birth defects were not increased in frequency among 50 infants born to women who used hydroxyzine during the first trimester (Heinonen *et al.*, 1977). Hydroxyzine has been shown to be a teratogen in rats (Giurgea and Puigdevall, 1968; King and Howell, 1966).

### CHLORAL HYDRATE

Chloral hydrate is an effective hypnotic and sedative agent. There is a paucity of information regarding the safety of chloral hydrate use during pregnancy. However, among 71 infants born to women who used chloral hydrate during the first trimester, the frequency of congenital anomalies was not increased (Heinonen *et al.*, 1977). No gross external defects were observed in pregnant mice with chloral hydrate in doses less than one to five times the human dose (Kallman *et al.*, 1984).

### ETHCHLORVYNOL

Ethchlorvynol is a tertiary acetylenic alcohol and is used as an oral hypnotic and sedative agent. No studies have been published regarding the frequency of congenital malformations among newborns of women exposed to ethchlorvynol during gestation. Symptoms of neonatal withdrawal were observed in the newborn of a woman who was treated with ethchlorvynol as a hypnotic during the last 3 months of gestation. Neonatal withdrawal symptoms observed were jitteriness, irritability, and hypotonia (Rumak and Walravens, 1973). No animal studies evaluating the teratogenic effects of ethchlorvynol are published, but behavioral changes were observed among the offspring of pregnant rats treated with ethchlorvynol in doses greater than those used in humans (Peters and Hudson, 1981).

### MEPROBAMATE

Meprobamate is a carbamate tranquilizer that is useful in the treatment of anxiety but seems to be less effective than the benzodiazepines. The most common side effect is drowsiness. Inconsistencies in studies of the possible teratogenic effects of meprobamate in humans make it difficult to assess the risk of congenital anomalies with exposure to the drug in therapeutic doses during embryogenesis. Reports of an association between maternal use of this drug during the first trimester of pregnancy and a variety of congenital defects in newborns have been published, but the association is weak, and in no two studies was the same defect present. Among 66 infants born to women exposed to meprobamate in the first 42 days after their last menstrual period, congenital anomalies were increased fourfold (Milkovich and van den Berg, 1974). No apparent pattern of congenital anomalies was identified, but there were five infants with congenital heart disease. The frequency of hypospadias was increased among the 186 male infants born to women treated with meprobamate during the first trimester of pregnancy (Heinonen *et al.*, 1977), but the finding was disregarded because of the small sample size. Accordingly, the relationship is probably a random finding, not representing a causal link. A third study had an increased frequency of major congenital anomalies among the newborns of more than 50 pregnant women given meprobamate during the first trimester (Jick *et al.*, 1981), but no other details are available. Other studies have failed to find an association between the first-trimester use of meprobamate and congenital malformations. Among 356 pregnant women given meprobamate during the first trimester, the frequency of congenital anomalies was not increased (Heinonen *et al.*, 1977). Another cohort study of congenital anomalies among 207 infants whose mothers used meprobamate during the first trimester failed to find an association (Belafsky *et al.*, 1969). However, it should be noted that these studies analyzed only therapeutic dose exposures for infants examined for birth defects.

The frequency of birth defects was not increased among the offspring of pregnant mice, rats, or rabbits given meprobamate in doses greater than those used in humans (range 2.5–16 times) (Brar, 1969; Clavert, 1963; Werboff and Dembicki, 1962). In other studies when doses 16 times greater than those used in humans were administered to rabbits, and doses 2.5 or 20 times the typical dose in humans were given to pregnant rats, fetal and neonatal loss was increased (Bertrand, 1960; Clavert, 1963; Werboff and Kesner, 1963).

## METHAQUALONE

Methaqualone (Quaalude, Sopor, Parest) is an effective hypnotic and sedative agent and is not presently commercially available. No clear medicinal advantage of methaqualone over the other available hypnotics can be shown and the drug is commonly abused by drug-dependent people. Tolerance to the drug develops in abusers. No published reports are available that analyze the possible association of the use of methaqualone during pregnancy with congenital malformations. However, its use during gestation is not recommended because of its abuse potential. The frequency of congenital anomalies was not increased among rats or rabbits whose mothers were administered 200 mg/kg methaqualone orally (rabbits) from days 1 to 29 or 100 mg/kg (rats) from days 1 to 20 (Bough *et al.*, 1963).

## ELECTROCONVULSIVE THERAPY

High-voltage electrical shock is used to treat some psychiatric disorders, although it may also occur in accidental electrocution. The mechanism of action of electroconvulsive therapy is unknown. However, it is clearly understood that the seizure produced by electroconvulsive therapy is necessary for therapeutic efficacy (Ottosson, 1962a, 1962b). Electroconvulsive therapy was used safely in the treatment of depression in a pregnant woman following expanded clinical guidelines that included the presence of an obstetrician during treatment, endotracheal intubation, low-voltage, non-dominant therapy with electrocardiographic and electroencephalogram monitoring, Doppler ultrasonography of fetal heart rate, tocodynamometer recording of uterine tone, arterial blood gases during and after treatment, glycopyrrolate (anticholinergic of choice) use during anesthesia, and weekly non-stress tests (Wise *et al.*, 1984). The frequency of birth defects among the newborns of 318 women who received electroconvulsive therapy during gestation has not increased (Impastato *et al.*, 1964).

Reports of uterine contractions, vaginal bleeding, and transient benign fetal cardiac arrhythmias have been published (Miller, 1994b; Rabheru, 2001). Miscarriage was reported following a third electroconvulsive therapy session in the first trimester of pregnancy (Moreno *et al.*, 1998). One infant was described with hydrops fetalis and meconium peritonitis after the mother received electroconvulsive therapy during the third trimester of pregnancy (Gilot *et al.*, 1999). As is usually the case with isolated reports, it is not possible to evaluate any causal links with anecdotal data.

No animal studies evaluating the teratogenic effects of high-voltage electrical shock have been published.

## SPECIFIC CONDITIONS

### DEPRESSION

Management of depression during pregnancy should be undertaken in consultation with a psychiatrist and/or psychologist (Yonkers, 2003). Although psychotherapy or hospitalization in a supportive environment is the first consideration in treatment (Spinelli, 2001; Yolles, 2001), antidepressant therapy may be necessary if these regimens are unsuccessful (Yolles, 2001; Robinson *et al.*, 1986). Indeed, antidepressant medications are indicated in the pregnant woman whose depression is so severe that it threatens her life and the life of her unborn child (Yolles, 2001; Yonkers, 2003). Since the medications used in the treatment of depression have potential fetal risks and may result in obstetric complications and long-lasting sequelae, the minimal effective antidepressant dose should be initiated and maintained. Most antidepressants have established therapeutic serum levels that can be monitored.

No antidepressant has proven safety for use during gestation, although some are better studied than others. Thus, the selection of an antidepressant is dependent upon a patient's past response, side effects, and potential teratogenic effects of the particular agent. However, it is recommended that the physician use an agent that has been relatively well studied during pregnancy and has relatively few side effects (Miller, 1994a, 1996). These include desipramine, nortriptyline, and fluoxetine. The older antidepressants may have lower efficacy in women than the newer SSRI drugs. Women seem to respond better to fluoxetine, sertraline, and other SSRIs (Yonkers, 2003).

The usual starting dosages for imipramine, amitriptyline, and desipramine are 25–50 mg daily at bedtime. The dose can be increased to 25–50 mg daily every week, if warranted, to a maximum dose of 300 mg daily. The initial dosage for nortriptyline is 10–25 mg PO q d and can be increased by 10 mg each week if necessary to a maximum dose of 150 mg daily (Bryant and Brown, 1986). However, if the pregnant patient's depression is not improved on these older drugs, it is recommended to use one of the SSRIs. In fact, it may be beneficial to begin therapy with a well-studied SSRI such as fluoxetine (Yonkers, 2003).

Therapeutic response usually occurs within 10–14 days and includes improved sleep and appetite, as well as return of normal routine activities and mood elevation (Bryant and Brown, 1986). If there is absolutely no response to therapy after 2–3 weeks, one should consider an alternative antidepressant. It is recommended that tapering of the antidepressant dose begin approximately 2–3 weeks prior to delivery, to minimize neonatal effects. To prevent anticholinergic withdrawal symptoms (chills, malaise, muscle aches, diarrhea, and nightmares) in the mother, the dose should be reduced by 50 mg every 3–4 days (Blackwell, 1981). The starting dose of fluoxetine is 10–20 mg/day (Yonkers and Cunningham, 1993).

### PSYCHOSIS

Management of psychosis during pregnancy frequently requires hospitalization because of the patient's confusion, hostility, disorientation, anxiety, and possible suicidal tendencies. Psychiatric consultation and psychological evaluation are mandatory for patients with psychosis. Antipsychotic agents are frequently necessary in the treatment of psychosis. The agent of choice for acute psychotic reactions is haloperidol 1–5 mg PO (or IM) every six to eight hours. Chlorpromazine is another agent that is used in the acutely psychotic patient with a starting dose of 100 mg PO every 8–12 hours. Upon achievement of a stable dose, chlorpromazine can be administered once daily at bedtime. Some authorities recommend high-potency agents, haloperidol or trifluoperazine, over the low-potency neuroleptics (Miller, 1994a, 1996). The daily dose of haloperidol (Haldol) is 5–10 mg/day and of trifluoperazine (Stelazine), 10–40 mg/day (Yonkers and Cunningham, 1993).

Lithium may be necessary for manic-depressive disorders or manic disorders. For acute mania, the initial dosage is 0.6–2.1 g/day in three divided doses. Monitoring of the serum levels is mandatory, with adjustments in the dosage as indicated to maintain serum levels of 0.8–1.5 mEq/L. Recently, reevaluation of lithium use during early pregnancy led to marked lower estimated risk for birth defects, specifically for Ebstein's anomaly. The drug is currently recommended for use during pregnancy, avoiding weeks 2–6 of embryonic development if possible (Yonkers *et al.*, 1998, 2004).

Electroconvulsive therapy is warranted when all else fails. Although carbamazepine and valproic acid are used effectively to treat mania, these drugs are not recommended for use during pregnancy.

# 11 Antihistamines, Decongestants, and Expectorants during Pregnancy

Approximately 15 percent of women take cold-flu-allergy medications for upper respiratory infections and nasal congestion (Haas *et al.*, 2018). The drug classes include decongestants, antihistamines, expectorants, and antitussives. The most frequent respiratory condition in pregnant women is the "common cold." It is also the most frequent indication for using an antihistamine, decongestant and/or expectorant regimen (Hornby and Abraham, 1996). These drugs are only treating symptoms because there is no cure for rhinovirus infections, and the illness runs its course.

A number of antihistamines and antihistamine preparations are available by prescription and over the counter. Most antihistamines are used in combination with a sympathomimetic amine (e.g., pseudoephedrine) for decongestant activity. Pregnant women take these agents for symptomatic relief. Dose level and possible untoward systemic effects are important concerns. Intranasal route administration is equally, if not more, effective compared to oral administration. Importantly, the nasal route reduces maternal systemic drug exposure, and lowers the dose potentially delivered to the fetus while adequately treating the patient's symptoms (Hornby and Abrahams, 1996; Haas *et al.*, 2018).

**ADVISORY:** This class of drugs is used to treat conditions that could themselves be harmful to pregnancy (e.g., hyperthermia, viral infection syndromes). Therefore, any significant relationship between birth defects and a cold-flu-allergy medication may be confounded by maternal fever or an infection. These conditions can be associated with congenital anomalies, and may be the etiologic agent in some cases.

## DECONGESTANTS

The most frequently used decongestants were assigned a risk category under the old FDA pregnancy risk rating (Table 11.1). The ratings are annotated with recent research on the drug.

### PSEUDOEPHEDRINE

Pseudoephedrine hydrochloride is the most commonly used agent for pregnant women who require a decongestant (Hornby and Abrahams, 1996; Stanley *et al.*, 2019). It is also the most frequently used sympathomimetic in pregnant and non-pregnant individuals, and is typically used as a decongestant. Pseudoephedrine is also part of a combination therapy and combined with different antihistamines in "common cold" or "sinus" medications. Epidemiological studies of more than 1,000 first-trimester human pregnancies exposed to pseudoephedrine indicate no association with congenital anomalies (Aselton *et al.*, 1985; Heinonen *et al.*, 1977; Jick *et al.*, 1981; Rosa, unpublished, Briggs *et al.*, 2021). Among 12,734 malformed newborns, the frequency of birth defects was not increased among 531 infants whose mothers used pseudoephedrine during organogenesis (Yau *et al.*, 2013).

**TABLE 11.1**

**Commonly Used Decongestants**

| Drug | Old FDA Class | |
|------|------|------|
| *Decongestants* | **FDA** | **Data** |
| Ephedrine[a] | C | |
| Naphazoline | C | |
| Oxymetazoline | C | |
| Phenylephrine | C | |
| Phenylpropanolamine | C | |
| Pseudoephedrine | C | **No risk** |
| Tetrahydrozoline | C | |
| Xylometazoline | C | |
| *Expectorants* | | |
| Guaifenesin | None | |
| Iodinated glycerol | X | |
| Potassium iodide | D | |
| Terpin hydrate | None | |
| Antitussives | | |
| Benzonatate | Ca | |
| Codeine | C | |
| Dextromethorphan | C | |

[a] See Chapter 7.

*Abbreviation:* FDA, Food and Drug Administration.

Research that is more recent has associated pseudoephedrine use during early pregnancy with an increased frequency of some birth defects. BUT these must be considered in the light of possible confounders that are correlated with medications used to treat potentially teratogenic maternal conditions (e.g., hyperthermia). For example, based upon only two birth defects cases exposed to pseudoephedrine in the first trimester, an increased risk for gastroschisis close to significance was reported (Raitio *et al.*, 2020). In an earlier study, pseudoephedrine use was weakly and non-significantly associated with ear and eye anomalies (Heinonen *et al.*, 1977), probably because the number of exposed cases was small; the anomalies were not observed in later studies.

It is generally accepted that pseudoephedrine is not associated with a significantly increased frequency of birth defects (Kallen, 2019; Werler, 2006). Ephedrine (Ephedra, Ma Huang, over-the-counter weight loss/energy pill) used in large doses is associated with sudden cardiac death in adults, and based upon anecdotal information should be avoided during pregnancy because of potential adverse maternal and fetal effects, including tachycardia and serious adverse cardiovascular events, such as heart attack, stroke, and fetal vascular disruption.

### PHENYLEPHRINE AND PHENYLPROPANOLAMINE

Phenylpropanolamine and phenylephrine are decongestants in wide use, and are commonly combined with various antihistamines in flu and cold over-the-counter preparations. Phenylephrine may also be used for the treatment of acute hypotension.

Phenylephrine is used in in nasal sprays, and it is known that it may interfere with uterine blood flow. Phenylpropanolamine has a similar warning, and should be used with caution in women with pre-existing conditions associated with diminished uterine blood flow (e.g., hypertension). A weak, possible association of phenylephrine and phenylpropanolamine with congenital anomalies was reported among 1,249 and 726 pregnancies exposed to these drugs, respectively (Heinonen *et al.*, 1977)

Among more than 225 infants exposed to phenylpropanolamine or phenylephrine during the first trimester, the frequency of birth defects was not increased (Aselton *et al.*, 1985; Jick *et al.*, 1981). No adverse effects were found among offspring in animal studies regarding the teratogenicity of these two agents. It is unlikely that either agent is causally related to congenital malformations in first-trimester exposed fetuses if therapeutic doses are used.

## Naphazoline, Oxymetazoline, and Xylometazoline

Naphazoline, oxymetazoline, and xylometazoline are sympathomimetic agents with decongestant in long-acting nasal sprays (Afrin, Allerest, Dristan, 4-Way). Birth defects were not increased in frequency among more than 250 infants born to women who used oxymetazoline during the first trimester (Aselton *et al.*, 1985; Jick *et al.*, 1981). The Swedish registry reported no increased frequency of birth defects (3.3 percent) among 3521 infants whose were exposed to oxymetazoline during organogenesis (Kallen, 2019). Likewise, the frequency of birth defects was not increased in 432 infants exposed to xylometazoline during embryogenesis (Aselton *et al.*, 1985; Jick *et al.*, 1981). The Swedish registry reported the frequency of birth defects was not increased among 1168 infants born to women who used xylometazoline during the first trimester (Kallen, 2019). An incidental observation is that xylometazoline was significantly protective against congenital anomalies in the analysis. No studies have been published regarding naphazoline monotherapy use during pregnancy. However, the combination antazoline—naphazoline ophthalmologic preparation was used during the first trimester among 3061 infants, and the rate of birth defects was not increased above background (3.0 percent) or compared to controls (3.5 percent) (Thomseth *et al.*, 2019).

## ANTIHISTAMINES

Antihistamine medications act primarily by competing with histamine for H 1-receptor binding (Table 11.2). Antihistamines are chemically related to local anesthetics, and are sometimes used for this effect. Effects of other antihistamines include sedation, antiemetic, anti-motion sickness, and anti-dyskinesia.

The sedative effect is the primary difference between first-generation and second-generation antihistamines. Second-generation antihistamines are also referred to as the non-sedating antihistamines.

The old FDA pregnancy risk categories for antihistamines (Table 11.3) with the percentage of congenital anomalies extracted recent reviews shows the generally accepted non-teratogenic designation of antihistamines in human exposure pregnancy (Gilbert *et al.*, 2005; Seto *et al.*, 1997; Li *et al.*, 2013; Etwell *et al.*, 2017). Most authorities consider antihistamines safe for use during pregnancy, but it is prudent to rely on research for *specific agents* rather than a broad declaration of safety about drug classes. One report suggested that antihistamines as a group may be associated with an increased frequency of retrolental fibroplasia in premature infants (Zierler and Purohit, 1986). In a cohort of 3015 low birth weight infants with retrolental fibroplasia, significant risk factors were maternal diabetes and antihistamine exposure during the last two weeks of pregnancy (Purhoit *et al.*, 1985).

## Propylamine Derivatives

Brompheniramine, chlorpheniramine, dexchlorpheniramine, and triprolidine are propylamine derivatives. Brompheniramine was weakly associated with birth defects in 65 offspring exposed during the first trimester, but the association is not likely causative (Heinonen *et al.*, 1977). In a larger study of 270 infants born following first-trimester exposure to brompheniramine, birth defects were not increased in frequency among 270 infants whose mothers took brompheniramine during embryogenesis (Aselton *et al.*, 1985; Jick *et al.*, 1981). Analysis of pheniramine (either

## TABLE 11.2
## Antihistamines

| Generation | Old FDA Class |
| --- | --- |
| *First generation* | |
| Azatadine (Optimine) | C |
| Bromodiphenhydramine (Ambenyl) | C |
| Brompheniramine | C |
| Buclizine (Bucladin) | C |
| Carbinoxamine (Clistin) | C |
| Chlorpheniramine | B |
| Clemastine (Tavist) | B |
| Cyclizine (Marezine) | C |
| Cyproheptadine (Periactin) | B |
| Dexchlorpheniramine (Polaramine) | B |
| Dimenhydrinate | C |
| Diphenhydramine | B |
| Diphenylpyraline (Hispril) | C |
| Doxylamine (Unisom) | B |
| Meclizine (Antivert, Bonine) | C |
| Methdilazine | B |
| Phenindamine (Nolahist) | C |
| Promethazine | C |
| Pyrilamine (Dormarex, Sommicaps, Sominex) | C |
| Terfenadine (Seldane) | C |
| Trimeprazine | C |
| Tripelennamine (PBZ) | B |
| Triprolidine (Actidil, Bayidy) | C |
| *Second generation* | |
| Astemizole | C |
| Cetirizine | B |
| Cromolyn sodium | B |
| Desloratadine | — |
| Ebastine | — |
| Fexofenadine | C |
| Ipratropium | B |
| Loratadine | B |

brompheniramine or chlorpheniramine) in the National Birth Defects Prevention Study found no causal relationship between birth defects and first trimester exposure to these pheniramines (Gilboa *et al.*, 2009). Meta-analysis of available data on brompheniramine indicate it is not a human teratogen (Seto *et al.*, 1993) and this finding is supported by a recent review (Gilbert *et al.*, 2005) that included more information than the meta-analysis (Table 11.3).

Chlorpheniramine use during the first trimester was not associated with an increased frequency of congenital anomalies in general, but based on 7 exposed infants a weak association with ear and eye abnormalities was found for this sub-group (Heinonen *et al.*, 1977). The closely related agent dexchlorpheniramine was not associated with an increased frequency of birth defects (Gilbert *et al.*, 2005; Heinonen *et al.*, 1977). The frequency of birth defects (4.4 percent) was not increased in the Swedish registry analysis of 656 infants were exposed to dexchlorpheniramine Of 275 infants exposed to chlorpheniramine during organogenesis the frequency of malformations was not increased (Gilbert *et al.*, 2005; Jick *et al.*, 1981). Chlorpheniramine was not associated with

**TABLE 11.3**
**Congenital Anomalies and First-Trimester Antihistamine Exposure**

| Antihistamine | Percent Congenital Anomalies (%) | n/N |
|---|---|---|
| *First generation* | | |
| Azatadine | 4.7 | 6/127 |
| Brompheniramine | 5.9 | 16/271 |
| Chlorphenamine (chlorpheniramine) | 6.9 | 96/1388 |
| Clemastine | 3.7 | 110/2847 |
| Cyproheptadine | 4.2 | 12/285 |
| Dexchlorpheniramine | 4.6 | 50/1080 |
| Diphenhydramine | 4.7 | 154/3286 |
| Hydroxyzine | 6.0 | 60/995 |
| Tripelennamine | 6.0 | 6/100 |
| Triprolidine | 1.4 | 9/628 |
| *Second generation* | | |
| Astemizole | 1.8 | 2/114 |
| Cetirizine | 4.0 | 38/950 |
| Loratadine | 3.8 | 81/2147 |
| Terfenadine | 4.0 | 88/2195 |

Most of these studies were controlled and only the numbers of exposed are shown here for illustrative purposes without odds ratios and comparative data.

*Abbreviations:* n, number of infants with a congenital anomaly who were exposed to antihistamine during the first trimester; N, number of mother-infant pairs exposed to antihistamine during the first trimester.

*Source:* Compiled from Gilbert *et al.*, 2005.

birth defects in rodents given the drug during embryogenesis (Manufacturer Information) but the study was not peer reviewed. The frequency of malformations was not increased in the offspring of 628 women who took triprolidine in the first trimester (Aselton *et al.*, 1985; Gilbert *et al.*, 2005; Jick *et al.*, 1981). In a case control study of 23 infants exposed to triprolidine the frequency of both defects was not increased in the exposed group (Hansen *et al.*, 2020). Animal teratology studies of triprolidine exposure during embryogenesis are published.

### ETHANOLAMINE/ETHYLAMINE DERIVATIVES

Clemastine is a mast cell inhibitor and an H2 antihistamine. The frequency of congenital anomalies was not increased among 2847 infants whose mothers took clemastine during organogenesis (Gilbert *et al.*, 2005). Among 7115 infants in the Swedish registry exposed to clemastine during the first trimester, the frequency of birth defects was not increased (Kallen, 2019).

Bromodiphenhydramine and carbinoxamine have not been studied during human pregnancy. Experimental animal teratology studies of bromodiphenhydramine are published. Malformations were not increased in frequency in one animal study of carbinoxamine (Maruyama and Yoshida, 1968). The Hungarian Birth Defects study of a large case-control sample (23,757 cases; 39,877 controls) found that the frequency of birth defects was not increased among 2640 infants whose mothers took dimenhydrate during embryogenesis (Czeizel and Vargha, 2005). The frequency of congenital anomalies was not increased in one animal study of dimenhydrinate exposure during embryogenesis (McColl *et al.*, 1965).

The frequency of birth defects was not increased among 865 infants born to women who used diphenhydramine during the first trimester (Aselton *et al.*, 1985; Heinonen *et al.*, 1977). No studies regarding the use of bromodiphenhydramine during pregnancy are published. Ten normal infants whose mothers were exposed to bromodiphenhydramine during early gestation were reported (Heinonen *et al.*, 1977), but this cannot be related to risk of birth defects. Ethanolamine derivatives are reported to have oxytocic-like effects when used parenterally (Hara *et al.*, 1980; Klieger and Massart, 1965; Rotter *et al.*, 1958).

## BENDECTIN®

Doxylamine was one of the main components of the popular antinausea drug, Bendectin (along with pyridoxine and dicyclomine). Several studies reported an association of Bendectin use in pregnancy and diaphragmatic hernias (Bracken and Berg, 1983), congenital heart disease, and pyloric stenosis (Aselton *et al.*, 1985; Eskenazi *et al.*, 1982). Other researchers did not find an increased frequency of congenital anomalies after exposure during embryogenesis (Mitchell *et al.*, 1981, 1983; Zierler and Rothman, 1985). Birth defects were not increased in frequency among more than 1,100 infants exposed to doxylamine during the first trimester (Heinonen *et al.*, 1977). Recall that doxylamine is an antihistamine component of Bendectin. In a case control study doxylamine was not associated with an increased frequency of congenital heart disease (Zierler and Rothman, 1985). Birth defects were increased in frequency in one animal teratology study of doxylamine (Gibson *et al.*, 1968). Considering the millions of women who have used Bendectin during the first trimester of pregnancy without scientific evidence of adverse fetal effects, it is extremely unlikely that doxylamine or the components of Bendectin are human teratogens. Drugs such as Bendectin do not cause birth defects but do cause other untoward outcomes. They are associated with lawsuits, and were aptly labeled "litogens" (i.e., lawsuit-inducing agents) by one of the world experts in human teratology, Dr. Robert Brent (Brent, 1983). Recently, an increased frequency of spina bifida was associated with the ingredients in Bendectin (doxylamine-pyridoxine-dicyclomine) (Bérard *et al.*, 2019). In stark contrast, a large study that used CDC birth defects surveillance data found no increased frequency of birth defects in a multi-state analysis, and directly addressed the Berard article (Schrager *et al.*, 2021).

In summary, doxylamine is a safe drug for use during pregnancy, and recent findings that claim an association of birth defects with Bendectin component (Berard *et al.*, 2019) are not well received (Biffi *et al.*, 2020). The Bendectin lawsuits hit at the heart of science because of the wide disparity in quality of evidence presented by purported experts, and led to a major US Supreme Court, the Daubert-Robinson ruling on what qualifies as evidence in court. The junk science that was used in the Bendectin lawsuits forced improved rules of evidence by requiring an hypothesis that can be tested, it was tested, and established that statistical probability of significance must be presented (i.e., the *p* value).

## PIPERIDINE DERIVATIVES

Piperidine was discovered in 1850 and is a substrate in the manufacture of several classes of drugs (SSRIs, antipsychotics, vasodilators), including antihistamines. Birth defects were not increased in frequency among 127 infants exposed to azatadine during the first trimester (Gilbert *et al.*, 2005). The frequency of congenital anomalies was not increased among 285 infants whose mothers took cyproheptadine during embryogenesis (Gilbert *et al.*, 2005; see Table 11.3). No epidemiological studies of birth defects or adverse fetal effects among infants born to mothers who took diphenylpyraline during pregnancy are published. Animal teratology studies of cyproheptadine are not consistent (de la Fuente and Alia, 1982; Rodriguez-Gonzalez *et al.*, 1983; Weinstein *et al.*, 1975), making it impossible to interpret the findings. No animal teratology studies of azatadine are published.

### ETHYLENEDIAMINE DERIVATIVES

The *ethylenediamines are used as H₁ antagonists to treat hypersensitivity reactions, coughs, and the common cold*.

The frequency of congenital anomalies was not increased in 100 and 112 offspring exposed to tripelennamine and pyrilamine during the first trimester, respectively (Heinonen *et al.*, 1977). In several animal studies, pyrilamine was associated with an increased rate of fetal loss at levels many times the usual human dose (Bovet-Nitti *et al.*, 1963; Naranjo and de Naranjo, 1968). No animal teratology studies on tripelennamine are published.

## SECOND-GENERATION ANTIHISTAMINES

### BUTYROPHENONE DERIVATIVES

Terfenadine (Seldane) is a medication derived from **butyrophenone. Butyrophenone derivatives are diverse, and range from antihistamines to antipsychotics**. The frequency of birth defects among 134 infants born following first trimester exposure to terfenadine was not increased (Schick *et al.*, 994). In a large review, the frequency of birth defects was not increased among 2,194 infants exposed to terfenadine during embryogenesis (Gilbert *et al.*, 2005; see Table 11.3).

Terfenadine is not recommended for nursing mothers because it was associated with decreased postnatal pup weight gain in rat teratology studies by the manufacturer (PubChem, 2020).

### OTHER SECOND-GENERATION ANTIHISTAMINES

Cetirizine is a selective peripheral H1-receptor antagonist antihistamine that acts by blocking histamine action. It is used to treat itching and redness symptoms caused by hives; however, it does not prevent hives or other allergic skin reactions.

The frequency of congenital anomalies was not increased among 196 infants whose mothers took cetirizine during the first trimester (Weber-Schoendorfer *et al.*, 2008). In a small series of 39 infants exposed to cetirizine during organogenesis, the frequency of birth defects was not increased (Einarson *et al.*, 1997). Similarly, astemizole exposure during the first trimester was not associated with an increased frequency of congenital anomalies among 114 infants. Loratadine, an FDA category B drug, exposure during the first trimester was not associated with a higher than expected frequency of congenital anomalies (see Table 11.3). These drugs seem safe for use during pregnancy, with greater confidence assigned to those drugs whose studies have the larger denominators (Gilbert *et al.*, 2005).

### PIPERAZINE DERIVATIVES

Piperazine derivatives are selective Histamine-1 antagonist drugs used to treat allergic rhinitis and chronic urticaria. They are also used to prevent and treat nausea and vomiting. These drugs are also effective to treat motion sickness and vertigo. Cyclizine, buclizine, and meclizine are used primarily as antiemetics, although they also have antihistamine action. One study reported 44 infants who were born following first-trimester exposure to buclizine, and no birth defects were reported (Heinonen *et al.*, 1977). Exposure to cyclizine during embryogenesis among 111 infants was not associated with an increased frequency of congenital anomalies (Milkovich and van den Berg, 1976). In the Swedish registry, 2185 infants were born following first-trimester exposure to cyclizine with no increased frequency of birth defects (Kallen, 2019). No studies have been published on the use of buclizine during pregnancy.

The frequency of congenital anomalies was not increased among over 1,000 infants exposed to meclizine in the first trimester (Heinonen *et al.*, 1977). The risk of birth defects was not increased by first trimester exposure to meclizine in one cohort and three case-control studies (Greenberg *et al.*, 1977; Mellin, 1964; Milkovich and van den Berg, 1976; Nelson and Forfar, 1971).

The frequency of craniofacial and skeletal anomalies was increased among rat fetuses exposed to meclizine during embryogenesis (King, 1963). No birth defects were found in the offspring of monkeys who received 10 times the usual human dose of meclizine during embryogenesis (Courtney and Valerio, 1968; Wilson and Gavan, 1967).

## Phenindamine

Phenindamine is an antihistamine and anticholinergic closely related to cyproheptadine. No studies regarding congenital anomalies and the use of phenindamine in pregnant women are published. One study included one exposed infant with major congenital anomalies (Mellin, 1964), but the meaning of this finding is unclear.

*Phenindamine* is closely related to chlorpheniramine, a better-studied drug that was found not to increase the frequency of birth defects (Table 11.4).

### TABLE 11.4
### Teratogen Information System (TERIS) Risk for Congenital Anomaly and Food and Drug Administration (FDA) Pregnancy Risk Category

| Drugs | TERIS Risk | Old FDA Risk Rating |
| --- | --- | --- |
| Astemizole | Unlikely | C |
| Azatadine | Undetermined | B |
| Bendectin | None | NA |
| Benzonatate | Undetermined | NA |
| Bromodiphenhydramine | Undetermined | C |
| Brompheniramine | None | C |
| Buclizine | Undetermined | C |
| Carbinoxamine | Undetermined | C |
| Chlorpheniramine | Unlikely | B |
| Chlorpheniramine | Unlikely | B |
| Clemastine | Undetermined | B |
| Cyclizine | Unlikely | B |
| Cyproheptadine | Undetermined | B |
| Dextromethorphan | None | C |
| Dicyclomine | None | B |
| Dimenhydrinate | Unlikely | B |
| Diphenhydramine | Unlikely | B |
| Diphenylpyraline | Undetermined | NA |
| Doxylamine | None | A |
| Guaifenesin | None | C |
| Hydroxyzine | Unlikely | C |
| Iodinated glycerol | Undetermined | X |
| Meclizine | Unlikely | B |
| Naphazoline | Undetermined | NA |
| Oxymetazoline | Unlikely | C |
| Phenindamine | Undetermined | C |
| Phenylephrine | None to minimal | C |
| Pseudoephedrine | None to minimal | C |
| Pyridoxine | None | NA |

| Drugs | TERIS Risk | Old FDA Risk Rating |
|---|---|---|
| Pyrilamine | None | C |
| Terfenadine | Unlikely | C |
| Triprolidine | Unlikely | C |
| Xylometazoline | Unlikely | NA |

*Abbreviation:* NA, not available.

*Sources:* Compiled from Friedman *et al.*, *Obstet Gynecol*, 1990; 75: 594; Briggs *et al.*, 2021; Friedman and Polifka, 2006.

## EXPECTORANTS AND ANTITUSSIVES

### EXPECTORANTS

Guaifenesin is a major expectorant in common use, and is an active component of most cough medicines. No animal teratology studies are published. Guaifenesin use during the organogenesis among more than 1,000 human pregnancies was not associated with an increased risk of birth defects (Aselton, 1985; Heinonen *et al.*, 1977; Jick *et al.*, 1981).

Other mucolytic agents or drugs that act as an expectorant include potassium iodide or iodinated glycerol, but should be considered contraindicated. Iodine-containing agents cross the placenta freely and may result in fetal goiter. Therefore, iodide-containing agents should be avoided for use anytime during pregnancy, but especially after weeks 11–12 of pregnancy when the thyroid begins to function.

### ANTITUSSIVES

Dextromethorphan is commonly used as an antitussive. The frequency of congenital anomalies was not increased among 300 infants born to women who tool dextromethorphan during the first trimester (Heinonen *et al.*, 1977).

Narcotics (opioids) are used for their antitussive properties in cough preparations, including codeine, hydrocodone, and hydromorphone. Chronic use of narcotic agents may result in neonatal addiction, withdrawal, and respiratory depression. Recently narcotics (opioids) were associated with an increased frequency of congenital anomalies (see Chapter 8). Importantly, acute use of narcotic antitussives is not associated with neonatal addiction, and after the first trimester is not associated with congenital anomalies.

Benzonatate (Tessalon) acts as an antitussive by anesthetizing the stretch receptors in the respiratory passage. No studies of benzonatate use during pregnancy are published.

**Caution Note:** A number of cough preparations contain ethyl alcohol, which may cause adverse fetal effects (i.e., fetal alcohol effects) if used chronically, and some cough preparations may contain iodine, which may be associated with fetal goiter. Case reports of fetal alcohol syndrome have been published in which the mother abused cough preparations during pregnancy. However, it is unlikely that short-term use carries significant risk. Alcohol is discussed in further detail in Chapter 16. Fetal goiter is described in Chapter 4.

## SPECIAL CONSIDERATIONS

### VIRAL UPPER RESPIRATORY INFECTIONS (COMMON COLD)

Women with a recognized pregnancy with colds usually do not require specific therapy, especially in the first trimester. Colds may occur during an unrecognized pregnancy and be treated. The review of the available data in this chapter have an underlying theme that is not clearly expressed. The major risk from cold and flu during pregnancy may be hyperthermia. High fevers are associated with an increased frequency of birth defects (Graham, 2020). If symptomatic therapy is indicated, pregnant women with the common cold may be treated with acetaminophen for fever. This may be combined with a decongestant, an antihistamine, and an antitussive/ expectorant combination. Pseudoephedrine and chlorpheniramine are the preferred treatments (Hornby and Abrahams, 1996). If a nasal spray is needed, agents containing oxymetazoline, xylometazoline, or naphazoline are reasonable, since minimal systemic absorption occurs. Antitussive compounds containing iodide are contraindicated. Other, non-iodinated preparations offer equally effective alternative medication (Tables 11.1 and 11.2).

## ALLERGIC RHINITIS/SINUSITIS

Treatment with the well-studied drugs during pregnancy is the reasonable approach to treatment of the common cold, occurring in between 10–20 percent of gravidas. Chlorpheniramine compounds may be used as first-line use in pregnant women because they are better studied. The histamine H-receptor antagonists astemizole (Hismanal), cetirizine, loratadine, and terfenadine (Seldane) used the first trimester in pregnant women (Table 11.3) were not associated with significant increased frequencies of birth defects.

## PRURITIS/URTICARIA

Antihistamines for treatment of pruritus during pregnancy include chlorpheniramine and diphenhydramine. Loratadine is the first choice and cetirizine the second choice among second-generation antihistamines (Bechtel, 2018). Diphenhydramine is well studied during pregnancy and is a safe agent to use (Table 11.3). Its oxytocic effects do not appear to be as pronounced as dimenhydrate (Hara *et al.*, 1980), and studies support its safety. Other medications found to be safe and effective in the treatment of pruritus are hydroxyzine or dexchlorpheniramine (Drugs and Pregnancy Study Group, 1994) (Table 11.3).

## MOTION SICKNESS/VERTIGO

Dimenhydrinate is a commonly used agent, although it may have some oxytocic properties. It has been studied during the first trimester of human pregnancy and was not associated with an increased frequency of congenital anomalies (Czeizel and Vargha, 2005). Among 358 infants exposed to dimenhydrinate or diphenhydramine, the frequency of birth defects was not increased (Kallen, 2019).

## DRUG-INDUCED DYSKINESIA

Diphenhydramine's antimuscarinic and sedative effects are the reason it is used to treat drug-induced dyskinesia in the pregnant patient. The studies cited earlier reported no adverse effects (Table 11.3).

# 12 Nutritional and Dietary Supplementation during Pregnancy

A balanced "nonfad" diet should provide pregnant women with an adequate complement of nutrients during pregnancy. Prenatal vitamin supplements are usually given, but there is no clear consensus that they are needed. Under the Hippocratic dictum of "do no harm," prenatal vitamin supplements are not harmful in recommended daily allowance (RDA) doses. Vitamin supplements for pregnant women should, along with dietary intake, approximate the RDA set by the FDA (Table 12.1). Iron is the only nutrient for which supplementation during pregnancy is invariably required because of ~40 percent blood volume expansion by term.

## PROTEIN-CALORIE REQUIREMENTS AND SUPPLEMENTS

1. During a normal pregnancy, women should gain between 22 and 27 lbs. Calories required during pregnancy increase (approximately 300–500 calories per day) only marginally above the needs of non-pregnant women (2,100 calories daily). Composition of the 2,400 to 2,600 calories should be comprised of 74 g of protein. A reasonably balanced diet provides adequate protein and calories during pregnancy (ACOG, 1993). Under special circumstances, protein-calorie supplementation is warranted. Gravidas who follow a vegetarian diet or are otherwise nutritionally restricted (e.g., gluten intolerant), may require supplementation. When considering the gravid vegetarian, it is extremely important to distinguish between the strictly vegetarian (e.g., Buddhist) and the lacto-ovo vegetarian (e.g., Seventh Day Adventists). Lacto-ovo vegetarians do not consume animal flesh–derived foods (i.e., meat and fish) in their diets, but do consume animal products (i.e., eggs and dairy products). Non-lacto-ovo vegetarians eat only plant-derived foods and are at high risk of inadequate protein-calorie nutrition. Special action from the clinician to ensure an adequate intake of the essential amino acids and folate must be taken. A professional nutritionist should be involved to help manage meal plans during pregnancy for the strict vegetarian. Non-lacto-ovo vegetarians may also suffer from various other nutrient deficiencies, specifically of vitamins of the A and B group.

## VITAMINS

Over-the-counter "super-vitamin" preparations or megadose regimens, such as Centrum, should not be used during pregnancy for reasons discussed in the following. A balanced diet should provide the necessary nutrients during pregnancy, except for iron, which is routinely prescribed.

### VITAMIN A

Vitamin A is an essential nutrient, and the recommended supplement of vitamin A (approximately 8,000 IU per day; Table 12.1) is usually consumed. The risk of birth defects and adverse fetal effects is likely not above population background risk with maternal intake of 10,000 IU or less of

DOI: 10.1201/9780429160929-12

**TABLE 12.1**

**National Institute of Medicine Recommended Daily Dietary Allowances for Women before and during Pregnancy and Lactation**

| Nutrient | Non-Pregnant[a] | Pregnant | Lactating |
|---|---|---|---|
| Kilocalories | 2200 | 2500 | 2600 |
| Protein (g) | 55 | 71 | 71 |
| Fat-soluble vitamins | | | |
| A (IU)[b] | 800 | 800 | 1300 |
| D (IU) | 500 | 600 | 600 |
| E (mg TE)[c] | 8 | 11.5 | 15 |
| K (µg) | 55 | 90 | 90 |
| Water-soluble vitamins | | | |
| C (mg) | 60 | 85 | 120 |
| Cobalamin, $B_{12}$ (µg) | 2.0 | 2.6 | 2.8 |
| Folate (µg) | 180 | 600 | 500 |
| Niacin (mg) | 15 | 18 | 17 |
| Pyridoxine, $B_6$ (mg) 1.6 | 1.9 | 2.0 | |
| Riboflavin (mg) | 1.1 | 1.4 | 1.6 |
| Thiamin (mg) | 1.3 | 1.4 | 1.4 |
| Minerals | | | |
| Calcium (mg) | 1200 | 1000 | 1000 |
| Iodine (µg) | 150 | 220 | 290 |
| Iron (mg) | 15 | 27 | 9 |
| Magnesium (mg) | 280 | 320 | 355 |
| Phosphorus (mg) | 1200 | 1200 | 1200 |
| Zinc (mg) | 12 | 15 | 19 |
| Choline (mg) | 450 | 450 | 450 |

[a] For non-pregnant females age 15–18 years.

[b] 1 µg retinol = 1 retinol equivalent (RE).

[c] TE, tocopherol equivalent.

*Sources:* From the Institute of Medicine (2006, 2011) and ACOG (2021) www.acog.org/womens-health/faqs/nutrition-during-pregnancy (Accessed May 19, 2021).

vitamin A daily. However, megadoses of vitamin A, taken by some individuals for undocumented health advantages, are often encountered in practice. No data to support large-dose vitamin A consumption are published in the scientific literature. Investigators analyzed the teratogenicity of high vitamin A intake of pregnant women and found that one in about 57 children had a malformation in cranial neural crest formation associated with high dose vitamin A (>10,000 IU supplements per day) (Rothman *et al.*, 1995). The prevalence of malformations among infants born to mothers who ingested 5,000 IU or less of food and supplements of vitamin A per day was significantly lower than the high-dose group (Rothman *et al.*, 1995). The vitamin A dose associated with an increased risk for congenital anomalies is unknown; however, more than 10,000 IU daily may significantly increase that risk (Bastos Maia *et al.*, 2019). Some over-the-counter preparations that contain very **high doses of vitamin A (e.g., 45,000 IU) are contraindicated for use during pregnancy**. The Swedish Birth Defects Registry included 39 infants born to women who took 50,000 IU of vitamin A during embryogenesis and 2 infants (5.1 percent) had a major congenital anomaly (Kallen, 2019).

*Important note*: Current RDA of 10,000 IU of vitamin A includes dietary intakes, not just supplementation.

Water-soluble vitamin A supplements are beta-carotene derived from vegetables. Other vitamin A supplements (retinoic acid, discussed earlier) are fat soluble, and usually fish liver derived.

Beta-carotene vitamin A probably has a higher clearance rate than retinoic acid because it is water soluble. Beta-carotene presumably poses much less, if any, teratogenic risk compared to similar amounts of retinoid acid-derived vitamin A (or Retinol).

Anecdotal data (case reports) support the hypothesized association of birth defects with high-dose retinoic acid-derived vitamin A. Case reports describe urinary tract and craniofacial complex congenital anomalies among infants whose mothers who took > 40,000 IU or more of vitamin A during pregnancy (Bernhardt et al., 1974; Mounoud et al., 1975; Pilotti and Scorta, 1965). Among infants born to women who used megadoses of vitamin A analogs (isotretinoin, etretinate) support the existence of a retinoic acid embryopathy (see Chapter 14). Importantly, the frequency of congenital anomalies (cleft lip, cleft lip and palate, cleft palate) was not increased in a large Japanese case control study of 98,787 infants whose mothers took supplemental retinoids during pregnancy (Yoshida et al., 2020).

Offspring of rats, mice, hamsters, pigs, and dogs whose mothers received vitamin A (doses up to 5,000 times RDA) during embryogenesis had dose-related increased frequencies of congenital anomalies (Cohlan, 1951; Kalter and Warkany, 1961; Kochhar, 1964; Marin-Padrilla and Ferm, 1965; Palludan, 1966; Wiersig and Swenson, 1967; Willhite, 1984). As with human case reports, anomalies in animal studies were heterogeneous (brain, cardiac, eye, and craniofacial anomalies) and not consistent with a constellation or cluster of birth defects that characterize a syndrome. An increased risk of congenital anomalies seems highly likely, although the data are purely anecdotal. On balance, information regarding the association of birth defects and high-dose vitamin A lacks of a pattern of congenital anomalies expected if there were a syndrome. The high frequency of congenital anomalies with isotretinoin and etretinate—vitamin A congeners—exposure during embryogenesis offers evidence that megadose vitamin A during pregnancy increases the risk of congenital anomalies, and comprises a syndrome (see Chapter 14).

## VITAMIN D

Vitamin D is produced by skin exposed to ultraviolet light and is integral to normal calcium metabolism. Notably, vitamin D deficiency is associated with rickets. Skeletal anomalies comparable to rickets in humans were found in rats born to mothers who were vitamin D deficient during gestation (Warkany, 1943). No congenital anomalies were observed in a clinical case series of 15 children born to hypoparathyroid women who took more than 200 times the RDA of vitamin D throughout pregnancy (Goodenday and Gordon, 1971). Vitamin D deficiency was associated with an increased frequency of congenital heart defects in a case-control study of 345 infants (Koster et al., 2018).

Birth defects associated with high-dose vitamin D parallel observations in Williams syndrome (supravalvular aortic stenosis, unusual facies, and infantile hypercalcemia) (Chan et al., 1979; Friedman and Mills, 1969; Friedman and Roberts, 1966). Williams syndrome was speculated to be caused by the use of megadoses of vitamin D during pregnancy (Friedman, 1968), but the available data do not support this (Forbes, 1979; Warkany, 1943). Interestingly, rats and rabbits born to mothers given several thousands of times the human RDA of vitamin D during gestation had cardiovascular and craniofacial anomalies (Friedman and Mills, 1969). The frequency of cleft lip, cleft lip and palate, or cleft palate only was not increased among infants whose mothers took vitamin D supplements during pregnancy in a recent Japanese study (Yoshida et al., 2020).

## VITAMIN B GROUP

### Niacin

Niacin is a B complex vitamin that is metabolized to niacinamide, the active form of $B_3$, in humans. Niacin is naturally present in a wide variety of foods. Treatment for hyperlipidemia with niacin usually is for doses 200–400 times the RDA. In a unique study of niacin deficiency, it was eloquently shown that niacin deficiency is associated with birth defects in humans and mice (Shi et al., 2017). No increased frequency of congenital anomalies was found in rats and rabbits born to mothers given large doses of niacin during organogenesis (Takaori *et al.*, 1973). The frequency of orofacial clefts was not increased in infants whose mothers took niacin during the first trimester in a large case-control study of 98,787 births (Yoshida *et al.*, 2020).

## Pantothenate

Pantothenate is an essential cofactor in metabolism of carbohydrates, proteins, and fats. It contributes to the composition of coenzyme A. Pantothenate is nearly ubiquitous in a well-balanced diet.

In a case control study that involved more than 98,000 infants, pantothenate use in the usual human dose range was not associated with increased frequencies of orofacial clefts, cleft lip, cleft lip and palate, cleft palate only (Yoshida *et al.*, 2020). Deficiency of pantothenate during pregnancy in rats, mice, and swine was associated with an excess of intrauterine deaths and brain, eye, limb, and heart defects in offspring exposed during organogenesis (Kalter and Warkany, 1959; Kimura and Ariyama, 1961; Lefebvres, 1954; Nelson *et al.*, 1957; Ullrey *et al.*, 1955).

## Pyridoxine

Pyridoxine (vitamin $B_6$), another essential nutrient, is an enzyme cofactor. Dietary pyridoxine requirements are increased among pregnant women (Table 12.1). The frequency of congenital anomalies was not increased among more than 170 infants whose mothers took pyridoxine during the first trimester in the Hungarian Case-Control Surveillance of congenital Anomalies (Czeizel *et al.*, 2004). Among more than 250,000 infants exposed to doxylamine and pyridoxine for pregnancy associated nausea, the frequency of birth defects was not increased (Biffi *et al.*, 2020).

No investigations have been published on the frequency of congenital anomalies among infants born to women who took megadoses of pyridoxine during pregnancy. In one animal study, congenital anomalies were not increased in frequency among rats born to mothers given many times the RDA for pyridoxine during pregnancy (Khera, 1975). Pyridoxine deficiency during pregnancy was associated with digital defects and cleft palate in mice and rats (Davis *et al.*, 1970; Miller, 1972).

## Thiamine

Vitamin B (thiamine) is an essential dietary component because it is a coenzyme. No studies of high doses of thiamine during human pregnancy are published. Thiamine multivitamin supplements were protective against orofacial clefts in the Dutch registry (Krapels *et al.*, 2004). Congenital anomalies were not increased in frequency among offspring of rats given up to 140 times the RDA of thiamine during pregnancy (Morrison and Sarett, 1959; Schumacher *et al.*, 1965) or about 50 times the rat daily requirement. Thiamine deficiency was associated with an increased frequency of fetal death and decreased fetal weight gain among pregnant rats (Nelson and Evans, 1955; Roecklein *et al.*, 1985). Among 98,787 infants born to women who took thiamine supplements during organogenesis, the frequency of orofacial clefts (cleft palate, cleft lip, cleft lip and palate) was not increased (Yoshida *et al.*, 2020).

## Cyanocobalamin

Vitamin $B_{12}$, cyanocobalamin, is an essential nutrient. Megadose cyanocobalamin (about 260 times RDA) is used to treat pernicious anemia. The frequency of congenital anomalies among infants whose mothers took megadoses of vitamin $B_{12}$ during pregnancy has not been published. Malformations were not increased in frequency among the offspring of mice treated during pregnancy with 5250–10 500 times the RDA of cyanocobalamin (Mitala *et al.*, 1978). Cyanocobalamin deficiency among offspring of rats treated with megadoses of cyanocobalamin had increased frequencies of hydrocephalus, eye defects, and skeletal anomalies (Grainger *et al.*, 1954; Woodard and Newberne, 1966). The frequency of birth defects was not increased among 5,675 infants whose mothers took cyanocobalamin during organogenesis at the recommended dose in Swedish Birth Defects Registry (Kallen, 2019). In a large case-control study of orofacial clefts (lip, palate, lip and palate), the frequency of exposure to cyanocobalamin was not significantly increased among babies with orofacial birth defects (Yoshida *et al.*, 2020).

## Vitamin C

Vitamin C (ascorbic acid) is an essential nutrient. Deficiency of vitamin C causes scurvy. No increase in the use of vitamin C was found in a case-control study of the use of vitamin C during the first trimester by mothers of 175 infants with major congenital anomalies and 283 with minor anomalies compared to the control group (Nelson and Forfar, 1971). Embryo-fetal effects of megadoses of vitamin C during pregnancy have not been published. Two infants born to women who took more than six times the RDA of vitamin C during pregnancy had scurvy (Cochrane, 1965).

The frequency of congenital anomalies was not increased among mice and rats born to mothers treated with hundreds to several thousand times the RDA of vitamin C during embryogenesis (Frohberg *et al.*, 1973). An increased frequency of fetal death was found in offspring of mice fed 4800 times the RDA of ascorbic acid during embryogenesis (Pillans *et al.*, 1990). Increased dietary requirements for vitamin C was found in guinea pigs born to mothers who were given several hundred times the RDA throughout pregnancy; increased clearance apparently caused the need for more vitamin C (Cochrane, 1965; Norkus and Rosso, 1975, 1981). The frequency of birth defects was not increased among 1907 infants whose mothers took the recommended dose of vitamin C during embryogenesis in the Swedish birth defects study (Kallen, 2019). In a Japanese case control study (n = 98,787) of cleft lip/palate, the frequency of exposure to vitamin C during embryogenesis was not increased (Yoshida *et al.*, 2020).

## Vitamin E

Vitamin E is another essential nutrient. If caloric intake is adequate, vitamin E deficiency is extremely rare. The frequency of birth defects was not increased among 322 infants whose mothers took vitamin E during organogenesis (Kallen, 2019).

Among rats and mice born to mothers given vitamin E in doses up to thousands of times the RDA, the frequency of congenital anomalies was not increased (Hook *et al.*, 1974; Hurley *et al.*, 1983; Krasavage and Terhaar, 1977; Sato *et al.*, 1973). In contrast, the frequency of cleft palate was increased among mice born to mothers given several-hundred times the human RDA of vitamin E during embryogenesis (Momose *et al.*, 1972).

## OTHER ESSENTIAL NUTRIENTS

### Folic Acid

Folic acid, a water-soluble vitamin B complex, is an essential nutrient. It is a coenzyme, and has been shown to be extremely important in normal embryonic development, the neural tube complex in particular. Pregnancy elevates the RDA for folic acid. And on "March 5, 1996, the US Food and Drug Administration (FDA) required that manufacturers fortify enriched cereal-grain products with 140 µg of folic acid per 100 g of cereal-grain product by January 1, 1998" (Grosse *et al.*, 2005). Subsequent analysis has shown a reduction in neural tube defects (NTDs) on a national scale of 20–30 percent, and a resulting associated monetary saving of $312–425 million annually ($426–$581 million in 2021 dollars). Direct cost avoidance was $88–145 million per year ($120–$198 million in 2021 dollars) for an annual investment of $23 million ($32 million in 2021 dollars). The return on investment (ROI) in dollars for the associated economic impact and direct cost avoidance had ROIs minimally 13.6 and 3.8, respectively.

The scientific background to a very effective public health intervention to reduce birth defects (neural tube defects) through improved population level nutrition intervention, providing needed folic acid supplementation indicates a simple solution worked well.

Numerous investigators published folic acid supplementation and deficiency during pregnancy with infant outcome, but results were inconsistent. No congenital anomalies were found among 44 treatment infants whose mothers took 15 times the RDA throughout pregnancy to prevent the recurrence of a NTD (Laurence *et al.*, 1981). However, there were two NTDs in the treatment non-compliance group and four in the placebo control group. Other studies have analyzed folic acid supplements at doses similar to the RDA, and the occurrence of neural tube defects was not more frequent than expected. Notably, small sample sizes confounded the analysis of a rare event (i.e., NTDs with an incidence of 0.2 to 2 in 1,000 or less).

Folic acid supplements given in prospective studies to prevent NTDs decreased the risk of neural tube defects (Bower and Stanley, 1989; Smithells *et al.*, 1980, 1983, 1989). Daily intake of folic acid reduced the occurrence and recurrence of NTDs in 5502 women in a randomized controlled study (Czeizel and Dudas, 1992; Czeizel *et al.*, 1994). Folic acid antagonists (e.g., aminopterin) are well-known human and animal teratogens. Numerous animal teratology studies (rats, mice) consistently show that folic acid deficiency is associated with an increased frequency of various congenital anomalies (Shepard and Lemire, 2010), including NTDs. Periconceptional daily intake of 0.4 mg of folic acid in a case-control study decreased the risk of NTD occurrence in their infants by 50 percent (Werler *et al.*, 1993). Conversely, retrospective studies do not show a reduced risk of neural tube defects with folic acid supplementation during pregnancy (Mills *et al.*, 1989; Milunsky *et al.*, 1989). Folic acid deficiency was associated with adverse pregnancy outcome in one study (Dansky *et al.*, 1987), but not in two others (Pritchard *et al.*, 1970, 1971). In 1992, the US Centers for Disease Control (CDC) issued the recommendation that childbearing age women should consume 0.4 mg of folic acid per day but should not exceed 1.0 mg per day. Untoward effects of hypervitaminosis $B_{12}$ are not well studied during pregnancy. Folate intake among women of childbearing age should regulate their intake to 0.4 mg or less than 1 mg per day (MMWR, 1992).

The frequency of birth defects was not increased among 4,055 infants born to women who took folic acid supplements during the first trimester in the Swedish Birth Defects Registry (Kallen, 2019). However, it was noted that folic acid was not significantly protective, merely neutral (i.e., not harmful).

## IRON

Iron is an essential dietary metal. Iron requirements during pregnancy increase as gestation age progresses. Iron deficiency anemia was related to low energy levels and a lower mean corpuscular volume among 800 pregnant women at their first prenatal care visit (Scholl *et al.*, 1992). Preterm delivery was doubled and the incidence of low birth weight was tripled among iron deficient, anemic women. Iron supplementation need emerges at 20–28 weeks gestation as maternal blood volume augments. Iron supplementation (60–100 mg daily) is needed because the normal diet cannot supply the required amounts. Iron supplement be given alone and not as a component of prenatal vitamins because iron is poorly absorbed from multivitamin preparations. Iron overdose is a common suicide attempt method during pregnancy (see Chapter 14). A prudent practice for patients at high risk of suicide is to prescribe only a 1-week supply at a time, thereby limiting access to toxic iron doses. Toxic iron doses are between 3 and 6 g. Iron supplement megadoses are among the more commonly used medications in suicide gestures, discussed in Chapter 14.

Congenital anomalies were not increased in frequency among 66 infants born to women who received parental iron supplementation during the first trimester. No complications or malformations were found among more than 1,800 infants whose mothers received iron supplementation at any time during pregnancy (Heinonen *et al.*, 1977). The frequency of birth defects or pregnancy complications was not different from the general population among 1,336 infants born to women who took iron supplements when they were anemic, or those gravidas women who took the supplement during the second and third trimesters of pregnancy (Hemminki and Rimpela, 1991).

No abnormalities were observed in a group of 19 children whose mothers had ingested overdoses of iron during the last two trimesters of pregnancy (McElhatton *et al.*, 1991), but first trimester exposures were not reported.

Iron use during pregnancy in animal models are not consistent. The frequency of birth defects was not increased in rat pups born to mothers given up to 100 times the usual human dose of iron during embryogenesis (Flodh *et al.*, 1977; Tadokoro *et al.*, 1979). The frequency of central nervous system anomalies were increased in frequency among mice and rabbits whose mothers were given large doses of iron during embryogenesis (Flodh *et al.*, 1977; Kuchta, 1982).

## CALCIUM

Calcium is an essential nutrient required for normal physiological function and fetal growth. A balanced diet provides the required amount of calcium.

The frequency of congenital anomalies was not increased among more than 1000 infants born to women who received calcium supplements during the first trimester, or among more than 3500 infants whose mothers took calcium supplements after the first trimester (Heinonen *et al.*, 1977). A slight, but significant excess of nonspecific central nervous system abnormalities was reported. The heterogeneity of the defects suggests that the association may be a chance occurrence of multiple comparisons.

Among rats, rabbits, and mice whose mothers were given twice the RDA of calcium during embryogenesis, the frequency of congenital anomalies was no greater than controls (McCormack *et al.*, 1979). Fetal death and growth retardation occurred more frequently in the offspring of pregnant rats given about 1600 mg/kg/day of calcium chloride (Hayasaka *et al.*, 1990).

## SPECIAL CONSIDERATIONS

### Neural Tube Defects

Highly compelling evidence supports occurrence and recurrence of NTDs can be decreased by folic acid supplementation, as discussed earlier. Risk of NTD recurrence was decreased in several different studies in England when a combination vitamin regimen that contained folic acid and seven other vitamins was given to women who had given birth to a child with a NTD in a previous pregnancy (Smithells *et al.*, 1980, 1983, 1989; MRC Vitamin Study Research Group, 1991). The group concluded that, 'Folic acid supplementation starting before pregnancy can now be firmly recommended for all women who have had an affected pregnancy and public health measures should be taken to ensure that the diet of all women who may bear children contains an adequate amount of folic acid,' (MRC Vitamin Study Research Group, 1991). This has led to a cost-effective and significant reduction in the occurrence of NTDs in the USA. Notably, the Swedish Birth Defects Registry specifically analyzed the possible presence of a protective effect and found no decreased risk for neural tube defects or any congenital anomaly (Kallen, 2019).

## NUTRITIONAL SUMMARY

In conclusion, iron supplements during pregnancy are definitely necessary. Folic acid supplements are also a universal necessity, despite ambiguous protection found by some authorities. The gravid vegetarian or one who is following a "fad" diet is a special concern and a nutritional assessment should be undertaken to assure adequate intake. Prenatal vitamins should probably be given, although there is no consensus on whether they are necessary. At RDA doses, such preparations will not cause harm and may be of benefit. Following Hippocrates, above all do no harm, prenatal vitamins should be given. Megadose regimens are clearly contraindicated.

# GASTROINTESTINAL MEDICATIONS DURING PREGNANCY

Gastrointestinal disorders occur frequently during pregnancy, often in response to the pregnancy-related physiological changes. Nausea, with or without vomiting is the most common gastrointestinal disorder of early pregnancy. In the extreme form (i.e., hyperemesis gravidarum), vomiting may result in significant weight loss and dehydration. Pyrosis or "heartburn" is a very common symptom in pregnancy and is related to increased gastroesophageal reflux secondary to decreased muscular tone in the lower esophagus. Gastrointestinal disorders that may be associated with pregnancy, but occur with about the same frequency in non-gravid women, include peptic ulcer disease, inflammatory bowel disease, and gallbladder disease—cholelithiasis and cholecystitis (Cunningham, 1994). Medications to treat gastrointestinal disorders, including antacids, anticholinergics, antiemetics, antiflatulents, and laxatives, are discussed in this section. Corticosteroids, which may be useful in the therapy of inflammatory bowel disease, are discussed in Chapter 4.

## ANTACIDS

Antacids are classified based on their content: aluminum, calcium, magnesium, magaldrate, sodium bicarbonate, and combinations of any of these. Antacids are the most common over-the-counter and prescribed gastrointestinal medications used by pregnant women. Combinations of aluminum hydroxide and magnesium hydroxide are used in popular commercial preparations (e.g., Maalox, Mylanta, Riopan, and Gelusil). Calcium carbonate is also a very popular antacid (e.g., Tums, Titralac, Rolaids, and Chooz).

No human or animal teratology studies have been published regarding antacids. Antacids are associated with little, if any, significant risk for congenital anomalies or fetal risk when used in moderation. Chronic use of high-dose antacids has been associated with adverse effects such as hypercalcemia, hypermagnesemia, or hypocalcemia.

## HISTAMINE RECEPTOR ANTAGONISTS

Histamine receptor antagonists are systemic agents used to reduce gastric acidity. Preparations include cimetidine, ranitidine, famotidine, and nizatidine (Table 12.2). Prophylaxis against aspiration is a routine use of these agents in pregnant women before general anesthesia. Histamine receptor antagonists are used to treat peptic ulcer disease, although the condition is uncommon in pregnant women. H-receptor antagonists (i.e., inhibitors of gastric acid production) are used to treat pregnant women with severe forms of reflux esophagitis that is unresponsive to the usual antacids. Histamine receptor antagonists are known to cross the placenta (Howe *et al.*, 1981; Schenker *et al.*, 1987).

Among 237 infants born to women who took cimetidine during the first trimester of pregnancy, the frequency of congenital anomalies was not increased (Ruigomez *et al.*, 1999). In another study, the frequency of congenital anomalies was increased among 113 infants exposed to cimetidine during the first trimester (Garbis *et al.*, 2005). First trimester ranitidine exposure

---

**TABLE 12.2**

**Histamine ($H_2$) Receptor Antagonists**

| Agent | Brand Name |
|---|---|
| Cimetidine | Tagamet |
| Famotidine | Pepcid |
| Nizatidine | Axid |
| Ranitidine | Zantac |
| Roxatidine | Roxit |

---

was reported in 335 infants and the frequency of congenital anomalies was not increased above controls (Garbis *et al.*, 2005). Similarly, congenital anomalies in infants born to 300 women who took ranitidine during embryogenesis were not increased over controls (Ruigomez *et al.*, 1999). Among infants born to 58 women who used famotidine in the first trimester, the frequency of congenital anomalies was no higher than that expected in the general population (Kallen, 1998). In one study of 75 infants whose mothers took famotidine during the first trimester, the frequency of congenital anomalies detected at birth was no higher than would be expected in the general population (Garbis *et al.*, 2005). However, two elective terminations occurred in the famotidine group because they had NTDs. The relevance of these data is unknown because of the small sample size; the authors felt that timing of famotidine exposure excluded a causal association with the neural tube defects (Garbis *et al.*, 2005). Data have been published on a small number of first-trimester exposures to nizatidine (n = 15) and roxatidine (n = 15) and there were no congenital anomalies (Garbis *et al.*, 2005). Nizatidine is closely related to cimetidine. The Swedish Birth Defects Registry include only seven infants born following maternal use of nizatidine during the first trimester (Kallen, 2019).

Histamine receptor antagonists were not associated with an increased frequency of malformations or adverse fetal effects in several animal teratology studies involving rodents (Brimblecombe *et al.*, 1985; Higashida *et al.*, 1983; Tamura *et al.*, 1983). Several reports regarding the use of these agents as premedications prior to Cesarean section found an increased frequency of complications (Gillett *et al.*, 1984; Hodgkinson *et al.*, 1983; Mathews *et al.*, 1986; Thorburn and Moir, 1987), but these exposures are not relevant to the risk for congenital anomalies.

Therefore, data suggest that histamine receptor antagonists may be used safely in the first trimester of pregnancy in humans, with apparent safety for both mother and fetus in the latter half of pregnancy.

## PROTON PUMP INHIBITORS

### Omeprazole, Lansoprazole, and Esomeprazole

Omeprazole (Prilosec) is a proton pump inhibitor (PPI). PPIs block the production of gastric acid. Among 295 infants whose mothers were exposed to omeprazole during embryogenesis, the frequency of congenital anomalies was no greater than among controls (Kallen, 1998). Additional information from the Swedish Registry reported 9607 infants exposed to omeprazole during the first trimester, among whom the frequency of birth defects was not significantly increased (Kallen, 2019). Ninety-one infants were born to women who took omeprazole during the first trimester and the frequency of congenital anomalies was no greater than expected (Lalkin *et al.*, 1998). Among 233 infants exposed during the first trimester to omeprazole, the frequency of congenital anomalies was not significantly greater than unexposed controls (Diav-Citrin *et al.*, 2005). A case report of an omeprazole overdose during pregnancy that resulted in a normal infant has been published (Ferner and Allison, 1993). A small case series (n = 3) in which mothers were treated with omeprazole chronically, resulted in three healthy infants in the neonatal period (Harper *et al.*, 1995). No congenital anomalies were found among rat pups born to mothers given many times the usual human dose of omeprazole during embryogenesis, although growth retardation was present (Shimazu *et al.*, 1988).

Among 55 infants exposed to lansoprazole during the first trimester, the frequency of congenital anomalies was not increased. In the same investigation, the frequency of congenital anomalies among infants exposed to pantoprazole during the first trimester was no greater than controls (Diav-Citrin *et al.*, 2005). The Swedish Registry reported 975 infants exposed to lansoprazole during organogenesis during the first trimester, and the frequency of congenital anomalies was not increased (Kallen, 2019).

Esomeprazole is the levorotatory racemate of omeprazole. Clinically, the advantage of esomeprazole over omeprazole is that the *S*-racemate isomer is cleared more slowly, decreasing dose frequency (Kendall, 2003). The frequency of birth defects was not increased among 542 infants born following first trimester esomeprazole exposure in the Swedish Registry (Kallen, 2019).

Proton pump inhibitors seem to be safe for use during pregnancy.

## ANTIEMETICS

Most pregnant women experience at least some degree of nausea during the first trimester; most can be managed without medication. A variety of medications can be used in women requiring therapy for protracted vomiting or vomiting resulting in dehydration.

## PHENOTHIAZINES

Phenothiazines are used for several medical indications (nausea, vomiting, psychotic disorders, mild pain). This drug class is also effective as an antidyskinetic and a mild sedative. Prochlorperazine, chlorpromazine, and promethazine are the most commonly used phenothiazine derivatives used to treat nausea and vomiting during pregnancy. Phenothiazine use during pregnancy may be associated with extrapyramidal symptoms in the mother as well as the fetus, but these adverse effects are uncommon. The phenothiazine class does not seem to be associated with an increased frequency of congenital anomalies when used during gestation. The frequency of birth defects was not increased among infants of 315 exposed to phenothiazines during the first trimester (Rumeau-Rouquette *et al.*, 1977).

## CHLORPROMAZINE

The frequency of birth defects was not increased among infants of more than 142 women who took chlorpromazine during embryogenesis (Heinonen *et al.*, 1977). No birth defects were observed among 36 infants whose mothers use chlorpromazine during the first trimester (Rosa, 1993, unpublished).

The frequency of congenital anomalies was not increased among rodents whose mothers were given large doses of the drug during embryogenesis (Beall, 1972; Jones-Price *et al.*, 1983; Robertson *et al.*, 1980).

## PROMETHAZINE

Promethazine is sold under several proprietary names. It is also used with meperidine during labor and for post-Cesarean section pain. Birth defects were not increased in frequency among 114 infants whose mothers took promethazine in the first trimester (Heinonen *et al.*, 1977). The frequency of malformations was not increased in two other studies that included several hundred women who used the drug during their first trimester (Aselton *et al.*, 1985; Farkas and Farkas, 1971). The frequency of congenital anomalies was not increased in frequency among 1,197 newborns whose mothers took promethazine during the first trimester (Briggs *et al.*, 2021).

The frequency of birth defect was not increased in the offspring of animals exposed to this agent (King *et al.*, 1965).

## PROCHLORPERAZINE

Published studies include over 3,000 women who took prochlorperazine during pregnancy. In one large study, 877 infants exposed to prochlorperazine during the first trimester (Heinonen *et al.*, 1977). No birth defects were observed among 50–99 infants whose mothers used prochlorperazine (Jick *et al.*, 1981). In the Swedish Medical Birth Registry, the frequency of birth defects was not increased among 145 infants exposed during the first trimester (Asker *et al.*, 2005. In 453 infants exposed during the first trimester to prochlorperazine, the frequency of birth defects was not increased (Milkovich and van den Berg, 1977). The frequency of congenital anomalies was not increased in the offspring of 704 women who took the drug in the first trimester (Briggs *et al.*, 2021).

The frequency of cleft palate was increased in the offspring of pregnant animals given large doses of prochlorperazine during embryogenesis (Roux, 1959; Szabo and Brent, 1974). The relevance of this finding in humans is unknown.

## PIPERAZINE DERIVATIVES

Piperazine derivatives (cyclizine, buclizine, meclizine) are used for their antiemetic and antihistamine properties. The frequency of congenital anomalies was not increased with exposure to cyclizine or meclizine during the first trimester in the Collaborative Perinatal Project in more than 1,000 infants (Heinonen *et al.*, 1977). Among 111 infants whose mothers took cyclizine in the first trimester, no increase in congenital anomalies was found (Milkovich and van den Berg, 1977). More detailed discussion of these agents is given in Chapter 11. No studies have been published on buclizine during pregnancy. The Swedish Birth Defects Registry reported no increased frequency of birth defects among 1,408 and 62 infants born to women who used meclizine and cyclizine, respectively, during organogenesis (Kallen, 2019).

## DOXYLAMINE-PYRIDOXINE

The combination of doxylamine-pyridoxine (Bendectin) has received considerable attention over the past decade as a possible teratogen. Until it was taken off the market, Bendectin was the most commonly prescribed antiemetic for hyperemesis during pregnancy.

There have been reports of an association of Bendectin use with diaphragmatic hernias (Bracken and Berg, 1983) and with congenital heart disease and pyloric stenosis (Aselton *et al.*, 1985; Eskenazi and Bracken, 1982). Reports refuting such an association (Mitchell *et al.*, 1981, 1983; Zierler and Rothman, 1985) have also been published. Among more than 1,100 infants exposed to doxylamine (Bendectin) during the first trimester of pregnancy, the frequency of congenital anomalies was not increased (Heinonen *et al.*, 1977). No statistically significant association was found between doxylamine and congenital heart disease in a large case-control study (Zierler and Rothman, 1985). Animal teratology studies are also negative (Gibson *et al.*, 1968).

Millions of women used Bendectin during the first trimester of pregnancy with no apparent epidemic of birth defects or adverse fetal effects. Therefore, it seems very unlikely that either doxylamine or pyridoxine is a significant human teratogen. It is generally accepted that neither Bendectin nor its components caused birth defects in human infants. Unfortunately, it does appear that Bendectin was a significant "litogen" (i.e., capable of inducing lawsuits) (Brent, 1983,; Holmes, 1983). A recent paper (Berard *et al.*, 2019) resurrected claims of the possible association of Bendectin components with birth defects, but was quickly followed by a Meta-Analysis (Biffi *et al.*, 2020) that showed no association between Bendectin ingredients and birth defects. The human teratology scientific community does not believe that this combination of drugs (Bendectin) is a cause of birth defects.

## OTHER

Ondansetron (Zofran) is a 5-hydroxytryptamine (5-HT) receptor agonist. It is a potent antiemetic, commonly used to treat severe nausea and vomiting associated with cancer chemotherapy, radiotherapy, and postoperative nausea. In addition, it has been used to treat severe hyperemesis gravidarum (World, 1993; Guikontes *et al.*, 1992. Among 169 infants born to women who used ondansetron during pregnancy, six (3.6 percent) major malformations occurred, not different from the control group (Einarson *et al.*, 2004). Among 55 pregnancies exposed to ondansetron during the first trimester, the frequency of birth defects was not increased. However, Anderka *et al.* (2012) reported an association between ondansetron and cleft palate among individuals exposed to ondansetron during the first trimester.

In unpublished studies, this agent was not teratogenic in animal studies (information provided by the manufacturer). It is an FDA pregnancy risk category B drug.

## PROKINETIC AGENTS

Prokinetic agents stimulate upper gastrointestinal tract motility and are used primarily for the treatment of gastrointestinal reflux. Two agents are currently available in this class: cisapride (Propulsid) and metoclopramide (Reglan). Among 88 infants born to women who used cisapride during the first trimester, the frequency of congenital anomalies was not increased (Bailey *et al.*, 1997). In Swedish Registry, 106 infants were exposed to cisapride during the first trimester, and the frequency of birth defects was not increased (Kallen, 2019).

Metoclopramide is used as an antiemetic, especially for postoperative nausea. Among 175 infants born to women who used metoclopramide during the first trimester, the frequency of congenital anomalies was 4.4 percent, which was no different from the control rate, 4.8 percent (Berkovitch *et al.*, 2002). Among 884 infants whose mothers used metoclopramide during the first trimester in the Swedish Registry, the frequency of congenital anomalies was not increased (Asker *et al.*, 2005). Unpublished data from the manufacturer, metoclopramide was not teratogenic in rats or rabbits (unpublished data). Interestingly, cisapride is listed as a category C drug and metoclopramide as a category B drug under the old system. In view of the data, both prokinetic agents appear safe for use during pregnancy, keeping in mind that metoclopramide has a number of patients and more statistical power.

## ANTICHOLINERGICS

Anticholinergics are mainly used as antispasmodics and in the therapy of gastrointestinal diseases (ulcer disease, irritable bowel disease). Some of these medications are utilized for other non-gastrointestinal indications, such as cardiac arrhythmias or urologic disorders. This class of preparations (Table 12.3) is known to cross the placenta.

**TABLE 12.3**
**Anticholinergics**

| Agents | Brand Name(s) |
| --- | --- |
| Atropine Belladonna | |
| Clidinium | Quarzan |
| Dicyclomine | Bentyl, Byclomine, Dibent, Di-Spaz |
| Glycopyrrolate | Robinul |
| Hexocyclium | Tral Filmtabs |
| Homatropine | Homapin |
| Hyoscyamine | Cystospaz, Levsinex, Levsin, Anaspaz, Neoquess, Bellafoline |
| Isopropamide | Darbid |
| Mepenzolate | Cantil |
| Methantheline | Banthine |
| Methscopolamine | Pamine |
| Oxyphenonium | Oxyphencyclimine |
| Propantheline | Norpanth, Pro-Banthine Scopolamine |
| Tridihexethyl | Pathilon |

## Atropine

Atropine is an anticholinergic that is utilized for a variety of indications, such as cardiac arrhythmias (especially bradycardia), Parkinsonism, asthma, biliary tract diseases, as an antidote for organophosphate insecticide poisoning, and as a preanesthetic agent. The frequency of congenital anomalies was not increased among 401 infants born to women who used atropine in early pregnancy (Heinonen et al., 1977). Only one birth defect occurred among 50–99 infants exposed to atropine during the first trimester, and this was not an increased frequency (1 percent to 2 percent) (Jick et al., 1981).

Skeletal anomalies were reported to be increased in one animal study (Arcuri and Gautieri, 1973). Such anomalies have not been reported to date in humans and the data suggest atropine is a safe drug for use during pregnancy.

## Scopolamine

Scopolamine is an anticholinergic agent similar to atropine, and like atropine, may be utilized as a preoperative medication. It may also be used as an antiemetic and for motion sickness. The frequency of congenital anomalies was no different from control in the offspring of 309 women who received this medication in early pregnancy (Heinonen et al., 1977). Unpublished data for 27 infants exposed to scopolamine found no birth defects (Briggs et al., 2021).

The frequency of birth defects was not increased among the offspring of rodents given doses much larger than the human dose during embryogenesis (George et al., 1987).

## Homatropine and Methscopolamine

No information has been published regarding the use of the anticholinergics homatropine (an ophthalmic preparation) or methscopolamine (used for cardiac arrhythmias, functional bowel disease, and ulcer disease) during pregnancy for experimental animals or humans.

## Belladonna

Belladonna is a naturally occurring anticholinergic and is used to treat several conditions: functional bowel disorders, motion sickness, dysmenorrhea. Among more than 500 infants born to women who took belladonna during the first trimester, the frequency of major congenital anomalies was not increased (Heinonen et al., 1977). There was an association with minor malformations, but the meaning of this finding is unknown. No animal teratology studies of this agent have been published.

## Glycopyrrolate

Glycopyrrolate is used for several indications: ulcer disease, functional bowel syndrome, and as a preanesthetic agent. No publications on human or animal exposure to this agent during pregnancy have been published.

## Dicyclomine

Used primarily for the treatment of spastic or irritable colon, dicyclomine was at one time used in combination with doxylamine and pyridoxine in the popular antiemetic preparation, Bendectin®. No increase in the frequency of congenital anomalies was found in the offspring of about 100 women who used this agent in early pregnancy (Aselton et al., 1985). The frequency of malformations was not increased in the offspring of animals given dicyclomine in doses several times that of the human dose during embryogenesis (Gibson et al., 1968).

## Hyoscyamine

Hyoscyamine is used to treat spasmodic bowel diseases and asthma. Over 300 women were exposed to hyoscyamine in early pregnancy, and their infants did not have an increased frequency of birth defects (Heinonen et al., 1977). No animal teratology studies have been published on hyoscyamine.

### Isopropamide

This agent is used as an adjunct to treat ulcer disease and is used for the treatment of spastic bowel disorders. Congenital anomalies were not increased in frequency in the offspring of 180 women who took the drug during early pregnancy (Heinonen *et al.*, 1977). No published animal teratology studies are available regarding isopropamide.

### Propantheline

Very little information is available regarding the use of this agent during early pregnancy. Only 33 women who took this drug during early pregnancy are included in the Collaborative Perinatal Project database, and the frequency of congenital anomalies in their infants was not increased (Heinonen *et al.*, 1977).

### Other Agents

No epidemiological studies of congenital anomalies in infants born to women who took clidinium, hexocyclium, mepenzolate, tridihexethyl, oxyphencyclimine, or methantheline during pregnancy have been published. No animal teratology studies of these agents have been published.

### APPETITE SUPPRESSANTS

Appetite suppressants are not indicated during pregnancy. Frequently, pregnant women use these medications during the first trimester before pregnancy is recognized because these agents are commonly used by women of reproductive age. Numerous available commercial preparations and some common appetite suppressants are listed (Box 12.1).

---

**BOX 12.1   APPETITE SUPPRESSANTS**

| | | |
|---|---|---|
| Amphetamine | Benzphetamine | Diethylpropion |
| Fenfluramine | Mazindol | Methamphetamine |
| Phendimetrazine | Phenmetrazine | Phentermine |

---

### Amphetamines, Dextroamphetamines, and Methamphetamines

These controlled substances are used in a variety of medications for the treatment of hyperactivity, short attention span syndrome, narcolepsy, and as an appetite suppressant for morbid obesity. They are not recommended for use during pregnancy or in breastfeeding mothers because of potential adverse effects. These stimulants are discussed in further detail in Chapter 16.

### Benzphetamine

**No information has been published on teratogenicity of the use of benzphetamine (Didrex) in pregnant women.**

### Diethylpropion

Use of diethylpropion (M-Orexic, Nobesine, Tenuate) in early pregnancy was not associated with an increased frequency of congenital anomalies among infants born to several-hundred women (Bunde and Leyland, 1965; Heinonen *et al.*, 1977). Diethylpropion was not teratogenic in one animal study (Cohen *et al.*, 1964).

Although appetite suppressants are generally not recommended for use during pregnancy, this agent is listed as an FDA old category B.

## Phendimetrazine

At least 36 different commercial preparations of this agent are available in the USA, but no epidemiological studies have been published of human infants born following its use during pregnancy. No animal teratology studies of phendimetrazine (Prelu-2) have been published. It should be listed as a category C drug because of lack of information.

## Phentermine and Fenfluramine

Among 98 infants born to women who took phentermine/fenfluramine during the first trimester, the frequency of both minor and major congenital anomalies was comparable to the control group frequency (Jones *et al.*, 2002).

## Mazindol

No human reproduction studies with mazindol (Mazanor) have been published.

## Dexfenfluramine

Dexfenfluramine is a dextroisomer of fenfluramine, a serotoninergic agent. Information on dexfenfluramine and exposure during pregnancy have not been published.

## ANTIFLATULENTS, LAXATIVES, AND ANTIDIARRHEALS

Gastric motility is decreased during pregnancy (Little, 1999) and constipation is a relatively common complaint in pregnant women. Various iron preparations may also contribute to constipation in the pregnant patient. Laxatives are frequently used during pregnancy. The majority of such agents are absorbed very little, if at all, from the gastrointestinal tract. Overall, they should have no systemic effects or pose any serious threat to the fetus.

### Antiflatulents

## Simethicone

Simethicone (Phazyme, Myliam, Gas-X, Gas Relief) is the most commonly used antiflatulent. There are no human or animal reproductive studies available. Simethicone is logically not expected to cause systemic effects or have access to the fetal-placental unit, because simethicone is not absorbed from the gastrointestinal tract. It is contained in several antacid preparations.

## Charcoal

No information has been published regarding the use of charcoal during pregnancy, although activated charcoal capsules and tablets are used for relief of gas. Notably, it is not absorbed systemically.

From a practical standpoint, it has no clear indications for use during pregnancy; neither does this agent offer any advantage over simethicone. However, *activated charcoal should be used without hesitation when it is needed in the treatment of acute poisoning*.

## Calcium Carbonate

This agent in combination with magnesium hydroxide (Mylanta) is utilized as both an antacid and an antiflatulent. This combination can be used safely in pregnancy, avoiding chronic high doses that pose a risk (hypercalcemia, etc.).

### Laxatives and Purgatives

Laxatives/purgatives can generally be divided into several classes depending on the mode of action: (1) Emollients and softeners, (2) bulk-forming agents, (3) stimulants, and (4) saline, hyperosmotic, or lubricant agents (Box 12.2). Fortunately, there are few side effects associated with the use of these agents. Allergic reactions are rare. Chronic use of the agents should be avoided because diarrhea and electrolyte imbalances may occur.

---

### BOX 12.2   LAXATIVES AND PURGATIVES

**Emollients and stool softeners**

- Docusate sodium (Colace plus numerous others) plus combinations
- Docusate calcium (Surfak, Pro-Cal-Sof) plus combinations
- Docusate potassium (Dialose, Diocto-K, Kasof)

**Bulk-forming agents**

- Psyllium (Metamucil, Konsyl-D, Pro-Lax, Serutan, plus several others)
- Methylcellulose (Citrucel, Cologel)
- Malt soup extract (Maltsupex)
- Polycarbophil (Fibercan, Equalactin, Mitrolan)

**Stimulants**

- Castor oil
- Bisacodyl (Dulcolax plus others) plus combinations
- Casanthranol (Black-Draught) plus combinations
- Cascara sagrada plus combinations
- Phenolphthalein (Ex-Lax plus others) plus combinations
- Senna (Senokot plus others) plus combinations
- Saline, hyperosmotic, or lubricant agents
- Mineral oil (Kondremul plus others) plus combinations
- Glycerin
- Lactulose (Chronulac plus others)
- Magnesium citrate (Citroma; Citro-Nesia)
- Magnesium hydroxide (Milk of Magnesia) plus combinations

---

## Docusate

This agent is an emollient-type laxative used either singly as a stool softener or in combination with other laxatives. Congenital anomalies were not increased in frequency among the offspring of over 800 women who utilized this agent in early pregnancy (Aselton *et al.*, 1985; Heinonen *et al.*, 1977; Jick *et al.*, 1981). Docusate is not absorbed systemically.

## Casanthranol and Cascara Sagrada

The anthraquinone cathartics belong to the stimulant class of laxatives. They are used as monotherapy or in combination with other laxatives. Congenital anomalies were not increased in frequency among offspring of mothers who utilized either casanthranol (21 patients) or cascara sagrada (53 patients) in early pregnancy (Heinonen *et al.*, 1977).

## Senna

Senna is also an anthraquinone laxative. No human reproduction studies have been published. It is very unlikely that it poses any risk to the fetus because this agent is minimally absorbed from the gastrointestinal tract.

## Phenolphthalein

Phenolphthalein (Ex-Lax, Feen-A-Mint, Atophen, Medilax, Modone, Espotabs) is a commonly utilized agent in commercial preparations. In one mouse study, decreased litter size and fertility were observed, but no somatic effects (Anonymous, 1997).

## Lactulose

This agent is utilized as a laxative and for lowering serum ammonia in cases of hepatic encephalopathy. Although there are no human reproduction studies, this agent is not absorbed from the gastrointestinal tract for the most part, and thus is unlikely to be associated with adverse fetal effects.

## Mineral Oil

Mineral oil is a lubricant laxative. There are no published human epidemiological or animal teratology studies with this agent. However, chronic use of mineral oil as a laxative might interfere with the absorption of fat-soluble vitamins such as vitamin K and D, and thus theoretically could have adverse fetal effects.

## Castor Oil

There are no published human epidemiological or animal teratology studies with this agent. There are also no reports of an association of adverse fetal effects with the use of castor oil during pregnancy. It has been a commonly held belief that this agent would stimulate labor and it is often utilized for this purpose in women close to term. However, little scientific data support the use of this agent as a potent stimulant of labor.

## ANTIDIARRHEAL AGENTS

Unlike constipation, diarrhea is an uncommon complaint of pregnancy and is usually secondary to medications (especially antibiotics), infections (bacterial, viral, and parasite), and abuse of laxatives or lactose intolerance. Fortunately, most cases of acute diarrhea are self-limited and require no specific therapy. Patients should maintain adequate hydration. Antidiarrheals can generally be divided into three major categories—bulk-forming agents, absorbents, and opiates (Box 12.3).

---

### BOX 12.3   ANTIDIARRHEAL MEDICATIONS

- Bulking agents
- Absorbents
- Kaolin and pectin (Kaopectate)
- Opioid agents

---

## Bulk-Forming Agents

These agents are utilized primarily for chronic diarrhea and are listed in Box 12.3. None of these agents is absorbed systemically. Therefore, embryo-fetal exposure does not occur and there is no associated risk.

## Absorbents

The combination of kaolin and pectin (Kaopectate) is probably the antidiarrheal agent most commonly used, including during pregnancy. Its main mode of action is absorbent action. No epidemiological studies regarding the use of this agent in pregnant women are published. However, since very little, if any, of the agents are absorbed from the gastrointestinal tract, it is highly unlikely this antidiarrheal poses a significant risk to either mother or fetus.

## Opioid Agents

Kaolin and pectin are combined with opium and belladonna (Amogel-PG, Donnagel-PG, Donnapectolin-PG, Quiagel-PG) and with paregoric (kapectolin with paregoric, parepectolin). The addition of belladonna and opioid agents results in decreased gastrointestinal mobility. Use of opioids in pregnant women may pose a risk of birth defects if used chronically in the first trimester (see Chapter 8). Only 36 women were exposed during early pregnancy were included in the Collaborative Perinatal Project database; no evidence of a significant increase in the frequency of congenital anomalies was found in this small sample (Heinonen *et al.*, 1977). Almost 100 women were exposed to paregoric in early pregnancy with no significant increase in frequency of congenital anomalies (Aselton *et al.*, 1985). However, the possibility exists of addiction and subsequent neonatal abstinence syndrome in neonates whose mothers use opioid agents chronically.

The combination of diphenoxylate and atropine (Lomotil and others) is another commonly used antidiarrheal. Diphenoxylate, a compound similar to meperidine, acts primarily to reduce intestinal motility. Atropine is included in this preparation in an effort to prevent abuse. A case report of an infant born with congenital heart disease whose mother used this agent during pregnancy is published (Ho *et al.*, 1975), but anecdotal reports cannot be used to establish causality. No large epidemiologic studies are published regarding its use during pregnancy. Fewer than 10 patients who used this agent in early pregnancy were included in the Collaborative Perinatal Project (Heinonen *et al.*, 1977). None of the offspring of these women had malformations.

## Loperamide

This antidiarrheal agent works by decreasing intestinal motility. No human reproduction studies have been published. According to its manufacturer, loperamide was not teratogenic in rats and rabbits. It is an FDA category B drug under the old system.

Teratogen Information System (TERIS) and FDA risk ratings for congenital anomalies

The TERIS and FDA risk ratings for drugs in this chapter provide a reasonable summary of risks that are supported by the medical literature. Most of the supporting literature for Table 12.4 has been discussed earlier.

---

## TABLE 12.4

## Teratogen Information System (TERIS) Risk Rating for Congenital Anomalies and Food and Drug Administration (FDA) Pregnancy Risk: Category Rating for Nutritional Supplements and Gastrointestinal Drugs

| Drugs | TERIS Risk | Old FDA Risk Rating |
|---|---|---|
| Aminopterin | Moderate to high | X |
| Amphetamine | Unlikely | C |
| Ascorbic acid (vitamin C) | None | A* |
| Beta-carotene | Low dose: None | C |
| Calcium salts | Unlikely | NA |
| Chlorpromazine | Unlikely | C |
| Cimetidine | Unlikely | B |
| Cisapride | Undetermined | C |
| Cyanocobalamin | Undetermined | NA |
| Dexfenfluramine | Undetermined | C |
| Diethylpropion | None | NA |

| Drugs | TERIS Risk | Old FDA Risk Rating |
|---|---|---|
| Famotidine | Unlikely | B |
| Fenfluramine | Undetermined | NA |
| Folic acid | None | A[*] |
| Iron | None | NA |
| Isotretinoin | High | X |
| Mazindol | Undetermined | NA |
| Methamphetamine | Unlikely | NA[*] |
| Metoclopramide | Unlikely | B |
| Niacin | Undetermined | A[*] |
| Nizatidine | Undetermined | B |
| Omeprazole | Unlikely | C |
| Pantothenate | Undetermined | NA |
| Phendimetrazine | Unlikely | NA |
| Phentermine | Undetermined | C |
| Prochlorperazine | None | NA |
| Promethazine | None | C |
| Pyridoxine | None | A |
| Ranitidine | Unlikely | B |
| Retinol (vitamin A) | Low dose: None | A[*] |
| High dose: NA, **probably high risk** | | |
| Thiamine | Undetermined | A[*] |
| Vitamin D | Unlikely | A[*] |
| Vitamin E | Undetermined | A[*] |

[*] Therapeutic dose.

*Abbreviation:* NA, not available.

*Sources:* Compiled from: Friedman *et al.*, *Obstet Gynecol*, 1990; 75: 594; Briggs *et al.*, 2021; Friedman and Polifka, 2006.

## SPECIAL CONSIDERATIONS

Most agents used for gastrointestinal disease may be used safely in pregnant women, especially after the first trimester.

### NAUSEA AND VOMITING

All pregnant women probably experience nausea to some degree in early pregnancy. "Morning sickness" or nausea and vomiting are common symptoms during the first trimester of pregnancy, but most pregnant women do not require antiemetic therapy. Frequent, small meals may prove beneficial in management of nausea without medical intervention. Fortunately, hyperemesis gravidarum, the most severe form of pregnancy-associated nausea and vomiting occurs in only a small percentage of gravidas. Women with hyperemesis gravidarum may require hospitalization and intravenous hydration, and antiemetic therapy. One of the most effective antiemetic agents for nausea and vomiting associated with pregnancy was doxylamine plus pyridoxine (Bendectin). However, this agent is no longer available because of the fear of litigation. When antiemetics are indicated, promethazine suppositories (or occasionally use of oral preparations) in doses of 25 mg should be used. Other agents that may prove useful for hyperemesis gravidarum are given in Box 12.4.

**BOX 12.4    THERAPY FOR NAUSEA AND VOMITING OF PREGNANCY[a]**

**Chlorpromazine**

- Suppositories            50–100 mg q 8 h
- Oral                     10–25 mg q 4 h
- Parenteral               2.5–25 mg IM q 4 h

**Ondansetron**

- Intravenous              32 mg as a single dose once a day
- Oral                     8 mg bid

**Prochlorperazine**

- Suppositories            5–10 mg two to three times per day
- Oral                     5–10 mg tid or gid
- Parenteral               5–10 mg IM q 4 h promethazine
- Suppositories            12.5–25 mg q 4 h
- Oral                     5–10 mg tid or gid
- Parenteral               25 mg IM q 4 h thiethylperazine
- Suppositories            10 mg gd to tid
- Oral                     10 mg qd to tid
- Parenteral               10 mg IM qd to tid

**Trimethobenzamide**

- Suppositories            200 mg tid or gid
- Oral                     250 mg tid or gid
- Parenteral               200 mg IM tid or gid

[a] See manufacturer's recommendations.

Agents such as prochlorperazine, promethazine, chlorpromazine, and thiethylperazine may be associated with extrapyramidal side effects, manifested as dystonia, torticollis, and oculogyric crisis. If extrapyramidal effects occur, the unusual syndrome of adverse effects can be treated with diphenhydramine (Benadryl). Importantly, chlorpromazine may be associated with significant hypotension when given intravenously. Therefore, suppositories are the preferred route of administration.

For severe cases of hyperemesis gravidarum in which other agents are largely ineffective, ondansetron (Zofran) 32 mg intravenously as a single dose may be effective. Ondansetron is also available in an oral form (8 mg b.i.d.). However, this route is much less likely to be effective in treatment of hyperemesis gravidarum because almost everything taken orally is vomited.

### REFLUX ESOPHAGITIS

Reflux esophagitis results in heartburn or pyrosis and esophageal erosion is very common in pregnancy. It is thought to be secondary to decreased gastroesophageal sphincter tone, with resultant gastric acid reflux. Reflux therapy consists primarily of one of the antacid preparations discussed in the previous section. Frequent small feedings and elevation of the head at night may be beneficial. $H_2$-receptor antagonists or PPI (omeprazole or esomeprazole) as well as metoclopramide may prove effective for severe forms of reflux. Esomeprazole and omeprazole are the most popular treatments for reflux esophagitis. Omeprazole and esomeprazole are sufficiently well studied during pregnancy to reasonably state they are safe.

## Peptic Ulcer Disease

Peptic ulcer disease is uncommon during pregnancy. Active ulcer disease may actually improve during pregnancy. Ulcer disease therapy in pregnant patients is concentrated on reduction of gastric acid production. Antacids or the $H_2$-receptor antagonists are effective, but the most popular treatment is PPIs.

The antacids described earlier can be used safely in pregnant women with peptic ulcer disease. However, preference should be given to the best studied agents during pregnancy (i.e., ranitidine or omeprazole/esomeprazole). Dosing after meals and at bedtime is the usual, most effective regimen. 'Prophylactic' antacids are not generally recommended for pregnant women with inactive or asymptomatic disease.

$H_2$-receptor antagonists (cimetidine, ranitidine) inhibit gastric acid secretion and may be used to treat peptic ulcer disease in pregnant women. Cimetidine is usually given in a dose of 300 mg orally four times a day; ranitidine is usually given in an oral dose of 150 mg b.i.d. Omeprazole or esomeprazole may also be used with once or twice daily dosing.

## Diarrhea

Acute diarrhea usually requires no specific therapy other than ensuring adequate hydration. When antidiarrheal therapy is necessary, the combination of kaolin and pectin (Kaopectate) may be safely used. If this first-line treatment fails indicating the need for a stronger regimen, opioid-like preparations may be used (Box 12.5). However, narcotic preparations should not be used chronically in pregnant women, and first trimester use of opioids should be avoided.

---

**BOX 12.5   THERAPY FOR UNCOMPLICATED DIARRHEA OF PREGNANCY**

- Diphenoxylate and atropine, 2.5–5 mg orally three to four times per day.
- Kaolin, pectin, belladonna, opium, 30 mL initial dose, followed by 15 mL q 3 h. Kaolin, pectin, 15–30 mL after each diarrheal episode.
- Kaolin plus pectin, 60–120 cc of regular strength orally after each diarrheal episode.
- Loperamide, 20 mL or two caplets after first diarrheal episode. Then 10 mL or 1 caplet after each diarrheal episode, not exceeding 40 mL or four caplets in 24 h.

---

Treatment of diarrhea with an infectious etiology (i.e., *Escherichia coli*, shigella, and salmonella) should employ traditional antidiarrheal medication cautiously because the underlying disease needs treatment. Infections may be increased in severity or prolonged when treated with traditional antidiarrheal agents.

Diarrhea secondary to bacterial infections may or may not need specific antimicrobial therapy. When necessary, therapy should be directed at the specific organism(s) (see Chapter 2).

Diarrhea secondary to protozoan disease (i.e., amebiasis and giardiasis) can be treated with metronidazole (500 or 750 mg t.i.d. for 5–10 days for the former, and 250 mg t.i.d. for 5–10 days for the latter). Therapy need not be delayed until after the first trimester as first-trimester use of metronidazole does not increase the risk for congenital anomalies (see Chapter 2).

## CELIAC DISEASE

Celiac disease is a characterized by diarrhea, bloating, anemia, weight loss, and gluten intolerance. In maternal celiac disease, folic acid, iron, and other essential nutrients are not adequately absorbed from the gastrointestinal tract. Patients usually improve when placed on a gluten-free diet. A series of 94 gravidas with celiac disease found that untreated celiac disease placed women at a nine-fold increased risk for miscarriages compared to pregnant women on a gluten-free diet. Low birth weight was increased approximately sixfold among untreated women, compared to gravidas maintained on a gluten-free diet. Severity of celiac disease during pregnancy was apparently not related to pregnancy outcome. Maintaining a gluten-free diet during gestation was the important determinant of pregnancy outcome, not severity of the disease (Ciacci *et al.*, 1996). This finding strongly implies that nutrient and micronutrient gut malabsorption in the gravid Celiac patient is related to pregnancy complications, although a nutrient profile was not analyzed in the referenced study.

## INFLAMMATORY BOWEL DISEASE

Ulcerative colitis and Crohn's disease are relatively common in pregnant women. Inactive inflammatory bowel disease worsened during pregnancy among approximately 30 percent of more than 1,000 pregnant women. The majority (n = 143, 45 percent) of 320 pregnant patients with active disease at the start of pregnancy became worse, while 84 (26 percent) remained the same, and 93 (29 percent) improved (Miller, 1986).

Ulcerative colitis, a chronic disease of unknown etiology, is associated with two life-threatening conditions: fulminant disease and adenocarcinoma of the colon. Ulcerative colitis therapy includes sulfasalazine (Azulfidine), glucocorticoids, azathioprine, and mercaptopurine. Sulfasalazine is comprised of sulfapyridine and aminosalicylic acid, and usually used for mild or moderate disease (Hanauer, 1996). Sulfapyridine, a sulfanilamide, crosses the placenta (Azad and Truelove, 1979) and theoretically could cause hyperbilirubinemia or kernicterus. However, no published cases of these theoretical complications are available. According to sulfapyridine's package insert, usual initial treatment dose is 0.5–1 g orally q.i.d. for active disease; for asymptomatic maintenance, doses are usually lower.

Glucocorticoids (e.g., prednisone) in large doses may be necessary for active disease. Azathioprine, an immunosuppressant (see Chapter 15), may be necessary in a minority of patients who do not respond to the usual regimen. Cyclosporine has also been used to treat patients refractory to intravenous steroids (Hanauer, 1996).

Aminosalicylate, metronidazole, corticosteroids, azathioprine, and cyclosporine may also be used to treat pregnant patients with Crohn's disease.

# 13 Use of Dermatologics during Pregnancy

Dermatologic disorders are frequent among pregnant women, but few conditions are unique to pregnancy. However, pruritic urticarial papules and plaques of pregnancy, herpes gestationis (pemphigoid gestationis), prurigo of pregnancy, intrahepatic cholestasis of pregnancy, impetigo herpatiformis, pruritic folliculitis, and papular dermatitis of pregnancy are unique to pregnancy. Various dermatologic preparations are available for local and systemic use, some of which are available over the counter. Most of these agents can be used with little or no risk to the unborn child, ***EXCEPT FOR THE RETINOIDS***. Two of the most potent known human teratogens, etretinate and isotretinoin, are dermatologic drugs. Six major categories of dermatologic preparations are reviewed in this chapter: (1) Vitamin A derivatives, (2) antibiotics, (3) antifungals, (4) antiseborrheics, (5) adrenocorticosteroids, and (6) keratolytics, astringents, and defatting agents. Dermatologic conditions unique to pregnancy and common dermatologic conditions that may occur during pregnancy are discussed under "Special Considerations."

## VITAMIN A DERIVATIVES

Three retinoic acid derivatives, vitamin A analogs (two oral agents and one topical agent), are available to treat cystic acne, acne vulgaris, or psoriasis. Isotretinoin (Accutane) and etretinate (Tegison) are oral preparations, and tretinoin (Retin-A) is a topical agent. Of 49 acne treatments available online, 26 of 49 (53 percent) contain vitamin A (retinoic acid). Three preparations may be teratogenic, and 4 have vitamin A doses higher than the RDA. Fifteen of the online acne medications have an unknown teratogenic risk. Six acne preparations contain >10,000 IU vitamin A. Two of these medicines do not have a pregnancy warning regarding possible adverse effects of hypervitaminosis A, including the preparation with the highest vitamin A dose found in this study. The ACOG recommendation is to avoid exposure to retinoids during pregnancy (2020).

### ISOTRETINOIN

Isotretinoin is the drug with greatest teratogenic potential of all the medications to which pregnant woman may be exposed in the first trimester, except for thalidomide. The "retinoic acid embryopathy" is a distinct pattern of anomalies that has been described in several reports encompassing over 80 offspring of women exposed to this agent during the first trimester of pregnancy (Coberly *et al.*, 1996; Lammer, 1985, Lammer *et al.*, 1987; Medical Letter, 1983; MMWR, 1984; Rizzo *et al.*, 1991; Rosa, 1983; Rosa *et al.*, 1986; Thompson and Cordero, 1989). Among 94 infants born to women who used isotretinoin in early pregnancy, 28 percent had major congenital anomalies, and 18 percent of the pregnancies resulted in spontaneous abortions (Chen *et al.*, 1990; Dai *et al.*, 1992). The constellation of anomalies observed in exposed infants is called retinoic acid embryopathy (Box 13.1). Postnatal intellectual development of retinoic acid exposed infants was subnormal at 5 years of age (IQ less than 85) in 47 percent of 31, although they were apparently unaffected (without major or minor congenital anomalies) at birth (Adams and Lammer, 1993; Adams *et al.*, 1991, 1992).

DOI: 10.1201/9780429160929-13

## BOX 13.1   CHARACTERISTIC ANOMALIES IN OFFSPRING OF MOTHERS EXPOSED TO ISOTRETINOIN (ACCUTANE)

- Anotia
- Cardiovascular defects
- Central nervous system anomalies
- Cleft palate
- Eye anomalies

- Limb reduction defects
- Micrognathia
- Microtia
- Thymic abnormalities

In a study based on TIS information in Canada, Italy, and Israel, 53 infants exposed in early pregnancy to isotretinoin were identified (Garcia-Bournissen *et al.*, 2008). Induced abortions were undertaken in 24 among 43 followed-up pregnancies (56 percent). Among 14 live-born infants, there were two with congenital malformations (anotia and heart defect). Bérard *et al.* (2007) in Canada reported 90 women pregnant during isotretinoin therapy. Among them 76 terminated the pregnancy (84 percent). There were three spontaneous abortions, one neonatal death due to obstetric trauma, and 10 live-born infants, among them one with congenital malformations of the face and neck. A study from the Berlin TIS (Schaefer *et al.*, 2010) identified 91 isotretinoin-exposed pregnancies of which 69 (76 percent) were terminated. Five spontaneous abortions occurred and 18 live infants were born, one of which had a small ventricular septum defect.

Risks are probably not associated with pregnancy among patients who discontinued taking isotretinoin before pregnancy, or close to the time of conception. This agent has a short half-life of 10–12 hours, and the risk of congenital anomalies is not increased in the offspring of women who discontinued this medication within days of conception (Dai *et al.*, 1989). The terminal elimination half-life of isotretinoin is 96 h.

Major and minor anomalies were increased in frequency in animal teratology studies with isotretinoin, similar to the pattern of malformations seen in human retinoic acid embryopathy (Agnish *et al.*, 1984; Kamm, 1982; Kochhar and Penner, 1987; Kochhar *et al.*, 1984; Webster *et al.*, 1986).

### ETRETINATE

Etretinate is an oral retinoid used to treat psoriasis. Etretinate may be detected in serum at therapeutic levels at least two years following therapy cessation (DiGiovanna *et al.*, 1984). Near-therapeutic levels of etretinate may be detected for three to seven years following cessation of therapy (Hoffman-LaRoche, personal communication). No epidemiological studies are published of infants born to women who used etretinate during pregnancy. Twenty-nine live-born infants were reported among 43 pregnancies exposed to etretinate, of whom six had major congenital anomalies; five infants had malformations similar to retinoid embryopathy (Geiger *et al.*, 1994). There are case reports of neural tube defects, other central nervous system malformations, and limb reduction defects in the offspring of mothers exposed to this drug during embryogenesis (Happle *et al.*, 1984; Lammer, 1988; Rosa *et al.*, 1986; Verloes *et al.*, 1990). In one published case report, a fetus with a hypoplastic leg was born to a mother who conceived several months after discontinuing etretinate (Grote *et al.*, 1985).

Conceptions after etretinate exposure may pose serious risks of birth defects because the drug has an indeterminate half-life. The published elimination half-life is at 100 to 120 days for etretinate. However, therapeutic levels of the drug have been detected as long as two years after discontinuation. The manufacturer has offered pro bono testing for etretinate in women of reproductive age who used this drug. In the ideal situation, this should be done preconceptually.

Studies of rats and mice born to mothers exposed to etretinate had an increased frequency of congenital anomalies consistent with the human retinoic acid embryopathy, including limb, genitourinary, neural tube, and cloacal defects (Mesrobian *et al.*, 1994). The implication of this with regard to human teratogenicity is unknown, but adds experimental support for the retinoic acid syndrome. Obviously, this drug should not be used for psoriasis during pregnancy.

## ACITRETIN

An active metabolite of etretinate, acitretin has an elimination half-life of approximately 60 hours, compared to 100–120 days for etretinate. Eight cases of acitretin exposure during pregnancy are published. One infant had multiple congenital anomalies consistent with the retinoic acid embryopathy, and one case of congenital hearing deficit was found (Geiger *et al.*, 1994). One case report of an infant born with features of the retinoic acid embryopathy was published. At 18 months' follow-up, the infants had microcephaly and significant neurodevelopmental delay (Barbero *et al.*, 2004). Notably, the dose of acitretin that the mother took from conception to the 10th week of pregnancy was low (10 mg/day) compared to other reports (e.g., Geiger *et al.*, 1994). Among 52 pregnancies where exposure to acitretin occurred after 6 weeks post-conception, no congenital anomalies were observed (Geiger *et al.*, 1994). The Swedish Birth defects registry included only 2 infants exposed to acitretin during the first trimester (Kallen, 2019). Speculation that paternal acitretin exposure may be associated with an increased frequency of birth defects was analyzed in a national (Norway) study. The frequency of birth defects was not significantly increased (Nørgaard *et al.*, 2019).

Animal models of acitretin teratogenicity have produced anomalies consistent with the retinoic acid embryopathy (Lofberg *et al.*, 1990; Turton *et al.*, 1992).

*Caution*: Acitretin can be metabolized back to etretinate through re-esterification. Therefore, it would be prudent to test serum for etretinate in addition to acitretin before any clinical recommendation (Almond-Roesler and Orfanos, 1996).

## TRETINOIN

### Topical Tretinoin

Tretinoin (Retin-A) is retinoic acid. It is usually prepared in liquid, gel, or cream for local application to treat acne vulgaris. Apparently, minimal amounts of this topical agent are absorbed systemically, and the theoretical teratogenic risk of tretinoin appears quite low (Kligman, 1988). Tretinoin is poorly absorbed topically. Also, skin metabolizes this agent, resulting in none to minimal amounts accumulating in maternal serum (DeWals *et al.*, 1991; Kalivas, 1992; Nau, 1993; Nau *et al.*, 1994).

Major congenital anomalies occurred among 2 percent of 212 pregnancies exposed to tretinoin during the first trimester, compared to 3 percent of controls (Jick *et al.*, 1993). In another study of 112 infants born to women who received prescriptions for tretinoin, there was no increased frequency of major anomalies (Briggs *et al.*, 2021). In a report confounded by isotretinoin exposure, among 45 pregnancies exposed to tretinoin, one infant had features of the retinoid embryopathy (Johnson *et al.*, 1994). However, the mother of the affected infant had also taken isotretinoin during pregnancy.

Major structural malformations in 106 infants and minor anomalies in a subset of 62 infants were examined by an experienced dysmorphologist to test the hypothesis that topical tretinoin during the first trimester might pose a risk for birth defects similar to those associated with the retinoic acid embryopathy. No differences in major or minor anomaly frequencies between the tretinoin and control groups were found (Loureiro *et al.*, 2005), offering reassurance for patients exposed to the drug during the first trimester. Most recently, among 39 infants exposed to tretinoin in the Swedish Registry there were no birth defects (Kallen, 2019). It was concluded in a review of the available evidence; the risk of birth defects is not increased with tretinoin exposure (Kallen, 2019).

Tretinoin administered to pregnant animals during embryogenesis in doses up to 50 times those used in humans was not associated with congenital anomalies or adverse fetal effects. In summary, tretinoin does not appear to be associated with an increased risk of congenital anomalies in infants born to women who used the drug *as directed* during pregnancy. ('As directed' is inserted here because we have encountered patients who ate—took orally—tretinoin cream.)

A recent review of tretinoin use in pregnancy stated:

> Although oral exposure of pregnant animals to high doses of third-generation retinoids results in significant systemic absorption with resultant retinoid embryopathies, topical administration of these molecules, as well as of the earlier generation retinoids formulated for dermal application, results in barely detectible changes in the normal concentrations of total retinoids in the blood. Substantial animal data exist to indicate the relative safety of topically applied retinoids in pregnancy and the limited epidemiologic data available to date support this conjecture
>
> (Williams *et al.*, 2020)

ACOG has a more conservative position, urging avoidance of retinoids in pregnancy when possible (ACOG, 2020).

### Systemic Tretinoin

Systemic tretinoin has been used to treat acute promyelocytic leukemia during pregnancy. Eleven case reports of systemic tretinoin use during pregnancy are reported (Harrison *et al.*, 1994; Simone *et al.*, 1995; Morton *et al.*, 1995; Nakamura *et al.*, 1995; Watanbe *et al.*, 1995; Lin *et al.*, 1996; Lipovsky *et al.*, 1996; Giagounidis *et al.*, 2000; Leong *et al.*, 2000; Consoli *et al.*, 2004).

## ANTIBIOTICS

Antibiotics are used to treat acne and other skin infections (Box 13.2), and often include clindamycin, erythromycin, meclocycline, tetracycline, sulfa-drug creams, and lotions. Systemic absorption of topical antibiotics through the skin is unlikely to result in significant serum concentration, and an association an increased risk of congenital anomalies is not plausible. Topical tetracycline preparations are not associated with yellow-brown discoloration of the teeth, unlike oral or parenteral tetracycline,

---

**BOX 13.2   TOPICAL ANTIBACTERIAL AGENTS TO
TREAT ACNE AND MINOR SKIN INFECTIONS**

- Chloramphenicol
- Clindamycin
- Clioquinol
- Erythromycin
- Gentamicin
- Meclocycline
- Metronidazole
- Mupirocin
- Neomycin
- Neomycin plus polymyxin B, bacitracin, gramicidin, and hydrocortisone
- Silver sulfadiazine
- Sulfur
- Tetracycline

Additional topical antimicrobial agents used to treat minor skin infections include neomycin (usually in combination with polymyxin B, bacitracin, gramicidin, and/or hydrocortisone). Some combinations of these agents are used to treat ophthalmic infections. No human epidemiological studies of polymyxin B are published. The frequency of congenital anomalies was not increased among 30 or 61 infants whose mothers used topical neomycin or gramicidin, respectively, during early pregnancy (Heinonen *et al.*, 1977).

Other topical antimicrobials used to treat local skin infections include chloramphenicol, gentamicin, and metronidazole. Topical use does not result in physiologically significant systemic concentrations of these agents. These agents are discussed in Chapter 2, and were not associated with an increased frequency of congenital anomalies.

Mupirocin (Bactroban), a topical antibacterial, is used to treat skin infections and folliculitis. Mupirocin was not teratogenic in several animal studies. No studies of mupirocin and congenital anomalies after exposure during embryogenesis are published.

Clioquinol is an antibacterial and antifungal agent. No studies are published on the use of this drug during human or experimental animal pregnancy. Mafenide (Sulfamylon) and silver sulfadiazine (Silvadene, Thermazene, Flint SSD, Sildimac) are topical antibacterial and antifungal agents used to treat infections secondary to skin burns. No human studies of these drugs in human pregnancy and birth defects are published. No animal teratology studies of mafenide are published. According to manufacturer information, silver sulfadiazine was not teratogenic in animal studies (unpublished).

## ANTIFUNGALS

Topical antifungal agents used to treat vaginitis include butoconazole, clotrimazole, econazole, miconazole, nystatin, and terconazole. Systemic preparations used for vaginitis include amphotericin B, griseofulvin, and ketoconazole. These agents are discussed in Chapter 2. Systemic antifungals are not associated with an increased risk of birth defects, except for griseofulvin (conjoined twinning is hypothesized with griseofulvin; see Chapter 2). Topical application of these agents on parts of the body is not associated with an increased frequency of congenital anomalies or other medical complications.

Antifungals used to treat tinea corpus, cruris, pedis, and versicolor include ciclopirox, haloprogin, naftifine, and tolnaftate. No human studies of use of these drugs during pregnancy are published, but manufacturers' information state that these antifungal agents were not teratogenic in several animal studies.

Tolnaftate (Aftate, Genaspore, NP27, Tinactin, Ting, Zeasorb-AF), another topical antifungal, is available as a powder, aerosol solution, spray solution, gel, or cream. It is used topically to treat tinea captis, corporis, cruris, versicolor, pedis, and barbae. No human or animal reproduction studies are published.

## ANTIPARASITICS

Topical antiparasitics are discussed in detail in Chapter 2.

## KERATOLYTICS, ASTRINGENTS, AND DEFATTING AGENTS

*Keratolytics, astringents, and defatting agents* are largely over-the-counter preparations, and are used to treat acne and related dermatologic conditions (Box 13.3). No human reproduction studies for any of these agents are published, nor are animal teratology data. Topical use of benzoyl peroxide, resorcinol, and salicylic acid may result in systemic absorption, but no cases of adverse fetal effects are documented related to the topical route of delivery. Salicylates are discussed in detail in Chapter 8, Analgesics during pregnancy. Manufacturer data on salicylic acid was reported to be teratogenic in animals when used in large doses, several times that used in humans.

> **BOX 13.3   KERATOLYTIC, DEFATTING, AND ASTRINGENT AGENTS**
>
> - Alcohol and sulfur (Liquimat, Transact, Xerac)
> - Alcohol and acetone (Seba-Nil, Tyrosum)
> - Benzoyl peroxide (Clearasil, Oxy-10, Acne-10, Benoxyl, Del-Aqua, Desquam, Dry & Clear, Fostex, Neutrogena, Acne Mask, Zeroxin-10)
> - Resorcinol (RA)
> - Resorcinol and sulfur (Acnomel, Clearsil, Rezamid, Sulforcin)
> - Salicylic acid (numerous brand names)
> - Salicylic acid and sulfur (numerous brand names)
> - Salicylic acid, sulfur, and coal tar (Sebex-T, Sebutone, Vanseb-T)

## ANTISEBORRHEIC AGENTS

Dandruff or seborrheic dermatitis is treated with antiseborrheic agents (Box 13.4). The mechanism of action is unknown. No animal or human reproduction studies are published. It is very unlikely that these agents have any effect on prenatal development because they are not absorbed systemically. Coal tar and salicylic acid are often used in combination with other agents, such as sulfa, and in combination with one another to treat seborrhea and seborrheic dermatitis.

> **BOX 13.4   ANTISEBORRHEIC AGENTS**
>
> - Chloroxine (Capitrol)
> - Coal tar (numerous brands)
> - Pyrithione (Danex, Head & Shoulders, Sebex, Sebulon, Zinolon)
> - Salicylic acid (numerous brands)
> - Selenium sulfide (Episel, Exsel, Glo-Sel, Selsun)

## RENOCORTICOSTEROIDS

A variety of topical adrenocorticosteroids is used to treat dermatologic disorders (Box 13.5), usually to treat localized dermatitis with associated inflammation and pruritis.

> **BOX 13.5   TOPICAL ADRENOCORTICOIDS FOR DERMATOLOGICAL CONDITIONS**
>
> - Alclometasone
> - Amcinonide
> - Betamethasone
> - Clobetasol
> - Clocortolone
> - Desonide
> - Desoximetasone
> - Dexamethasone
> - Diflurasone
> - Flumethasone
> - Fluocinolone
> - Fluocinonide
> - Flurandrenolide
> - Halcinonide
> - Hydrocortisone
> - Methylprednisolone
> - Mometasone
> - Triamcinolone: NOT Recommended

Fourteen observational studies of topical steroid use during pregnancy were reviewed, and included unpublished data from Hungary, Sweden, and other research registries. The European Dermatology Forum Guideline on Topical Corticosteroids in Pregnancy summary of pregnancy outcomes among 1,601,515 women who used topical steroids during the first trimester concluded that the risk of birth defects was not increased (Chi *et al.*, 2017).

Topical steroids are very unlikely to be associated with significant risk to the human fetus, except triamcinolone (see later).

A small number of systemic adrenocorticosteroids are indicated to treat dermatologic diseases in limited circumstances, and there is a small collection of these agents (Box 13.6). The two adrenocorticosteroids agents most commonly used systemically are prednisone and prednisolone. The frequency of congenital anomalies was not increased among 43 infants born to women who took prednisone during early pregnancy (Heinonen *et al.*, 1977). Perinatal deaths were increased in frequency among infants born to women who took this prednisone throughout pregnancy, but the disease being treated (e.g., lupus) may in itself be etiologic, rather than prednisone per se (Warrell and Taylor, 1968). Fetal growth retardation was associated with prednisone use during gestation by one research group (Reinisch *et al.*, 1978), but not several others (Lee *et al.*, 1982; Walsh and Clark, 1967).

---

### BOX 13.6   COMMONLY USED SYSTEMIC ADRENOCORTICOIDS

- Betamethasone
- Cortisone
- Dexamethasone
- Hydrocortisone
- Methylprednisolone
- Prednisone
- Prednisolone
- Triamcinolone: NOT recommended

---

#### PREDNISONE AND PREDNISOLONE

Prednisone is an active adrenoglucocorticoid, and prednisolone is an active metabolite of prednisone. Numerous animal studies reported an increase in the frequency of cleft palate with prednisolone (as well as other steroids) when given in large doses (e.g., Ballard *et al.*, 1977; Pinsky and DiGeorge, 1965; Shah and Killistoff, 1976; Walker, 1967). Among 111 infants exposed to prednisone during the first trimester, the frequency of birth defects (5/111, 4.5 percent) was not increased (Park-Wyllie *et al.*, 2000).

The association between oral clefts and prednisone exposure was assessed among humans using data from well-regarded case-control studies (Carmichael and Shaw, 1999; Rodriguez-Pinilla and Martinez-Frias, 1998) and it was concluded that the risk of non-syndromic cleft palate might be associated with prednisone/prednisolone and other glucocorticoid exposure during embryogenesis. However, if such a risk exists it is less than 1 percent (Shepard *et al.*, 2002). Note that most oral clefts can be surgically corrected and this isolated defect is not associated with other physical or mental abnormalities.

#### HYDROCORTISONE

Hydrocortisone, another glucocorticoid, is the main steroid produced by the adrenal glands. The frequency of congenital anomalies was not increased among infants whose mothers took hydrocortisone during early pregnancy, including the first trimester (Heinonen *et al.*, 1977). As with prednisone/prednisolone, an increased frequency of cleft palate was found among the offspring of experimental animals whose mothers were given hydrocortisone during embryogenesis (Chaudhry and Shah, 1973; Harris *et al.*, 1980). This is similar to experimental findings with other glucocorticoids. It is possible that a small risk for cleft palate in humans exists with hydrocortisone use during embryogenesis, but it is likely that the risk is small at less than 1 percent (Shepard *et al.*, 2002).

## DEXAMETHASONE AND BETAMETHASONE

These agents (dexamethasone and betamethasone) are glucocorticoids that are closely related to prednisone (see "Prednisone and Prednisolone"). No human teratology studies of dexamethasone or betamethasone are published. These drugs are commonly used in the late second and early third trimesters to promote fetal lung maturation, preventing respiratory distress syndrome (Collaborative Group on Antenatal Steroid Therapy, 1984; Liggins, 1976; Liggins and Howie, 1974). Consistent with other corticosteroids, dexamethasone and betamethasone are reported to be associated with an increased frequency of cleft palate in the offspring of pregnant animals that received these agents during embryogenesis (Mosier *et al.*, 1982; Pinsky and DiGeorge, 1965). Fetal body and organ weight were decreased in several animal studies with exposure to these glucocorticoids during pregnancy (Barrada *et al.*, 1980; Epstein *et al.*, 1977; Johnson *et al.*, 1981; Mosier *et al.*, 1982).

As with other glucocorticoids, it is possible that a small risk for cleft palate in humans exists with dexamethasone and betamethasone use during early pregnancy. However, the risk is very likely small, less than 1 percent (Shepard *et al.*, 2002).

## TRIAMCINOLONE

No human epidemiological studies of triamcinolone use during early pregnancy are published. Published case-control studies are confounded, and it is not possible to interpret triamcinolone exposures from them. Triamcinolone exposure during embryogenesis is associated with an increased frequency of congenital anomalies among offspring of three species of non-human primates given this corticosteroid during embryogenesis (Bacher and Michejda, 1988; Hendrickx and Tarara, 1990; Hendrickx *et al.*, 1980; Jerome and Hendrickx, 1988; Parker and Hendrickx, 1983). The collection of congenital anomalies included neural tube defects, craniofacial malformations, and skeletal anomalies. Therefore, triamcinolone should be avoided during pregnancy, especially during the first trimester (Friedman and Polifka, 2006). Triamcinolone exposure during embryogenesis is probably associated with an increased risk of birth defects in humans. This warning is issued to attempt a reduction of the number of infants who will be damaged, i.e., exposed to this drug, before official warnings are issued.

Maternal intranasal triamcinolone during the first trimester was associated with an increased frequency of respiratory birth defects (OR = 2.71, p<0.01) among 30 and 238 malformed infants (Berard *et al.*, 2016). It is unclear how systemic levels of triamcinolone differ between topical and intranasal use, but it is prudent to observe the warnings to avoid triamcinolone during pregnancy published by Friedman and Polifka (2006), especially the first trimester.

## CORTISONE

The risk of congenital anomalies among women who used cortisone during pregnancy and its possible adverse fetal effects cannot be assessed with the available published data. The frequency of congenital anomalies was not increased among 34 infants exposed to cortisone during early pregnancy, (Heinonen *et al.*, 1977). Cortisone is a glucocorticoid, and as noted earlier, speculated to be associated with a very small increased frequency of cleft palate in humans, based on some epidemiological evidence and several animal models, including non-human primates (Biddle and Fraser, 1976; Walker, 1971). The non-human primate association, even with small sample sizes, is an ominous indicator. Primarily based on primate data, these agents will predictably be shown to be associated with a small increased frequency of isolated cleft palate in human infants exposed to glucocorticoids during embryogenesis (<1 percent).

## GLUCOCORTICOIDS SUMMARY

In summary, limited human data are published of adrenocorticosteroid use during early human pregnancy and possible association with congenital anomalies or other possible adverse fetal effects. These agents were used for many years in pregnant women without apparent adverse effects, but no systematic studies are published. Analyses of reputable case-control studies indicate that a low risk (<1 percent) for cleft palate may be associated with glucocorticoid exposure during the first trimester. Triamcinolone effects are likely more severe than any glucorticoid, indicating it should be avoided drug during pregnancy, especially during early gestation. However, the consequence of not treating certain conditions during pregnancy, such as systemic lupus erythematosus and asthma, generally outweigh any theoretical risk of these medications. Failure to treat lupus and asthma during pregnancy may result in congenital heart block or maternal death, respectively.

Follow-up studies of children whose mothers received betamethasone and dexamethasone are reassuring because they show no growth delay or development deficits. Emphasis should be placed on the <1 percent of infants born following exposure during the first trimester who may have isolated cleft palate. Among infants exposed to triamcinolone during the first trimester, a cluster of congenital anomalies may occur given the evidence from non-human primate studies, suggesting a 'fetal triamcinolone syndrome' will be discovered, comprised of debilitating congenital anomalies (neural tube defects, characteristic facies, and skeletal dysplasias).

Therefore, triamcinolone—and other glucocorticoids—should be avoided in early pregnancy (first trimester), if possible.

# OTHER AGENTS

## ANTHRALIN

Anthralin (Anthra-Derm, Drithocreme, Lisan) is a topical agent that has been used since 1916 to treat psoriasis. Anthralin is used as a hair growth stimulant. No animal or human reproduction studies are published. Based upon related medication and the assumption of topical administration, a panel of experts inferred that if there is any risk of congenital anomalies associated with first-trimester exposure to anthralin, it must be very small (Friedman and Polifka, 2006). This may be interpreted to mean that the risk may be so small that it is indiscernible from the background risk of congenital anomalies (3.5–5 percent).

## METHOTREXATE

Methotrexate is a folate antagonist and is frequently used as an antineoplastic agent, but is effective to treat psoriasis. Methotrexate is similar to the well-known teratogen, aminopterin (see Chapter 7, Antineoplastic drugs during pregnancy). Anomalies associated with methotrexate and aminopterin include ossification and skeletal anomalies, hydrocephalus, and cleft palate (Milunsky et al., 1968; Reich et al., 1977; Warkany, 1978). Methotrexate should not be used to treat psoriasis during pregnancy. However, its benefits in the treatment of leukemia and other neoplastic diseases may outweigh its risk. For most dermatologic disorders, other less potentially dangerous therapies are available.

## PODOPHYLLIN

Podophyllin is a topical agent used to treat condyloma acuminata. A solution of 20 percent podophyllin solution in tincture of benzoin is used to treat condyloma. Use of podophyllin during pregnancy is associated with significant edema, skin irritation, and discomfort. The frequency of birth defects was not increased in frequency among 14 infants whose mothers used podophyllin during the first trimester (Heinonen *et al.*, 1977), but this sample was too small to interpret. Several anecdotal reports of maternal and fetal toxicity include a case of fetal demise in a mother who experienced systemic toxicity following the topical application of podophyllin (Gorthey and Krebs, 1954) and others that reported similar adverse effects (Chamberlain *et al.*, 1972; Slater *et al.*, 1978).

One case report of major congenital anomalies associated with podophyllin has been published (Karol *et al.*, 1980), but a causal link cannot be inferred from a single case report. It seems prudent to avoid podophyllin use during pregnancy because safer, equally efficacious therapies are available (e.g., laser removal of warts) (see "Condyloma" under "Special Considerations").

Among 33,151 controls (no birth defects) and 22,843 cases (with birth defects), 25 mothers had condyloma with no birth defects, and six were treated with podophyllum. In the case group, 17 infants had birth defects, and three of their mothers were treated with podophyllum (Banhidy *et al.*, 2011). Among 839 infants whose mothers used podophyllin during the first trimester, the frequency of major congenital anomalies (29/839, 3.5 percent) was not increased (Andersson *et al.*, 2020). Nonetheless, safer alternatives exist, and it may be best to avoid podophyllin during pregnancy.

## TRICHLOROACETIC ACID

Another topical chemical compound used to treat condyloma acuminate is trichloroacetic acid (TCA). It is a caustic and astringent agent that primarily causes sloughing of skin. The rate of congenital heart defects was increased in two studies of the offspring of rats fed TCA during embryogenesis (Smith *et al.*, 1989; Johnson *et al.*, 1998).

# SPECIAL CONSIDERATIONS

Few dermatologic diseases in pregnant women require emergency or extensive therapy during the first trimester. Most conditions can be treated with topical agents with little systemic effects.

## ACNE AND PSORIASIS

Acne is common in young women and young gravidas. Infrequently, psoriasis complicates pregnancy (<1 percent of gravidas), and may actually improve during pregnancy. Three vitamin A congeners, isotretinoin (for acne), acitretin (for psoriasis), and etretinate (for psoriasis) are contraindicated for use during pregnancy (Table 13.1). Women inadvertently exposed to these agents during early pregnancy should be counseled regarding the serious risk of major congenital anomalies in their babies. The patient should also be informed that even if the child does not have a major congenital anomaly at birth, intellectual development might likely be impaired. The best counseling option is to contact TERIS (see Chapter 1) and purchase the comprehensive summary on isotretinoin to (1) use in counseling, (2) place in the medical record, and (3) share with the patient. The option of pregnancy termination should be discussed. On the other hand, topical tretinoin (Retin-A) poses no known risk to the developing conceptus, and pregnancy termination discussion is not part of the consult.

Safe agents to treat acne during pregnancy are available and include topical agents, (such as topical erythromycin), keratolytics, and astringents. They may be safely used to treat acne during pregnancy. Topical steroids may also be safely used for the treatment of psoriasis during pregnancy. **The major exception is triamcinolone, which should be avoided during pregnancy**.

**TABLE 13.1**

**Teratogen Information System (TERIS) Risk for Congenital Anomalies and Food and Drug Administration (FDA) Pregnancy Risk Category**

| Drugs | TERIS Risk | Old FDA Pregnancy Risk Category Rating |
|---|---|---|
| Acitretin | High | X |
| Aminopterin | Moderate to high | X |
| Amphotericin B | Undetermined | B |
| Anthralin | Undetermined | NA |
| Bacitracin | Undetermined | C |
| Betamethasone | Undetermined | C* |
| Butoconazole | Undetermined | C |
| Ciclopirox | Undetermined | B |
| Chloramphenicol | Unlikely | C |
| Clindamycin | Undetermined | B |
| Clioquinol | Undetermined | NA |
| Clotrimazole | Unlikely | B |
| Dexamethasone | Minimal | C* |
| Econazole | Undetermined | NA |
| Erythromycin | None | B |
| Etretinate | High | X |
| Gentamicin | Undetermined | C |
| Gramicidin | None | NA |
| Griseofulvin | Undetermined | C |
| Haloprogin | Undetermined | NA |
| Hydrocortisone | Unlikely | C* |
| Isotretinoin | High | X |
| Ketoconazole | Undetermined | C |
| Mafenide | Undetermined | NA |
| Meclocycline | Undetermined | NA |
| Methotrexate | Moderate to high | X |
| Metronidazole | None | B |
| Miconazole | Undetermined | C |
| Mupirocin | Undetermined | NA |
| Naftifine | Undetermined | NA |
| Neomycin | None | C |
| Nystatin | None | C |
| Podophyllum | Undetermined | C |
| Prednisone/prednisolone | Oral clefts: Small | C* |
| | Other congenital anomalies: Unlikely | |
| Terconazole | Undetermined | C |
| Tetracycline | Unlikely | D |
| Tolnaftate | Undetermined | NA |
| Tretinoin | Topical use: unlikely | D |
| | Systemic administration: Undetermined | |
| Triamcinolone | Undetermined, but high potential | C * |

*Abbreviation:* NA, not available.

*Sources:* Compiled from Friedman *et al.*, *Obstet Gynecol*, 1990; 75: 594; Briggs *et al.*, 2021; Friedman and Polifka, 2006.

## Abnormalities of Pigmentation and Striae Gravidarum

Abnormal pigmentation and striae may be especially worrisome to the pregnant patient. Chloasma (increased pigmentation along the linea nigra or areola of the nipple) and melasma (brownish discoloration of areas of the face) are the two most common forms of abnormal pigmentation. No specific therapy is available or required for these conditions, other than possibly cosmetic makeup. It is especially important to the patient to know that striae and pigmentation usually regress and spontaneously disappear in a short time following delivery.

Striae gravidarum, or stretch marks, may be especially unsettling to pregnant women. Numerous creams and ointments (including "mink oil" or vitamin E) are available in the over-the-counter market to treat stretch marks. However, there is no medical therapy known to be effective. Most striae, which are hyperemic during pregnancy, will diminish in appearance (often becoming small, silvery lines). Most patients simply require reassurance.

## Condyloma Acuminata

Condyloma acuminate (wart-like growths) may proliferate rapidly during pregnancy. Local application of podophyllum (20 percent solution of podophyllin in benzoin) is a frequent therapy in nonpregnant patients. Based upon anecdotal evidence, podophyllin is contraindicated in pregnancy because of the potential for maternal and fetal toxicity. TCA is another local agent for topical use that is not associated with serious maternal or fetal side effects. TCA is not highly effective in the eradication of condyloma, especially during pregnancy. Topical application of 5-fluorouracil is probably not safe because it is an antineoplastic agent, and has known systemic absorption. No human studies of the topical TCA administration of this agent during pregnancy are published.

For small, isolated lesions, surgical excision, electrocautery, and cryotherapy are generally effective. A $CO_2$ laser is an effective tool for treatment of large or massive vulvar condyloma acuminata (Ferenczy, 1984; Hankins *et al.*, 1989; Malfetano *et al.*, 1981).

## Atopic/Allergic Dermatitis

Atopic dermatitis/allergic dermatitis is characterized by a pruritic rash, and is usually secondary to a variety of aggravating factors, such as stress, soap (especially with aroma additives), and irritants.

Atopic/allergic dermatitis is usually treated by (1) removal of the inciting factors and (2) topical or systemic steroids. Topical steroids are recommended during pregnancy and generally prove satisfactory.

## Erythema Multiforme

The etiology of erythema multiforme, another dermatitis, is virtually unknown. Erythema multiforme is characterized by erythematous "target lesions." An increased frequency of outbreaks occurs during pregnancy among women with erythema multiforme. The condition can be treated with antihistamines during pregnancy. If antihistamines are not sufficient, steroids may be effective in some cases. **Triamcinolone should not be used during pregnancy**.

## Papular Dermatitis of Pregnancy

Papular dermatitis is very rare (<1 percent of gravidas) and is limited to pregnancy (Spangler *et al.*, 1962). Pregnancy loss rate was 37 percent. Recurrence in subsequent pregnancies is known and it is associated with an increased frequency of pregnancy loss. Papular dermatitis is characterized by small, erythematous papules that usually involve all skin surfaces. High dose systemic steroids, such as prednisone, are used to treat this dermatitis. **Triamcinolone should not be used**.

## Pruritic Urticarial Papules and Plaques of Pregnancy

PUPPP, or pruritic urticarial papules and plaques of pregnancy, are common during gestation. Papular dermatitis of pregnancy may occur any time during gestation, but PUPPP usually occurs in late pregnancy. PUPPP recurrence in subsequent pregnancies is rare. Pruritis and erythematous papules and plaques characterize PUPPP. Unlike papular dermatitis, PUPPP is ___not___ associated with an increase in pregnancy loss. The rash usually starts on the abdomen and spreads to the extremities, with facial sparing (Alcalay *et al.*, 1988; Yancy *et al.*, 1984). Topical steroids are used to treat PUPPP, although oral prednisone may be required for severe cases intractable to topical therapy. **Triamcinolone should not be used**.

## Herpes Gestationis

Herpes gestationis is another rare dermatologic disease of unknown etiology. Erythematous papules and large, tense bullae, usually on the abdomen and extremities characterize herpes gestationis. It is not a viral infection, contrary to the name's implication. Herpes gestationis is an autoimmune disease. Peculiar to pregnancy, herpes gestationis may recur in subsequent gestations. An increased frequency of pregnancy loss is associated with this condition in some studies (Lawley *et al.*, 1978), but not in others (Katz *et al.*, 1976). Treatment consists primarily of oral prednisone (30–50 mg daily). **Triamcinolone should not be used**.

# 14 Drug Overdoses during Pregnancy

Drug and other substance poisoning or overdoses during pregnancy are often a suicide gesture or, less frequently, an attempt to induce abortion. Accidental overdoses are rare. Quinine overdoses during pregnancy are usually (>90 percent) an attempt to induce abortion, but overdoses of the drug in non-pregnant adults are suicide attempts. Fatalities due to suicide gestures during pregnancy are rare approximately one in every 88,000–400,000 live births (Rayburn et al., 1984). For example, of 6,888 pregnant women, 0.33 percent of all poisonings reported, who suffered a poisoning during pregnancy, three maternal deaths occurred (Gummin et al., 2019). Among 162 cases, 86 percent of pregnant women who presented with an indication of poisoning were overdoses (78 percent suicide attempts, 8 percent induced abortion attempts) (Czeizel et al., 1984). Among 211 maternal deaths in Colorado from 2004 to 2012, 63 (30 percent) were associated with intended self-harm overdoses (Metz et al., 2016). Maternal death associated with suicide gestures occurs in approximately 1 percent of gravid women and more than 95 percent of suicide gestures involve ingestion of a combination of drugs (Rayburn et al., 1984). In New York City, suicide was identified as the cause of 13 percent of maternal deaths (Dannenberg et al., 1995). In 2018, 3/6888 (0.00044 percent) of maternal poisonings were fatal. Of the 6888 poisonings during pregnancy, 6484 were of known gestational age: 45.3 percent occurred in the first trimester, 29.4 percent second trimester and 25.3 percent third trimester (Gummin et al., 2019).

Potentially lethal drug megadoses in pregnant women involves two patients: mother and fetus. Pregnant women who have potentially toxic (megadoses) amounts of drugs or other substances on board must begin with laboratory evaluation of the substance(s) ingested (i.e., serum levels), supplemented by any information from the patient (if conscious) or accompanying individuals.

The top three drugs used in suicide gestures in the United States from the late 1970s through 2015 were nonnarcotic analgesics, vitamins or iron, and sedatives/antianxiolytics (Figure 14.1). The pattern in Finland in the late 1990s was similar, with the top three substances used in suicide attempts being benzodiazepines, analgesics, and psychotropics (antipsychotics/antidepressants) (Table 14.2). In 2018, the top eight drug classes used in suicide gestures were analgesics (8.6 percent), sedative/hypnotic/antipsychotics (2.5 percent), antidepressants (2.8 percent), vitamins (3.5 percent), antihistamines (2.5 percent), antimicrobials (2.2 percent), stimulants/street drugs (1.6 percent), and hormones/antagonists (Gummin et al., 2019).

If the patient is still conscious, she will likely provide the most accurate information on drugs taken. Notably, drug overdoses are usually premeditated. Frequently, the patient will recall estimates of how many pills were taken of which substances. Family members significant, if present at the time of clinical evaluation, they should be able to provide corroborative information (i.e., presence of medicine bottles, known prescriptions, patient statements, etc.). Toxicology samples for drug screens should be collected with frequency (i.e., every hour or two) to provide serial evaluation. Toxicology screens should be ordered as soon as possible to determine (1) what substances were ingested, (2) whether or not levels are rising or falling, and (3) whether or not levels are toxic or approaching toxicity. However, a generalized treatment plan may be undertaken before toxicology results are available.

## CLINICAL MANAGEMENT

Samples (blood, urine) are obtained for toxicological analysis as soon as possible. Orogastric lavage with normal saline should be begun, if the patient still has a gag reflex. Following lavage,

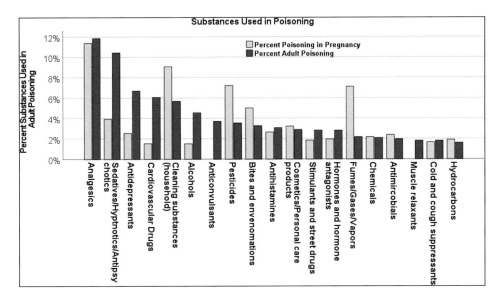

**FIGURE 14.1**    Distribution of substances used in poisoning among adults and pregnant women.

### TABLE 14.2
### Suicide Attempts by Pregnant Women in Finland: 1977 to 1999[a]

|  | n | Percentage |
|---|---|---|
| *Analgesics* | 21/43 | 49 |
| Acetaminophen (paracetamol) | 6 | |
| Acetylsalicylic acid (aspirin) | 5 | |
| Carisoprodol | 1 | |
| Codeine | 1 | |
| Ibuprofen | 2 | |
| Indomethacin | 1 | |
| Phenobarbital | 2 | |
| Salicylamide | 3 | |
| Diazepam | 8 | |
| Estazolam | 1 | |
| Flunitrazepam | 2 | |
| Nitrazepam | 2 | |
| Oxazepam | 1 | |
| Triazolam | 1 | |
| Antipsychotic | 2/43 | 5 |
| Benzodiazepines | 15/43 | 35 |
| Flupentixol | 1 | |
| Fluphenazine | 1 | |
| *Antidepressants* | 2/43 | 5 |
| Doxepin | 1 | |
| Nomifensine | 1 | |
| Iron supplement | 1/43 | 2.3 |
| *Appetite suppressant* | 1/43 | 2.3 |
| Benzodiazepines | 15/43 | 35 |

[a] 272 attempted suicides; 177 excluded for complicating factors (e.g., carbon monoxide), 43 of 122 were suicide gestures during pregnancy; the remainder were suicide attempts in the months of preconception.
*Source:* Compiled from Flint *et al.*, 2002.

administer an Activated charcoal slurry regimen (the nonspecific antidote regimen) should be administered following saline gastric lavage. In some drug overdose, whole-bowel irrigation has been used successfully to clinically significantly lower serum drug levels (Gei *et al.*, 2018; Diaz, 2014; Olson, 2018).

Fetal heart rate evaluation should begin as soon as possible, especially in cases in which the fetus is viable. Information on antidote regimens for given substances may be obtained from several sources when toxicological screens become available to document what drugs and/or chemicals were ingested and may be in potentially toxic doses. The authoritative source consulted by certified poison control centers (listed in the *Physician's Desk Reference*) is PoisIndex. It includes specific data on pregnancy from Teratogen Information System (TERIS). PoisIndex contains a detailed specific management plan for each substance, where available. An overview of a treatment plan for the drug overdose exposure in pregnancy is outlined in Box 14.1.

---

### BOX 14.1   MANAGEMENT PLAN FOR THE PREGNANT PATIENT WITH AN ACUTE OVERDOSE

**Acute stabilization**

- Establishment of an open airway
- Assisted ventilation, if needed
- Circulatory assistance, if needed

**Fetal monitoring**

- Fetal heart rate
- Ultrasound of target organs

**Supportive care**

- As needed to maintain stabilization

**Obtaining toxicological samples (serial measurements)**

- Blood, once per hour
- Urine, once per hour
- Amniotic fluid, twice in 48 h

**Medical history**

- This suicide gesture
- Past history of suicide gestures
- Other medical history

**Physical examination**

- Special attention to central nervous system function
- Special attention to cardiac function

**Nonspecific antidote therapy**

- Prevent absorption
- Orogastric lavage
- Whole-bowel irrigation

- Activated charcoal PO
- Enhance elimination
- Increase liquid intake
- Increase plasma volume
- Balance electrolytes

**Antidote administration**

- Administer specific antidotes after positive identification of drug(s) involved

Management plans for specific patients should be formulated in consultation with a certified poison control center. They are available 24 hours per day, and handle international calls. Maternal and fetal sequelae for specific antidote regimens are provided in Table 14.3 for the 14 drug classes most frequently taken in suicide gestures or other instances of overdose by pregnant women. Some instances of overdose are characterized as "unintentional" or "accidental" (Thornton and Minns, 2012; Franko *et al.*, 2013).

**TABLE 14.3**
**Selected Antidotes Available (see Appendix I for Complete List)**

| Overdose of Drug/Toxin | Antidote |
| --- | --- |
| Acetaminophen | Acetylcysteine |
| Anticholinergics | Physostigmine |
| Atropine | Cholinesterase inhibitors |
| Benzodiazepines | Flumazenil |
| Beta-blockers | Glucagon |
| Cholinesterase inhibitors | Hyoscyamine |
| Curare | Edrophonium |
| Curare | Neostigmine |
| Curare | Pyridostigmine |
| Cyanide | Amyl nitrate |
| Cycloserine | Pyridoxine |
| Digoxin/digitalis | Fab antidigoxin antibody fragments (Digoxin immune Fab) |
| Ergot alkaloids | Prazosin[a] |
| Folic acid antagonists (methotrexate, pyrimethamine, others) | Leucororin |
| Heavy metals (except iron) | Penicillamine |
| Heparin | Protamine |
| Iron | Deferoxamine |
| Isoniazid | Pyridoxine |
| Nonspecific substance(s)/No specific antidote | Activated charcoal |
| Nitroprusside[a] | Ergot alkaloids |
| Opioids | Naloxone: Nalmefene |
| Organophosphate poisoning | Muscarine |
| Quinidine | None |
| Specific for negatively charged medications | Cholestyramine |

[a] Nitroprusside is another antidote to ergot alkaloid overdoses, **but it conjugates to cyanide in fetal liver and should not be used in pregnancy**.

## NONNARCOTIC ANALGESIC OVERDOSES

### ACETAMINOPHEN

Acetaminophen is the most frequently used drug in suicide gestures during pregnancy (Czeizel *et al.*, 1984; Rayburn *et al.*, 1984; Mowry *et al.*, 2015). Clinical course of select cases of acetaminophen overdose are shown in Table 14.4. Ninety-four cases of acetaminophen overdose in suicide gestures during pregnancy have been reported (Appendix II). The salient clinical features of these cases are that early administration of the specific antidote *N*-acetylcysteine (NAC) can prevent maternal hepatotoxicity if the antidote is tolerated and fetal hepatotoxicity is uncommon.

In a case series of 60 acetaminophen overdoses during pregnancy from a multicenter study in which 24 mothers had serum acetaminophen levels in the toxic range (Riggs *et al.*, 1989), only one case of fetal hepatotoxicity and maternal death occurred. In addition, there were four spontaneous abortions. The distribution of these cases across trimesters of pregnancy is given in Table 14.4. No evidence of teratogenicity of NAC was found in one study (Janes and Routledge, 1992). Delays in the administration of the NAC treatment apparently increases the risk of spontaneous abortions, fetal death, and serious maternal liver damage. It is known that NAC crosses the placenta (Horowitz *et al.*, 1997), and rapidly reaches and exceeds maternal levels (Wiest *et al.*, 2014). Experience in treating fetal and neonatal acetaminophen overdoses was associated with favorable outcomes (Crowell *et al.*, 2008; Ibister *et al.*, 2001).

Among 29 case series and reports of 94 women who took an overdose of acetaminophen indicate that overdose treatment during pregnancy is associated with the most favorable outcome when the NAC is given as early as possible (Table 14.4). NAC administered as soon as the overdose is verified by toxicology is the most effective treatment (Table 14.5). Details of 450 paracetamol (acetaminophen) overdoses during pregnancy followed prospectively (McElhatton *et al.*, 1997, 2001) are described. The outcomes of this large cohort support treatment of acetaminophen overdose during pregnancy with NAC immediately, with either oral or intravenous NAC according to the protocols provided in the manufacturer's insert. Delay in administering the antidote increases the risk of maternal and fetal hepatotoxicity, hepatorenal failure, and death (Kozer and Koren, 2001).

## TABLE 14.4
## Case Reports of Acetaminophen Overdose during Pregnancy

| Amount Ingested (g) | EGA (weeks) | Treatment | Outcome | Maternal | Fetal | Source |
|---|---|---|---|---|---|---|
| < 20 | | Nonspecific | Hepatotoxicity | Elective abortion[a] | | Silverman and Carithess, 1978 |
| 32.5 | 36 | *N*-acetylcysteine | Uncomplicated | Normal | | Byer *et al.*, 1982 |
| 32.5 | 29 | Nonspecific | Hepatotoxicity | Normal[b] | | Lederman *et al.*, 1983 |
| 26 | 38 | *N*-acetylcysteine | Uncomplicated | Normal | | Ruthnum and Goel, 1984 |
| 25 | 18 | *N*-acetylcysteine | Hepatotoxicity | Normal | | Stokes, 1984 |
| 20 | 36 | *N*-acetylcysteine | Uncomplicated | Normal | | Roberts *et al.*, 1984 |
| 29.5 | 28 | *N*-acetylcysteine[d] | Hepatotoxicity[c] | | Fetal death | Haibach *et al.*, 1984 |
| 36 | 16 | *N*-acetylcysteine | Uncomplicated | Normal | | Robertson *et al.*, 1986 |
| 64 | 15 | *N*-acetylcysteine | Hepatotoxicity | Normal | | Ludmir *et al.*, 1986 |
| 50 | 32 | *N*-acetylcysteine | Uncomplicated | Normal | | Rosevear and Hope, 1989 |
| 35 | 31 | None | Hepatorenal failure | Death | Death | Wang *et al.*, 1997 |
| 19 | 40 | *N*-acetylcysteine | Uncomplicated | Normal | Normal | Sancewicz-Pach *et al.*, 1999 |

[a] Not autopsied.

[b] Hyaline membrane disease pursuant to preterm delivery.

[c] Maternal outcomes were not listed.

[d] Antidote not tolerated.

*Abbreviation:* EGA, estimated gestation age.

**TABLE 14.5**

**Outcome of 450 Acetaminophen Overdoses during Pregnancy**

|  | n |  | Outcome | Authors |
|---|---|---|---|---|
| Toxic | 33 (11%) | *N*-acetylcysteine | 24 normal, 1 malformed, 3 sp ab, 5 el ab | McElhatton *et al.*, 1997 |
| Toxic | 16 (5%) | Methionine | 11 normal, 5 el ab |  |
| Toxic | 52 (17%) | Ipecacuanha | 42 normal, 1 malformed, 2 sp ab, 7 el ab |  |
| Toxic | 16 (5%) | Charcoal | 13 normal, 1 sp ab, 2 el ab |  |
| Toxic | 42 (14%) | Gastric lavage | 28 normal, 4 malformed, 2 sp ab, 8 el ab |  |
| Toxic | 3 (1%) | Miscellaneous | 1 normal, 1 malformed, 1 el ab |  |
| Subtoxic | 81 (27%) | No treatment | 62 normal, 1 malformed, 5 sp ab, 14 el ab |  |
| Unknown | 59 (20%) | Treatment not recommended | 40 normal, 3 malformed, 5 sp ab, 12 el ab |  |

Acetaminophen levels measured at times post-ingestion can broadly predict whether or not hepatotoxicity should be expected (Figure 14.2). The Rumack-Matthews nomogram (Figure 14.2) is based in part on clinical observations made on 662 non-pregnant adults with acetaminophen overdose (Rumack *et al.*, 1981).

Importantly, acetaminophen per se is not the toxic agent in overdoses, it a proximate metabolite that is toxic, and preventing the drug's metabolism is key to antidote treatment, and the reason for urgency in NAC administration. In acetaminophen overdose, metabolic pathways (sulfation and glucuronidation) become saturated, causing an increased metabolic demand on cytochrome P-450 oxidases. The P-450 system oxidizes the drug and produces a highly reactive intracellular metabolite (N-acetyl-p-benzoquinone imine, or NAPBQI) that complexes with hepatic glutathione. The P-450 metabolite NAPBQI binds to hepatocellular macromolecules when glutathione is depleted and hepatotoxicity ensues (Andrews *et al.*, 1976; Davis *et al.*, 1976). Normally, NAPBQI is produced in small amounts and degraded by the liver almost immediately. Fetal P-450 has <10 percent of adult activity, resulting in negligible production of the toxic metabolite. Some authorities speculate that the increased risk of maternal hepatotoxicity compared to fetal hepatotoxicity may be related to the largely inactive fetal enzyme complement, i.e., fetal liver has a much lower capacity to metabolize the drug to NAPBQI. As the fetal liver matures, it is likely fetuses of more advanced gestational age are at greater risk for acetaminophen toxicity than less mature fetuses. In the largest series published, this relationship was not readily apparent (Table 14.6). Maternal-fetal outcomes are generally better with expedient NAC administration following acetaminophen overdose.

In summary, expeditious administration of NAC for acetaminophen overdose treatment is most effective if the antidote is administered as early as possible. Gravidas given NAC within 10 hours of ingesting large doses of acetaminophen had the best pregnancy outcomes (Table 14.6).

## Aspirin

Aspirin was the second most frequently used drug in attempted suicide or gestures among pregnant women (Rayburn *et al.*, 1984), but in 2018 it ranked 13th among substances on which gravidas overdosed (Gummin *et al.*, 2019). Clinical details are reported for several cases of intentional aspirin overdose during pregnancy (Table 14.7). Average aspirin half-life is approximately 20 hours, and

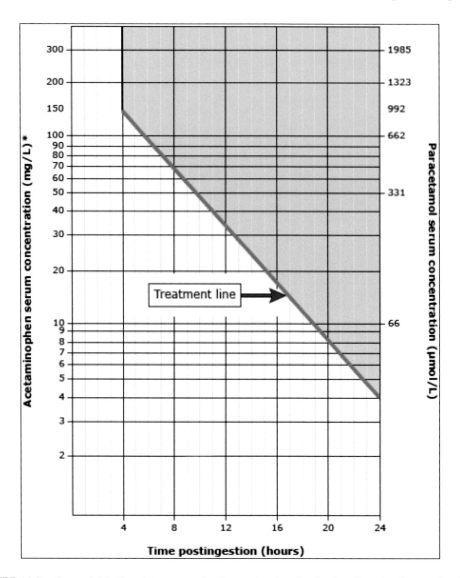

**FIGURE 14.2**    Rumack-Matthew Nomogram for Acetaminophen levels plotted against hours after intake and chances of of liver toxicity (shaded area).

(From www.emboardbombs.com.)

**TABLE 14.6**

**Acetaminophen Toxicity and Treatment with *N*-Acetylcysteine in One Large Series**

| Time of Treatment | n | Maternal Deaths | Maternal Hepatotoxic | Infant/Fetal Hepatotoxic | Stillbirths/ Spontaneous Abortion | Elective Abortions | Viable Infants | Viable Preterm |
|---|---|---|---|---|---|---|---|---|
| Less than 10 h after overdose | 10 | 0 | 0 | 0 | 0 | 2 | 7 | 1 |
| 10–16 h after overdose | 10 | 0 | 2 | 0 | 3 | 2 | 4 | 1 |
| 16–24 h after overdose | 4 | 1 | 3 | 1 | 2 | 1 | 1 | 0 |
| Total | 24 | 1 | 5 | 1 | 5 | 5 | 12 | 2 |

*Source:* Adapted from Riggs *et al.*, 1989.

**TABLE 14.7**

**Case Reports of Aspirin Overdose during Pregnancy**

| Amount Ingested | EGA (weeks) | Treatment | Outcome Maternal | Fetal | Author |
|---|---|---|---|---|---|
| 32.5 g | 37 | Bicarbonate, IV fluids, glucose | Tinnitus, C-section | Neonatal deafness, meconium aspiration | Farid et al., 2011 |
| 50 tablets | 37 | Urinary alkalization, hemodialysis, FFP, vitamin K | Uncomplicated | Macerated stillborn, 2360 g | Palatnick and Tenenbein, 1998 |
| 100 · 5 grain tablets | 24 | 300 ml mg citrate | Tinnitus, hyperventilated state | Stillborn, anomalies* | Rejent and Baik, 1985 |
| 8 · 365 mg tablets daily for several days until delivery | 37 | Not mentioned | Not mentioned | Tachypnea, compensated metabolic acidosis | Ahlfors et al., 1982 |
| Megadose | First trimester | Not mentioned | Not mentioned | Metanephric adenoma | Bove et al., 1979 |
| Unknown | 32 | Not mentioned | Uncomplicated | Generalized hypertonia, increased reflex, irritability | Lynd, 1976 |
| 5–6 g daily | 0–40 | Not mentioned | Abruptio placenta; C-section | Unremarkable | Levy et al., 1975 |
| 15–18 g | 40 | Exchange | Not mentioned | Hyperpnoea, intercostal and suprasternal retractions present | Earle, 1961 |

* Anomalies not causally related to aspirin overdose.

elimination of salicylate from the circulation in the post-absorptive period (approximately six hours after ingestion) is a first-order reaction (Done, 1968). No specific antidote to aspirin exists, and non-specific antidote treatment (i.e., activated charcoal, gastric lavage, whole bowel irrigation) and supportive therapy are traditional management. Urinary alkalinization using intravenous bicarbonate significantly increases renal excretion of salicylic acid, and enhances ionization of salicylate in plasma, assisting elimination of the drug from the central nervous system (Done, 1968). These strategies help shorten the toxicity duration.

Congenital anomalies are not meaningfully higher among children of women who used aspirin during pregnancy, but this is based on therapeutic dose amounts and duration. In a cohort of 41 infants whose mothers took greater than therapeutic aspirin doses at various times during pregnancy, one infant had a congenital anomaly and there was one fetal death (McElhatton *et al.*, 1991b). Aspirin overdose during pregnancy may pose a greater risk of fetal death than acetaminophen, probably because an antidote exists for the latter drug. In addition, aspirin per se is the toxic agent, and not a metabolite. Aspirin is transferred across the placenta to reach fetal concentrations higher than those in the mother (Garrettson *et al.*, 1975; Levy *et al.*, 1975). Salicylate poisoning in pregnancy reports support the same conclusion as acetaminophen overdoses: early therapy (activated charcoal, lavage, bowel irrigation) is associated with better outcomes (Table 14.9).

---

**TABLE 14.9**

**Recommended Management of Aspirin Overdose**

1. Early management

    Adult: >120 mg/kg: give 50 g activated charcoal. Child: for >120 mg/kg give activated charcoal.

    Consider charcoal even for late-presenting patients; peak absorption may be delayed up to 12 h post-ingestion especially with enteric coated tablets.

    Adults only: > 500 mg/kg.

    Consider gastric lavage followed by 50 g activated charcoal, if patient presents within 1 h. Contact National Poison Information Service (NPIS) in the UK on 0870 600 6266 and in the US on 1-800-222-1222

2. Maintenance management

    Check salicylate concentration 4 h post ingestion, then every 2–3 h until peak concentration achieved and is falling consistently. If history is reliable for an ingestion >120 mg/kg and tablets are enteric coated, consider measuring levels for minimum 12 h post ingestion even if no salicylate is detected initially. Monitor and correct urine and electrolytes, arterial blood gases and pH, blood sugar, prothrombin time.

    Rehydrate with oral or IV fluids; large volumes may be necessary to correct dehydration (care required with the elderly or those with cardiac disease). Moderate or severe cases may require central venous pressure monitoring particularly patients with cardiac disease or elderly people Repeat doses of activated charcoal (RAC) (adult, 25–50 g; child, 1 g/kg) every 4 h until salicylate level has peaked and is consistently falling. RAC is effective in preventing excessive delayed absorption.

3. Urinary alkalinization

    For salicylate level, 500–700 mg/L in adults or salicylate level 350–600 mg/L in children/elderly where patients have moderate clinical effects. In the presence of alkaline urine (optimum pH 7.5–8.5), renal elimination of salicylate is enhanced (10- to 20-fold with an increase from a urine pH of 5 to 8). Forced alkaline diuresis is not recommended.

    Adult: 1 L of 1.26 percent sodium bicarbonate (isotonic) + 40 mmol potassium IV over 4 h and/or 50 mL boluses of 8.4 percent sodium bicarbonate IV (ideally via a central line).

    Child: 1 ml/kg 8.4 percent sodium bicarbonate saline infused at 2–3 mL/k/.h 1 mmol/kg potassium diluted in 10 mL/kg hypokalemia prevents urinary excretion of alkali so must be corrected. Check urinary pH hourly aiming for pH 7.5–8.5, the rate of bicarbonate administration alone (avoiding hyperkalemia) may need to be increased if pH remains <7.5.

    Check urine and electrolytes every 2–4 h and keep potassium between 4.0 and 4.5.

*Sources:* From Kamanyire, 2002; Karalliedde and Gawarammana, 2012.

---

## Naproxen

No specific antidote to naproxen exists. In one case of 5 g naproxen taken in overdose during pregnancy, at 35 weeks gestation, nonspecific and supportive antidote therapy was initiated eight hours later Non-specific therapy was given, and spontaneous labor ensued with a preterm infant delivered. The neonate had severe hyponatremia and water retention, but subsequently recovered with no apparent sequelae at follow-up. The mother recovered, and had no signs of hepatotoxicity or other adverse sequelae (Alon-Jones and Williams, 1986).

Another case of naproxen overdose (8.25 g) use at 26 weeks was treated with supportive therapy, and the patient discharged from ICU 3 days later. A normal infant was delivered at 40 weeks with no complications reported (Ozturk and Ugras, 2018).

In contrast to the pharmacokinetics of salicylate elimination, high doses of naproxen (1–4 g) are associated with a disproportionate increase in renal excretion of the drug without saturation of excretory mechanisms or metabolic pathway (Erling and Strand, 1977; Runkel *et al.*, 1976). Increased renal elimination apparently contributed to lower acute toxicity compared with salicylate overdose.

## Ibuprofen

Ibuprofen overdose during pregnancy has not been described in case studies and no specific antidote exists. Therefore, nonspecific antidote and supportive therapy should be given. Symptoms of ibuprofen toxicity include nausea, epigastric pain, diarrhea, vomiting, dizziness, blurred vision, and edema. The half-life of ibuprofen is 0.9–2.5 hours in the post-absorptive period (Baselt, 2017). Among 67 cases of ibuprofen overdose, 36 percent occurred among children. Fifty reports of ibuprofen overdose during pregnancy were published, with mothers and infants suffering no untoward effects (i.e., hepatorenal failure, etc.) among those followed prospectively (Barry *et al.*, 1984). Forty-three cases of ibuprofen overdose during pregnancy were followed prospectively in post-marketing surveillance, and 23 live birth normal infants were born after maternal supportive therapy because no antidote exists. Nine elective terminations and one spontaneous abortion occurred, and one stillbirth. Nine were still pregnant at the time of publication (Barry *et al.*, 1984). More than 150 infants born following ibuprofen overdose in pregnancy were reported to have no increased frequency of birth defects, although the course of pregnancy was not reported in detail (Schaefer, 2007). These cases are from the UK TIS, and were followed prospectively, but no details were published.

# NUTRITIONAL SUPPLEMENT OVERDOSES

## Prenatal Vitamins

Prenatal vitamin overdose in pregnancy is not published. No specific antidote to prenatal vitamins, nonspecific and supportive antidote therapy should be given. It is reasonable to think that most cases of vitamin overdose would probably result in little, if any, risk to either mother or fetus. Two concerns are raised: iron and retinoic acid content. Iron and retinoic acid content of the vitamins should be determined from the manufacturer's labeling to determine the level of exposure to each to estimate the total exposure. Megadose vitamin A may be involved, in which case Chapter 13, Use of dermatologics during pregnancy, should be consulted. High iron doses are discussed in the following.

## Iron

Iron overdose during pregnancy is published for 10 cases (Table 14.10). Importantly, non-specific treatment (i.e., charcoal, gastric lavage, whole bowel irrigation) is associated with adverse outcomes more frequently than with treatment. Outcomes of iron overdose also associated with the amount ingested, with poorer outcomes occurring at higher doses. Gastrointestinal hemorrhage,

**TABLE 14.10**

**Cases of Iron Overdose during Pregnancy**

| Amount | EGA (weeks) | Treatment | Outcome Maternal | Fetus | Author |
|---|---|---|---|---|---|
| 99 Prenatal vitamins (8.8 g iron) and 10 ondansetron | 6 | Whole bowel irrigation | Uncomplicated | Uncomplicated | Geraci and Heagney, 2012 |
| 50 Ferrous gluconate tablets | 27 | Lavage, Deferoxamine | Uncomplicated | Uncomplicated | Tran et al., 1998 |
| 40 Ferrous sulfate tablets | 25 | Deferoxamine | Uncomplicated | Uncomplicated | Schauben et al., 1990 |
| 5 g Elemental iron (25 g ferrous sulfate) | 36 | Deferoxamine | Hepatic necrosis, coma and subsequent expiration in cardiac failure | Uncomplicated | Olenmark et al., 1987 |
| 50 300 mg Ferrous sulfate (30–50 mg/kg Elemental iron) | 15 | Deferoxamine | Temporary abdominal tenderness and mild metabolic acidosis | Uncomplicated | Blanc et al., 1984 |
| Unknown amount, along with prenatal vitamins | 34 | Deferoxamine | Brief episodes of vomiting and mild pain | Uncomplicated | Rayburn et al., 1983 |
| Unknown amount | 34 | Deferoxamine | ? | Uncomplicated | Rayburn et al., 1983 |
| 95 tablets of Fer-In-Sol | 14 | Deferoxamine | Died on the third day; pulmonary edema and hypotension | Spontaneous abortion | Strom et al., 1976 |
| 90 325 mg Ferrous sulfate capsules | 16 | Deferoxamine | Metabolic acidosis, depressed mental status; subsequent death 80 h post admission | Spontaneous abortion | Manoguerra, 1976 |
| 4–6 g Elemental iron with 1–5 Sodium amytal, 6 g Aspirin | 10 | DPTA | Brief episode of abdominal pain, drowsiness, a systolic BP fall to 60 mmHg | Uncomplicated | Dugdale and Powell, 1964 |

*Abbreviations*: EGA, estimated gestation age; DPTA, diethylenetriaminepentaacetic acid.

physiological shock, acidosis, hepatic failure, and coagulopathies are major sequelae of iron over-dose over time (Table 14.11). Death is usually the result of liver failure or cardiac collapse. Serum iron concentrations peak within four hours of ingestion. Serum iron levels in excess of 500 µg/100 mL at four hours are at highest risk of severe poisoning (James, 1970). Thus, these patients should be treated aggressively.

The specific antidote to iron overdose is deferoxamine. Clinical experience clearly indicates that early administration of the deferoxamine is essential efficacious therapy.

Liver function tests, thrombin and prothrombin (INR) times, and total iron-binding capacity should be routinely monitored in iron overdose patients The gravida with an iron overdose should be managed similarly to the non-pregnant adult, as is described in detail elsewhere (Friedman, 1987; Diaz, 2014; Gei *et al.*, 2018; Olson, 2018). Guidelines for treatment according to ingested dose (if dose is known) are given in Table 14.12. There were 43 live births from 49 pregnancies complicated by iron overdose. Three infants had congenital anomalies, but are not causally related to the iron overdose or deferoxamine because exposure(s) occurred after the first trimester. Aggressive treat-ment of iron overdose with the specific antidote to prevent maternal death or organ toxicity should be initiated as soon as practicable (McElhatton *et al.*, 1991a; Gei *et al.*, 2018). Review of 61 pregnan-cies indicated that in Iron poisoning in 61 gravidas indicate (1) peak maternal serum iron levels (~4 hrs post-ingestion) are associated with iron toxicity, and (2) deferoxamine should be administered without hesitation (Tran *et al.*, 2000).

Unpublished animal studies suggest deferoxamine may cause significant fetal effects; human clinical experience does NOT parallel these findings. The cause of adverse fetal outcomes in humans are associated with maternal iron overdose-associated pathophysiological effects, and not the direct result of iron overdose or antidote. No congenital anomalies were noted among infants whose moth-ers consumed high doses of iron during pregnancy (Lacoste *et al.*, 1992; Tenenbein, 1989). It appears

**TABLE 14.11**
**Time Course of Iron Overdose**

| Phase | Time to Onset | Symptoms |
| --- | --- | --- |
| I | 0–3 h | Vomiting, hematemesis, abdominal pain, diarrhea, lethargy, restlessness |
| II | Up to 12 h | Quiescent period, symptoms subside |
| III | 12–48 h | Shock, acidosis, hepatic necrosis, renal tubular necrosis, increasing lethargy, coma, seizures, hypotension, cyanosis, pulmonary edema, hypoglycemia, coagulopathies |
| IV | 2–4 weeks | Gastric scarring, gastric/pyloric strictures |

*Sources:* Adapted from Friedman, 1987; Karalliedde and Gawarammana, 2012.

**TABLE 14.12**
**Sequelae of Iron Overdose Based on Amount Ingested**

| Amount | Risk of Toxicity |
| --- | --- |
| Less than 20 mg/kg | Minimal risk, no action required |
| 20–60 mg/kg | Moderate risk, monitor for symptoms, induce vomiting |
| More than 60 mg/kg | High risk, requires treatment, gastrointestinal decontamination, chelation |

*Sources:* Adapted from Friedman, 1987; Karalliedde and Gawarammana, 2012.

as though the placenta acts as a partial barrier to iron (Olenmark *et al.*, 1987; Rayburn *et al.*, 1983; Richards and Brooks, 1966). Chemical properties of the deferoxamine molecule strongly suggest it may not cross the placenta in large amounts because it is a large molecule (molecular weight, 657) and is highly polarized. Deferoxamine's molecular weight is within the range for placental transfer (i.e., <1,000 m.w.), but high polarity moieties generally are impeded from transfer.

## ANXIOLYTIC OVERDOSES

### BENZODIAZEPINES

The most frequently used psychotropic medication in suicide gestures is the benzodiazepines, and in the top 10 medications used in overdoses (Gummin *et al.*, 2019). US Food approved a benzodiazepine receptor antagonist, flumazenil, and Drug Administration (FDA) approved in 1992 for the management of benzodiazepine overdose (Flumazenil in Benzodiazepine Intoxication Multicentre Study Group, 1992). Flumazenil efficacy in reversing the clinical signs and symptoms of a benzodiazepine overdose was shown in several studies (Krisanda, 1993; L'Heureux *et al.*, 1992; Spivey *et al.*, 1993). Flumazenil complications (e.g., seizures) were observed among patients with clinically high, but who had subtoxic antidepressant poisoning or those who are taking benzodiazepines to therapeutically control seizures (Flumazenil in Benzodiazepine Intoxication Multicentre Study Group, 1992; L'Heureux *et al.*, 1992). Reversal of fetal benzodiazepine intoxication using flumazenil was published (Stahl *et al.*, 1993). A 22-year-old primipara ingested between 50 and 60 5 mg diazepam tablets at 36 weeks EGA, and was given flumazenil intravenously in two small doses (0.3 mg). No adverse effects or withdrawal symptoms were noted in the patient or in the infant, who was born spontaneously two weeks later.

The "floppy infant syndrome" associated with benzodiazepine use late in pregnancy indicates that the drug (1) crosses the placenta, and (2) has a depressive effect on the fetus. Warnings signs of complications in benzodiazepine overdoses in pregnancy are bradycardia, hypothermia, hypotonicity and other symptoms typical of benzodiazepines'' depressive physiologic effects on mother and fetus.

### HYDROXYZINE

Clinical course of pregnancy after hydroxyzine overdoses are not published. Hypersedation and hypotension are the most frequently observed abnormalities with hydroxyzine overdose in nonpregnant adults (Phua and Ang, 2010). Hydroxyzine counteracts epinephrine's pressor effect. Therefore, **hydroxyzine overdose-associated hypotension should not be treated with epinephrine**. Intravenous fluids and other pressor agents (levarterenol or metaraminol) should be used instead of epinephrine to treat hypotension. A total of 1 to 2 g of hydroxyzine pamoate usually produces drowsiness and lethargy, possibly progressing to coma (Magera *et al.*, 1981). Hydroxyzine elimination half-life of is 2.5–3.4 hours for a single dose of the drug (Baselt, 2017). No specific antidote to hydroxyzine is available. Therefore, nonspecific, supportive antidote therapy should be given (Marino, 2018).

## HYPNOTIC AND SEDATIVE OVERDOSES

### PHENOBARBITAL AND SECOBARBITAL

A large series of 367 women who attempted suicide during pregnancy was evaluated (Timmerman *et al.*, 2008). The course of pregnancy following barbituric-acid-derivative overdoses during gestation was complicated by use of other substances (diazepam, aminophenazone, ethanol abuse). Among 10 infants born to mothers who attempted suicide during pregnancy (6 during organogenesis), there were features of fetal alcohol syndrome (FAS). Barbituric acid derivatives have no specific antidote, and nonspecific and supportive antidote therapy were indicated (see Table 14.8).

**TABLE 14.8**

**Barbiturate Overdose in Pregnancy**

| Drug | Among ingested Aminophenazone | EGA (weeks) | | Birth Weight | Maternal Outcome | Fetal Outcome |
|------|-------------------------------|-------------|---------|--------------|------------------|---------------|
| | | Overdose | Delivery | | | |
| **Barbital** | | | | | | |
| 520 mg | 1136 mg | 15 | 30 | 2150 | Uncomplicated | Normal |
| 2600 mg | 5680 mg | 9 | 38 | 3180 | Uncomplicated | Normal[*] |
| 3900 mg | 8520 mg | 23 | 32 | 2650 | Uncomplicated | Normal[**] |
| 1300 mg | 2840 mg | 12 | 27 | 1450 | Uncomplicated | Normal |
| 2600 mg | 5680 mg | 7 | 34 | 2450 | Uncomplicated | Normal |
| **Hexobarbital** | | | | | | |
| 2500 mg | — | 9 | 33 | 2950 | Uncomplicated | Normal |
| 2500 mg | — | 6 | 33 | 2750 | Uncomplicated | Normal |
| 2500 mg | Diazepam | 23 | 36 | 3200 | Uncomplicated | Normal |
| 2500 mg | Diazepam | 10 | 30 | 2750 | Uncomplicated | Normal[***] |
| 2500 mg | — | 8 | 32 | 2900 | Uncomplicated | Syndromic[****] |

[*] Tibial exostosis.

[**] Maternal alcoholism, multiple nevi, mental retardation at follow-up.

[***] Enamel hypoplasia at follow-up.

[****] Maternal alcoholism, features of FAS (low nasal bridge, lingual phrenulum).

*Source:* Adapted from Timmerman *et al.*, 2008.

Barbituric acids cross the placenta and these drugs may induce fetal hepatic enzymes. No congenital anomalies have been observed in several studies of children born to women treated with phenobarbital at usual therapeutic doses during pregnancy (Bertollini *et al.*, 1987; Heinonen *et al.*, 1977). Five clinical stages of intoxication have been described in adults with acutely toxic levels of phenobarbital (i.e., in nontolerant individuals) (Sunshine, 1957), as shown in Box 14.2.

**BOX 14.2   PHENOBARBITAL OVERDOSE STAGES**

**Stage I:** Awake, competent, and mildly sedated. Average blood level of 3.5 mg/100 mL.

**Stage II:** Sedated, deep tendon reflexes (DTRs) present, prefers sleep, answers questions when aroused, does not cerebrate properly. Average blood level of 4.4 mg/100 mL.

**Stage III:** Comatose, DTRs present. Average blood level of 6.5 mg/100 mL.

**Stage IV:** Comatose, no DTRs obtainable. Average blood level of 10.0 mg/100 mL.

**Stage V:** Comatose, no DTRs obtainable, and with circulatory and/or respiratory difficulty. Half-lives of phenobarbital and secobarbital range from 2 to 6 days and 22 to 29 h, respectively (Baselt, 2017).

## PYRILAMINE

Pyrilamine does not appear in the 2018 national poison control report, and seems rare. No reports of pregnancy following pyrilamine overdoses are published. No specific antidote to pyrilamine is available. Non-specific and supportive antidote therapy should be given because no specific antidote exists.

## NARCOTIC ANALGESIC OVERDOSES

### OPIOID NARCOTICS

Opioid narcotics are derivatives of opium, or are chemically synthesized. Available preparations include morphine, codeine, hydrocodone, oxycodone, and hydromorphone. They are metabolized to monoacetyl-morphine. Approximately 6 percent of suicide gestures in one study involved opioid analgesic preparations (Rayburn et al., 1984) and 2.5 percent in another (Flint et al., 2002). Analgesics are the leading substances used in suicide gestures, and opioid pain relievers are the second most frequent analgesic used in attempted suicides (Gummin et al., 2019).

Naloxone, an opioid-specific antagonist, is available and used as antidote. Naloxone competitively binds to opioid receptors and opioid analgesics, blocking uptake. Naloxone causes an almost immediate onset of withdrawal symptoms in patients addicted to opioids. In those patients not addicted to opioids, naloxone reverses the CNS and respiratory depression. Most narcotic analgesic preparations also contain other substances, such as acetaminophen and/or aspirin. In documented opioid overdose is encountered, naloxone should be given according to directions in the manufacturer's package insert. Opioids cross the placenta freely and affect the fetus. Accordingly, naloxone acts as a fetal antidote as well. Therefore, treatment of maternal overdose will treat the fetal overdose.

Nalmefene is an opiate antagonist with an 11-hour half-life, and has potential benefits over naloxone (Kaplan and Marx, 1993). Naloxone has a shorter half-life (one to two hours). Nalmefene is longer acting, and period of withdrawal is longer and less abrupt in opioid-dependent patients (Kaplan and Marx, 1993). Overdose of other non-opioid constituents (e.g., acetaminophen) must be considered in formulating the antidote regimen and treatment plan. For opioid preparations that contain acetaminophen, serious hepatic and renal toxicities require immediate attention. Use of the acetaminophen antidote (NAC) should be given as soon as possible after toxicology documents toxic serum levels. Half-life in the post-absorptive period for morphine is 1.3–6.7 hours, and for codeine, 1.9–3.9 hours; oxycodone, 4.0–5.0 hours; and hydromorphone, 1.5–3.8 hours. Opioid analgesics are ultimately excreted (Baselt, 2017).

### PROPOXYPHENE AND PENTAZOCINE

Propoxyphene is no longer commercially available, but may be obtained through the black market.

Propoxyphene and pentazocine are synthetic narcotic preparations. However, naloxone and nalmefene are not antidotes to either drug. Lethal doses of propoxyphene are estimated at 500–800 mg, or higher (Baselt, 2017). Whole-blood concentrations of 1 mg/L indicate serious toxicity and 2 mg/L or more of propoxyphene are associated with death (Baselt, 2017). Pentazocine overdose fatalities usually occur with blood concentrations in the 1–5 mg/L range, with brain concentrations often exceeding blood levels except in cases of intravenous administration (Baselt, 2017).

Propoxyphene or pentazocine overdose during pregnancy is not published. Nonspecific and supportive antidote therapy should be given because the effectiveness and safety of nalmefene for narcotic overdose have been demonstrated only in a pilot study. Naloxone and pentazocine combinations are used to treat moderate pain. Synthetic narcotic drugs are known to cross the placenta, and chronic use during pregnancy exposes the fetus to sufficient amounts to produce neonatal abstinence syndrome. Narcotics may cause fetal hepatic enzyme activity, and hasten liver enzyme maturation. Effects of potentially toxic doses of pentazocine are unknown. Adult half-lives of propoxyphene and pentazocine in the post-absorptive period are 8–24 hours and 2.1–3.5 hours, respectively (Baselt, 2017).

# ANTIBIOTIC OVERDOSES

### CEPHALEXIN, AMOXICILLIN, AND TRIMETHOPRIM SULFAMETHOXAZOLE

In one study three decades ago, antibiotics were used in 7 percent of suicide gestures during pregnancy. In 2018, 2.2 percent of poisonings in pregnancy were overdoses of antimicrobials, ranking 13th among agents used in suicide gestures (Gummin et al., 2019). Antibiotic overdoses in pregnancy are not published. Non-specific and supportive antidote therapy should be given because no specific antidote to antibiotic overdoses is available. Appreciable amounts of these drugs cross the placenta and expose the fetus to high drug doses, but the effects of potentially toxic doses on the fetus are unknown. Overdoses of antimicrobial substances known to lower folic acid concentrations (e.g., trimethoprim-sulfamethoxazole, pyrimethamine), folic acid supplementation should be given in the therapeutic range.

# ANTIHISTAMINE AND DECONGESTANT OVERDOSES

Six percent of attempted suicides by pregnant women included large doses of antihistamines and/or decongestants in one study from 1984 (Table 14.1), but not another in Finland in 2000 (Table 14.2). In 2018, antihistamines ranked ninth among substances used in poisoning among pregnant women, or approximately 2.5 percent (Gummin et al., 2019; Figure 14.1). One pregnancy following antihistamine overdose, diphenhydramine (35 Benadryl pills), in a suicide gesture at 26 weeks estimated gestation age (EGA) has been published. In the emergency room with palpable contractions, preterm labor was successfully treated with intravenous magnesium sulfate for tocolysis. Diphenhydramine overdose was treated with activated charcoal slurry because no specific antidotes exist. After 3 days, the patient was released from the hospital in good health (Brost et al., 1996).

Preterm labor was attributed to the oxytocin-like effects of diphenhydramine (Brost et al., 1996). Hence, nonspecific and supportive antidote therapy should be given. It is known that considerable amounts of these drugs cross the placenta to reach the fetus. However, the effects of a potentially toxic dose are unknown.

# ANTIPSYCHOTIC OVERDOSES

### THIORIDAZINE AND TRIFLUOPERAZINE

Approximately 3 percent of pregnant women who attempted suicide during pregnancy used antipsychotic preparations (Flint et al., 2002; Rayburn et al., 1984). In 2018, 2.5 percent of suicide gestures during pregnancy employed antipsychotics and psychoactive drugs (Gummin et al., 2019; Figure 14.1). One case report is published regarding overdose of trifluoperazine (including misoprostol) during pregnancy (Bond and Van Zee, 1994). Fetal death was the outcome, but the authors noted misoprostol as the probable cause of fetal death.

Antipsychotic overdose therapy includes non-specific supportive therapy because there are no specific antidotes. These drugs cross the placenta and achieve near-therapeutic fetal concentrations. Large doses of these drugs cause hypersedation in the non-pregnant adult and are expected to have the same effect on the gravida and fetus. The clinical course of potentially toxic doses during pregnancy are not published. Thioridazine and trifluoperazine half-lives in the post-absorptive period are 26–36 hours and 7–18 hours, respectively (Baselt, 2017).

# ANORECTIC OVERDOSES

### SYMPATHOMIMETIC AMINES, PHENYLPROPANOLAMINE

In one study, anorectic agents were used by approximately 2 percent of pregnant women in suicide gestures (Table 14.1). In the 2018 report from poison controls centers in the US, anorectics were

**TABLE 14.1**

**Drugs Used in Suicide Gestures among 111 Pregnant Women in the United States**

| Drug class | Percent |
|---|---|
| Nonnarcotic analgesics (acetaminophen, aspirin, ibuprofen) | 26 |
| Nutritional supplements (prenatal vitamins, iron) | 12 |
| Antianxiolytics (diazepam, hydroxyzine, other benzodiazepines) | 11 |
| Hypnotics and sedatives (phenobarbital, flurazepam, and others) | 10 |
| Narcotic analgesics (codeine, propoxyphene, and others) | 8 |
| Antibiotics (cephalexin, amoxicillin, trimethoprim sulfamethoxazole) | 7 |
| Antihistamines (diphenhydramine, others) | 6 |
| Antipsychotics (thioridazine, trifluoperazine) | 3 |
| Anorectics (sympathomimetics, phenylpropanolamine) | 2 |
| Hormonal agents (corticosteroids, oral contraceptives) | 2 |
| Antidepressants (doxepin, amitriptyline) | 2 |
| Anticonvulsants (phenytoin, carbamazepine) | 2 |
| Other drugs (miscellaneous drugs from other classes) | 6 |
| Nondrug chemicals (turpentine, camphorated oil, ammonia) | 2 |

*Source:* Compiled from Rayburn *et al.*, 1984.

used in about 2 percent of suicide gestures, but were not in the top 20 substances used in overdoses during pregnancy (Gummin *et al.*, 2019). The course of pregnancy following anorectic agent overdoses has not been published. Therapy consists of nonspecific antidote and supportive therapy. The drugs cross the placenta and reach near therapeutic levels in the fetus. Oral doses of 50–75 mg produce anxiety, agitation, dizziness, and hallucinations (Dietz, 1981). Higher doses (85–400 mg) are associated with severe headaches, hypertensive crisis, and occasionally vomiting (Frewin *et al.*, 1978; Horowitz *et al.*, 1979; Ostern, 1965; Salmon, 1965; Teh, 1979).

Potentially toxic dose effects on the fetus are unknown. The half-life of phenylpropanolamine is 5.6 h (Dowse *et al.*, 1987).

## HORMONAL AGENT OVERDOSES

### CORTICOSTEROIDS AND ORAL CONTRACEPTIVES

An estimated 2 percent of pregnant women used large doses of hormonal agents in their suicide attempt (Rayburn *et al.*, 1984). In 2018 approximately 2 percent of suicide poisonings in pregnancy used hormonal agents (Gummin *et al.*, 2019). The course of pregnancy following hormonal agent overdoses has not been published. Nonspecific supportive therapy should be given because no specific antidote to hormonal agents is available. Near-therapeutic amounts of these drugs cross the placenta and can be detected in the fetus. The effects of a potentially toxic dose of hormonal agents are unknown, but fetal adrenal suppression should be anticipated based upon known pharmacology and physiology.

One overdose of misoprostol and trifluoperazine has been reported (Bond and Van Zee, 1994). Signs of toxicity included hypertonic uterine contraction with fetal death, hyperthermia, rhabdomyolysis, hypoxemia, respiratory alkalosis, and metabolic acidosis. The clinical impression was that misoprostol was being used as an illegal abortifacient. In another misoprostol overdose in the first trimester, the drug was being used as an abortifacient (42 pills). The patient was given supportive antidote therapy (gastric lavage, activated charcoal) and a dilatation and curettage. She recovered within

6 h and was sent home (Bentov *et al.*, 2004). A third case report of a patient who took 60 pills (~12 mg *misoprostol*) in an attempt to induce an abortion, complained of upper gastrointestinal bleeding. She developed multiorgan failure, acute abdominal signs, and hemodynamic instability. Gastric and esophageal necrosis developed later, followed by several cardiac arrests events, and death (Henriques *et al.*, 2007). An attempted abortion using 8 mg misoprostol (1 mg orally and 7 mg vaginally) to induce abortion at 5 weeks gestation presented as agitation, tremors, hallucinations, tachycardia, fever, rhabdomyolysis, acute renal failure, elevated liver enzymes and metabolic acidosis. 48 hours after hospital admission, the abortion was complete (Barros *et al.*, 2011). In another case, there was an attempted abortion with 10.8 mg of misoprostol over 6 weeks starting at 5 weeks gestation. The patient presented with mild to moderate pelvic pain. An ultrasound at 16 weeks showed no detectable congenital anomalies; a normal infant was born at 38 weeks gestation (Rouzi, 2010).

## ANTIDEPRESSANT OVERDOSES

### DOXEPIN AND AMITRIPTYLINE

Approximately 2 percent of pregnant women used antidepressants in suicide gestures in two studies (Flint *et al.*, 2002; Rayburn *et al.*, 1984). In 2018, antidepressants were 2.8 percent of (7th most frequently used) substances in suicide attempts (Gummin *et al.*, 2019). The clinical details of the course of pregnancy in a 34-week gestation gravida who took 30–40 amitriptyline and 20–30 chlorpheniramine is published. Therapy was supportive, and consisted of increased fluid volume (Tang, 2018). The toxic systemic effects (tachycardia, dry mouth, dilated pupils, and urinary retention) as well as the central nervous system effects (agitation, hallucinations, and hyperpyrexia) are anticholinergic in nature (Burks *et al.*, 1974). For this reason, physostigmine (an anticholinesterase) has been used in the diagnosis and antidotal therapy of poisoning with amitriptyline and other tricyclic antidepressants (Burks *et al.*, 1974; Slovis *et al.*, 1971). Large doses of antidepressants are associated with coma in non-pregnant adults and cardiac toxicity has been reported with acute ingestion of high doses of these drugs. Although these drugs cross the placenta to reach the fetus, the effects of a potentially toxic dose are unknown. Half-lives in the post-absorptive period for doxepin and amitriptyline are 8–25 hours and 8–51 hours, respectively (Baselt, 2017). In one case reported with doxepin overdose at 34 weeks, the mother recovered and delivered a normal infant (birth weight 3,650 g). No details of the time after or drug concentration were given (Flint *et al.*, 2002).

### SSRI OVERDOSE

An overdose of escitalopram (280 mg) at 31 weeks pregnancy presented as acute serotonergic intoxication. At 5 hours post-ingestion, the patient was treated with activated charcoal. She experienced regular uterine contractions, signaling a possible premature delivery. The patient was given intravenous nicardipine and an intramuscular corticosteroid in addition to activated charcoal. After 24 hours, contractions subsided. Spontaneous vaginal delivery at 37 weeks resulted in a normal infant who was extremely agitated. Irritability and nervousness continued for several days (Tixier, 2008), but it seems unlikely that escitalopram persisted for 5 weeks given the half-life of 27–33 hours and six days for terminal clearance.

### LITHIUM OVERDOSE

Lithium was used in <1 percent of suicide gestures in 2018 (Gummin *et al.*, 2019), but none of these cases occurred in pregnancy. A gravida presented at 33 weeks gestation with signs of lithium toxicity (Nausea, vomiting, ataxia, myoclonic twitches, confusion). The patient was given intravenous fluids, but lithium concentration increased anyway (Zimani *et al.*, 2017).

## ANTICONVULSANT OVERDOSES

### PHENYTOIN AND CARBAMAZEPINE

An estimated 2 percent of pregnant women who attempted suicide used large doses of anticonvulsants (Rayburn *et al.*, 1984). In 2018, less than 1 percent (0.8 percent) of suicide gestures involved anticonvulsants (Gummin *et al.*, 2019). Pregnancy outcome after anticonvulsant carbamazepine overdose is published of a first trimester case report and a third trimester case report. Carbamazepine megadose in attempted suicide with > 10 g of carbamazepine during organogenesis resulted in a large meningomyelocele and frontal lobe necrosis in the fetus that was electively aborted. The mother recovered without complication following non-specific therapy and coma for 5 days (Little *et al.*, 1993). At 33 weeks gestation, a gravida in coma arrived in the emergency department following carbamazepine overdose (serum level was 10 times normal). The patient was treated with activated charcoal slurry by nasogastric tube, and by exchange plasmapheresis (19 units) (Saygan-Karamursel *et al.*, 2005). The patient indicated she had taken 40,200 mg carbamazepine tablets 12 hours prior to admission attempting to commit suicide. Steroids were given to promote fetal lung maturity, and on day two spontaneous labor began, with a vaginal delivery of a 2,300 g health infant delivered.

No cases of phenytoin overdose during pregnancy are published.

A cautionary anecdote regarding overdoses of anticonvulsants indicates that damage to the embryo or fetus is probable during organogenesis because the phenytoin and carbamazepine are known human teratogens. Anticonvulsant agents have no specific antidote, and supportive therapy should be given as soon as possible.

Near-therapeutic amounts of these drugs cross the placenta and achieve significant concentrations in the fetus. For example, the third trimester fetus had therapeutic levels of carbamazepine by the third day (Saygan-Karamursel *et al.*, 2005).

Phenytoin may induce fetal hepatic enzymes, but the effects of a potentially toxic dose are unknown. Phenytoin's half-life ranges from 8–60 hours and is dose dependent because each individual has a threshold plasma concentration beyond which the drug exhibits zero-order kinetics (Arnold and Gerber, 1970; Kostenbauder *et al.*, 1975). Carbamazepine half-life after a single dose is 18–65 hours (Baselt, 2017).

## OVERDOSES OF OTHER DRUGS

Miscellaneous other drugs (Bendectin, docusate, cimetidine, methyldopa) were used by about 6 percent of pregnant women in their suicide gestures (Table 14.1). Subsequent studies did not classify substances in this fashion, but miscellaneous substances used in suicide gestures in pregnancy may comprise as high as 8 percent of the agents used (Gummin, 2019). Details of the clinical course of pregnancy after overdoses of these agents are not published. No specific antidotes to these agents are available. It is known that significant amounts of these drugs cross the placenta to reach near-therapeutic levels in the fetus. Megadose effects on mother or fetus are unknown.

## OVERDOSES OF NONDRUG CHEMICALS

Approximately 2 percent of pregnant women who attempted suicide used nondrug chemicals in one study (Rayburn *et al.*, 1984). In the 2018 Poison Control National Report, household/cleaning agents were used in 8.4 percent of suicide gestures during pregnancy, and 3.4 percent used chemicals (nonspecific) in suicide gestures (Gummin *et al.*, 2019).

### CAMPHORATED OIL

Camphor, a gastrointestinal irritant and central nervous system stimulant. Camphor is a component in over-the-counter medications intended for external use only. It is available in drugstores. The substance is highly toxic and has a rapid onset of symptoms. It was used in five suicide attempts during pregnancy that are published (Blackmon and Curry, 1957; Jacobziner and Raybin, 1962; Riggs *et al.*, 1965; Weiss and Catalano, 1973; Rabl *et al.*, 1997). In an admitted attempt, a 16-year-old took 30 g of camphor dissolved with 250 ml wine for an abortifacient. Vomiting began 45 min after ingestion, possibly saving the gravida's life. The pregnancy was legally terminated 3 days after this episode (Rabl *et al.*, 1997). Estimated human lethal dose is 50 to 500 mg kg, and it is still used in suicide gestures (Gummin *et al.*, 2019).

Camphor is sometimes used as an abortifacient, and crosses the placenta. Fetuses lack the hydroxylase enzymes to hydroxylate and conjugate with glucuronic acid to clear camphor. The inability to metabolize camphor results in a toxic reaction (Rabl *et al.*, 1997).

Maternal seizures should be expected with camphor ingestion, but did not occur in one instance (Rabl *et al.*, 1997). Three of the five infants survived with no obvious abnormalities. The fourth pregnancy was compromised by preeclampsia, abruptio placenta, and other serious complications, and the infant died less than one hour after delivery. Clearly, the death cannot be directly attributed to megadose camphor oil.

Clinical experience with camphor overdose is limited to five cases, but it is still used in suicide gestures and as an abortifacient. No specific antidote is available. Nonspecific antidote regimens should be given and supportive therapy provided. Limited experience with gravid women who took camphor is sufficient to begin antiseizure medication as a component of the antidote regimen, anticipating seizures associated with ingestion of this substance.

## Turpentine and Ammonia

The course of pregnancy following poisoning with these nondrug chemicals are not reported. No specific antidote to these substances is available. Nonspecific antidote regimens and supportive therapy should be given.

## Quinine Overdose

Attempted abortion should be suspected when quinine overdose is encountered in pregnant women. Quinine has not been used in suicide attempts based upon published experience, and does not appear in the 2018 Poison Control Centers National Report (Gummin *et al.*, 2019). Outcomes of 70 pregnant women who took high-dose quinine in an attempt to induce abortion, findings suggest the drug may be teratogenic (Dannenberg *et al.*, 1983). Eleven women died because of quinine overdose, and most who survived experienced toxic effects of the drug (tinnitus, visual disturbance). Forty-one infants with major congenital anomalies were born to women who took large doses of quinine during pregnancy. Causality cannot be shown with these data because it contains only case reports. It is clear that large doses of quinine are associated with an increased risk of specific congenital anomalies that parallel the drug's ototoxicity from the drug observed in adults. Eighteen of 60 infants (30 percent) born to women who ingested large amounts of quinine during pregnancy had congenital deafness (Dannenberg *et al.*, 1983). Ototoxicity is a common and well-documented complication of quinine therapy in adults.

Large doses of quinine during the first trimester of pregnancy are anecdotally associated with major congenital anomalies, including central nervous system anomalies (especially hydrocephalus or otolithic damage), limb defects, cardiac defects, and gastrointestinal tract anomalies (Nishimura and Tanimura, 1976). No characteristic pattern of anomalies or syndrome was identified. The association of these congenital anomalies with maternal quinine ingestion remains empirically uncertain because the data are anecdotal case reports, but the association is biologically plausible.

Non-specific antidote treatment and supportive therapy should be given because no specific antidote for quinine overdose is available.

## Ergotamine Overdose

Overdose of ergotamine during pregnancy was published in a case report of a woman at 35 weeks' gestation who took 10 tablets of ergotamine tartrate in a suicide gesture. Two hours later uterine contractions began with no relaxation between contractions. Fetal death occurred approximately eight hours after the overdose. Two weeks after the overdose, a macerated stillbirth with no gross abnormality was delivered. Impaired placental perfusion and fetal anoxia associated with ergotamine was speculated to have caused the fetal death (Au *et al.*, 1985). Ergot compound exposure during pregnancy was reviewed for non-overdose use, and reported eight pregnancies exposed during organogenesis. Birth defects reported in these case reports are consistent with increased vascular resistance, spasm, and ischemia (Raymond, 1995). Ergot contaminated animal food results in peripheral gangrene, a result of vascular disruption. A similar etiologic mechanism is suggested for the congenital anomalies observed in cases of non-overdose ergot therapy (Raymond, 1995).

Ergot compounds have an oxytocin-like action and stimulates uterine contractions. Spontaneous onset of preterm labor following ingestion of ergot also occurred with therapeutic levels of the drugs, but at usual therapeutic levels prematurity was the only complication, and there were no fetal deaths. Two antidotes to ergot alkaloid overdose (prazosin and nitroprusside) are now available that were unavailable to treat patients described earlier (Au *et al.*, 1985). Nitroprusside should be avoided during pregnancy because it conjugates to cyanide and accumulates in the fetal liver. Therefore, prazosin is the preferred antidote for use during pregnancy.

## SUMMARY

Early aggressive treatment of attempted suicide during pregnancy is associated with better outcomes than late or passive treatment. Fetal monitoring should begin as early as possible. If a specific antidote exists, it should be given as soon as possible. If there is no specific antidote, a nonspecific aggressive treatment should be instituted as early as possible (see Appendix II). Toxicology should be ordered as soon as possible to empirically ascertain the exposure(s) and potential toxicity. Time since ingestion is a very important data point, but it is infrequently published (e.g., see Appendix II for Acetaminophen overdoses for paucity of reporting).

Most drug overdoses may be managed with supportive care, including airway management, IV fluids, gastric lavage, whole bowel irrigation, and electrolyte balance. Sedatives and anticonvulsants are commonly associated with loss of consciousness, and may require airway assistance. Other drugs (salbutamol, theophylline) stimulate the sympathetic nervous system, often presenting with hypertension and tachycardia.. Fluid replacement and sedation (e.g., benzodiazepines) may be used to manage hyperirritability. Serotonin syndrome may be induced by SSRI overdoses, and have hyperthermia and muscle rigidity. Hydration and cooling are warranted.

In general, overdoses with not-sustained-release drugs should be monitored for 6–8 hours. Signs and symptoms should appear by this time lag. However, sustained-release drugs may produce symptoms as late as 18–24 hours post-ingestion.

## APPENDIX I
## List of Antidotes Available 2021

| Antidote | Used for Drug Overdose, Poison, or Toxin |
|---|---|
| N-Acetylcysteine or NAC (Mucomyst, Acetadolte) | Acetaminophen |
| | Carbon tetrachloride |
| | Other hepatotoxins |
| Amyl nitrite, sodium nitrite, and sodium thiosulfate (Cyanide Antidote kit) | Acetonitrile |
| | Acrylonitrile |
| | Bromates (thiosulfate only) |
| | Chlorates (thiosulfate only) |
| | Cyanide (e.g., HCN, KCN, and NaCN) |
| | Cyanogen chloride |
| | Cyanogenic glycoside natural sources (e.g., apricot pits and peach pits) |
| | Hydrogen sulfide (nitrites only) |
| | Laetrile |
| | Mustard agents (thiosulfate only) |
| | Nitroprusside (thiosulfate only) |
| | Smoke inhalation (combustion of synthetic materials) |
| Antivenin, Crotalidae Polyvalent (equine origin) | Pit viper envenomation (e.g., rattlesnakes, cottonmouths, timber rattlers, and copperheads) |
| Antivenin, Crotalidae Polyvalent Immune Fab – Ovine (CroFab) | Pit viper envenomation (e.g., rattlesnakes, cottonmouths, timber rattlers, and copperheads) |
| Antivenin, *Latrodectus mactans* (black widow spider) | Black widow spider envenomation |
| Atropine sulfate | Alpha$_2$ agonists (e.g., clonidine, guanabenz, and guanfacine) |
| Antimyesthenic agents (e.g. pyridostigmine) | Alzheimer drugs (e.g., donepezil, galantamine, rivastigmine, tacrine) |
| | Bradyarrhythmia-producing agents (e.g., beta-blockers, calcium channel blockers, and digitalis glycosides) Cholinergic agonists (e.g., bethanechol) |
| | Muscarine-containing mushrooms (e.g., Clitocybe and Inocybe) |
| | Nerve agents (e.g., sarin, soman, tabun, and VX) |
| | Organophosphate and carbamate insecticides |
| Calcium disodium | Lead |
| EDTA (Versenate) | Zinc salts (e.g., zinc chloride) |
| Calcium chloride & Calcium gluconate | Beta-blockers |
| | Calcium channel blockers |
| | Fluoride salts (e.g., NaF) |
| | Hydrofluoric acid (HF) |
| | Hyperkalemia (not digoxin-induced) |
| | Hypermagnesemia |
| Deferoxamine mesylate (Desferal) | Iron |
| Digoxin immune Fab (Digibind, Digifab) | Cardiac glycoside-containing plants (e.g., foxglove and oleander) |
| | Digitoxin Digoxin |
| Dimercaprol (BAL in oil) | Arsenic |
| | Copper |
| | Gold |
| | Lead |
| | Lewsite (organic arsenic) |
| | Mercury |
| Ethanol | Ethylene glycol |
| | Methanol |

## List of Antidotes Available 2021

| Antidote | Used for Drug Overdose, Poison, or Toxin |
| --- | --- |
| Flumazenil (Romazicon) | Benzodiazepines |
| | Zalepion |
| | Zolpidem |
| Folic acid and Folinic acid (Leucovorin) | Methanol |
| Folic acid and Folinic acid (Leucovorin) | Methotrexate trimetrexate |
| | Pyrimethamine |
| | Trimethoprim |
| Carbopeptidase G2 (Voraxase®) | Methotrexate trimetrexate |
| Fomepizole (Antizol) | Ethylene glycol |
| | Methanol |
| Glucagon | Beta-blockers |
| | Calcium channel blockers Hypoglycemia Hypoglycemic agents |
| Hyperbaric oxygen (HBO) | Carbon monoxide Carbon tetrachloride Cyanide |
| | Hydrogen sulfide Methemoglobinemia |
| Methylene blue | Methomoglobin-inducing agents including aniline dyes |
| | Dapsone Dinitrophenol |
| | Local anesthetics (e.g., benzocaine) Metoclopramide |
| | Monomethylhydrazine-containing mushrooms (e.g. Gyromitra) |
| | Naphthalene |
| | Nitrates and nitrites Nitrobenzene Phenazopyridine |
| Nalmefene (Revex) and Naloxone | ACE inhibitors (Narcan) |
| | Alpha agonists (e.g., clonidine, guanabenz and guanfacine) |
| | Coma of unknown cause |
| | Imidazoline decongestants (e.g., oxymetazoline and tetrahydrozoline) |
| | Loperamide |
| | Opioids (e.g., codeine, dextromethorphan, diphenoxylate, fentanyl, heroin, meperidine, morphine, and propoxyphene) |
| D-Penicillamine (Cuprimine) | Arsenic |
| | Copper |
| | Lead |
| | Mercury |
| Physostigmine salicylate (Antilirium) | Anticholinergic alkaloid-containing plants (e.g., deadly nightshade and jimson weed) Antihistamines Atropine and other anticholinergic agents Intrathecal baclofen |
| Phytonadione | Indandione derivatives |
| Vitamin K (AquaMEPHYTON, Mephyton) | Long-acting anticoagulant rodenticides (e.g., brodifacoum and bromadiolone) |
| | Warfarin |
| Pralidoxime chloride | Antimyesthenic agents (e.g., pyridostigmine) |
| (2-PAM) | Nerve agents (e.g., sarin, soman, tabun and VX) |
| (Protopam) | Organophosphate insecticides Tacrine |
| Protamine sulfate | Enoxaparin |
| | Heparin |
| Pyridoxine hydrochloride | Acrylamide |
| (Vitamin B$_6$) | Ethylene glycol |
| | Hydrazine Isoniazid (INH) |
| | Monomethylhydrazine-containing mushrooms (e.g., Gyromitra) |

## List of Antidotes Available 2021

| Antidote | Used for Drug Overdose, Poison, or Toxin |
|---|---|
| Sodium bicarbonate | Chlorine gas |
| | Hyperkalemia |
| | Serum alkalinization: |
| | Agents producing a quinidine-like effect as noted by widened QRS complex on EKG (e.g., amantadine, carbamazepine, chloroquine, cocaine, diphenhydramine, flecainide, propafenone, propoxyphene, tricyclic antidepressants, quinidine and related agents) |
| | Urine alkalinization: |
| | Weakly acidic agents (e.g., chlorophenoxy herbicides), chlorpropamide, phenobarbital, and salicylates) |
| Succimer (Chemet) | Arsenic Lead Lewisite Mercury |
| Benztropine mesylate (Cogentin) mesylate (Parlodel) | Medications causing a dystonic reaction Bromocriptine Medications causing neuroleptic malignant Syndrome (NMS) |
| L-Carnitine (Carnitor) | Valproic acid |
| Cyproheptadine HCL (Periactin) | Medications causing serotonin syndrome |
| Dantrolene sodium (Dantrium) | Medications causing NMS |
| | Medications causing malignant hyperthermia |
| Diazepam (Valium) | Chloroquine and related antimalarial drugs NMS Serotonin syndrome |
| Diphenhydramine HCL (Benadryl) and dextrose | Medications causing a dystonic reaction |
| | Insulin |
| | Beta-blockers |
| | Calcium channel blockers (diltiazem, nifedipine, verapamil) |
| Octreotide acetate (Sandostatin) | Sulfonylurea hypoglycemic agents (e.g., glipizide, glyburide) |
| Phentolamine mesylate (Regitine) | Catecholamine extravasation |
| | Intradigital epinephrine injection |
| Thiamine | Ethanol |
| | Ethanol glycol |
| Calcium-diethylenetriamine penaacetic acid (Ca-DTPA; Pentetate calciumdisodium injection) | Internal contamination with transuranium elements americium, curium, plutonium |
| Zinc-diethylenetriamine pentaacetic acid (Zn-DTPA: pentetate zinc trisodium injection) | |
| Potassium Iodide, Kl tablets (Iostate, Kl liquid (Thyroshield) | Prevents thyroid uptake of radioactive iodine (I-131) Thyro-Block, Thyrosafe) |
| Prussian blue, ferric hexacyanoferrate (Radiogardase) | Radioactive cesium (Cs-137), radioactive thallium (TI-201), and nonradioactive thallium) |
| Idarucizumab Praxbind® | Dabigatran |
| PPSB | Vitamin K antagonist anticoagulants Direct oral anticoagulant |
| Sugammadex | Rocuronium |
| | Vecuronium |

ACE, angiotensin-converting enzyme

DTPA, diethylenetriaminepentaacetic acid

EDTA, ethylenediaminetetraacetic acid.

Compiled from Gei *et al.*, 2018; Olson, 2018; Diaz, 2014.

## APPENDIX II
## Acetaminophen OD in Pregnancy

| Dose | Treatment | Blood Concentration | Other Exposures | EGA | Maternal Outcome | Fetal Outcome | Source |
|------|-----------|---------------------|-----------------|-----|------------------|---------------|--------|
| Unknown | N-acetylcysteine | 293 | Acetylsalicylate | 26 | Uncomplicated | C-section, Preterm birth | Pavlak *et al.*, 2018 |
| <20 | Nonspecific | Not reported | Diazepam, chlorpheniramine, phenylp | Not reported | Hepatotoxicity | Unknown | Silverman and Carithess, 1978 |
| >35 g | N-acetylcysteine | 40.43 mg/L | None | 31 weeks | Hepatic necrosis, | Premature delivery, neonatal death | Wang *et al.*, 1997 |
| >4 g/day, chronic | N-acetylcysteine | 234 mg/L | None | 27 weeks | Recovered | Discharged w/o evidence of liver injury | Horowitz *et al.*, 1997 |
| >4 g/day, chronic | N-acetylcysteine | Undetectable 48 h late | None | 22 weeks | Recovered | Previable delivery, died no evid liv injury | Horowitz *et al.*, 1997 |
| 0.2 g | Nonspecific | Not reported | Salicylamide, aspirin, caffeine, chlorph | Early pregnancy | Not reported | Harelip, cleft palate | McNeil, 1973 |
| 1 g | Nonspecific | Not reported | Nimesulide | 37 weeks | Not reported | Constricted ductus arteriosus, nl at 6 weeks | Simbi *et al.*, 2002 |
| 1 g | Nonspecific | Not reported | Diazepam, avomine, vallergan | 12 weeks | Not reported | Normal | McElhatton *et al.*, 1997 |
| 1.2 g/day, chronic | Nonspecific | Not reported | Codeine, carisoprodol, aspirin, phenyto | 35 weeks | Hepatic injury, recovered | Preterm delivery, hepatic injury, coagulopat | Kurzel, 1990 |
| 1.2 g/day, chronic | Nonspecific | Not reported | Salicylamide, aspirin, caffeine, multivit | 0–12 weeks | Not reported | Hand and foot deformities | McNeil, 1973 |
| 1.3 g/day | Nonspecific | Not reported | None | All of pregnancy | Normal | Polyhydramnios; neonatal renal failure and d | Char *et al.*, 1975 |
| 1.95–3.25 g/day | Nonspecific | Not reported | None | 0–38 weeks | Not reported | Minor anomalies | Golden and Perman, 1980 |
| 10 g | Nonspecific | Not reported | Not reported | 18 days | Not reported | Term delivery | Flint *et al.*, 2002 |
| 10 g | Nonspecific | Not reported | None reported | 12 weeks | Not reported | Elective abortion | McElhatton *et al.*, 1997 |
| 10 g | Nonspecific | Not reported | None | 6 weeks | Not reported | Normal | McElhatton *et al.*, 1997 |
| 10 g | Nonspecific | Not reported | Methyldopa, ethanol | 12 weeks | Not reported | Normal | McElhatton *et al.*, 1997 |
| 10 g | Nonspecific | 75 mg/L | None | 16 weeks | Not reported | Normal | McElhatton *et al.*, 1997 |
| 10 g | Nonspecific | 170 mg/L | None | 20 weeks | Not reported | Normal | McElhatton *et al.*, 1997 |

| | | | | | | | |
|---|---|---|---|---|---|---|---|
| 10 g | Nonspecific | Not reported | Codeine | 28 weeks | Not reported | Normal | McElhatton et al., 1997 |
| 10–13 g | Nonspecific | Not reported | None reported | 21 weeks | Not reported | Elective abortion | McElhatton et al., 1997 |
| 12 g | Nonspecific | Not reported | None | 17 weeks | Not reported | Normal | McElhatton et al., 1997 |
| 12–15 g | Nonspecific | 105 mg/L | Dihydrocodeine | 28 weeks | Not reported | Term delivery, cleft lip and palate | McElhatton et al., 1997 |
| 12.5 g | Nonspecific | Not reported | Not reported | 18 weeks | Not reported | Term delivery | Flint et al., 2002 |
| 12.5 g | Nonspecific | 115 mg/L | None | 28 weeks | Not reported | Normal | McElhatton et al., 1997 |
| 12.5 g | Nonspecific | Not reported | None | 28 weeks | Not reported | Normal | McElhatton et al., 1997 |
| 14 g | Nonspecific | 125 mg/L | None | 35 weeks | Not reported | Normal | McElhatton et al., 1997 |
| 15 and 50 g | Nonspecific | 448 mg/L | N-acetylcysteine | 31 and 32 weeks | Hepatic injury | Induced premature deliv, jaundice, hypog; yc | McElhatton et al., 1997 |
| 15 g | Nonspecific | Not reported | Not reported | 18 days | Not reported | Term delivery | Flint et al., 2002 |
| 15 g | Nonspecific | Nor reported | Dihydrocodeine, methionine, polyphar | 34 weeks | Not reported | Term delivery, | McElhatton et al., 1997 |
| 15 g | Nonspecific | 60 mg/L | None | 7 weeks | Not reported | Normal | McElhatton et al., 1997 |
| 15 g | Nonspecific | 290 mg/L | None | 18 weeks | Not reported | Normal | McElhatton et al., 1997 |
| 19 | N-acetylcysteine | Not reported | N-acetylcysteine | 40 | Uncomplicated | Normal | Sancewicz-Pach et al., 1999 |
| 19 g | Nonspecific | Not reported | None prior to delivery | Term | Anemia | No evidence of | Sancewicz-Pach et al., 1998 |
| 2 g | Nonspecific | Not reported | Phenylpropanolamine | 12 weeks | Not reported | Normal | McElhatton et al., 1997 |
| 2.6 g/day chronically | Nonspecific | Not reported | Dextropropoxyphene, OCPs, prrednison | All of pregnanc | Not reported | Elective abortion of | McElhatton et al., 1997 |
| 20 | N-acetylcysteine | Not reported | None | 36 | Uncomplicated | Normal | Roberts et al., 1984 |
| 20 g | Nonspecific | 280 mg/L | Ethanol | 36 weeks | Normal | Normal | Roberts et al., 1988 |
| 22.5 g | Nonspecific | 200 mg/L | None | 36 weeks | Normal | Normal | Byer et al., 1982 |
| 23 g | Nonspecific | Not reported | None | 4 weeks | Not reported | Normal | McElhatton et al., 1997 |
| 24 | N-acetylcysteine | 55 mg/L | None | 31 | Uncomplicated | Normal, emergency c-section, preterm, RSD | Payen et al., 2011 |
| 24 g | Nonspecific | 222 mg/L | None | 12 weeks | Not reported | Normal | McElhatton et al., 1997 |
| 25 | N-acetylcysteine | Not reported | None | 18 | Hepatotoxicity | Term delivery | Stokes, 1984 |
| 25 g | Nonspecific | Not reported | Not reported | 19 weeks | Not reported | Term delivery | Flint et al., 2002 |
| 25 g | Nonspecific | Not reported | None | 16 weeks | Not reported | Elective abortion at 21 weeks, normal fetus | McElhatton et al., 1997 |

## Acetaminophen OD in Pregnancy

| Dose | Treatment | Blood Concentration | Other Exposures | EGA | Maternal Outcome | Fetal Outcome | Source |
|---|---|---|---|---|---|---|---|
| 25 g | Nonspecific | 121 mg/L | None | 36 weeks | Not reported | Normal | McElhatton et al., 1997 |
| 25 g | Nonspecific | 236 mg/L | vitamin K | 20 weeks | Jaundice, resolve | Normal delivery at 41 weeks, jaundice | Stokes, 1984 |
| 26 | N-acetylcysteine | Not reported | None | 38 | Uncomplicated | | Ruthnum and Goel, 1984 |
| 29.5 | N-acetylcysteined | Not reported | None | 28 | Hepatotoxicityc | Fetal death | Haibach et al., 1984 |
| 29.5 g | N-acetylcysteine | 56 mg/L (20 h later) | Note: NAC given after fetal demise | 27–28 weeks | Hepatic injury, recovered | Fetal demise; fetal liver acetaminophen | Haibach et al., 1984 |
| 3 g | Nonspecific | Not reported | Diphenhydramine | 32 weeks | Not reported | Normal | McElhatton et al., 1997 |
| 3.25 g | Nonspecific | Not reported | None | 7 weeks | Not reported | Normal | McElhatton et al., 1997 |
| 3.6 g | Nonspecific | Not reported | None | 12 weeks | Not reported | Normal | McElhatton et al., 1997 |
| 30 g | N-acetylcysteine | 210 mg/L | None | 26 weeks | Not reported | Normal | McElhatton et al., 1997 |
| 30 g | Nonspecific | 64 mg/L | None | 34 weeks | Not reported | Normal | McElhatton et al., 1997 |
| 32.5 | N-acetylcysteine | Not reported | None | 36 | Uncomplicated | | Byer et al., 1982 |
| 32.5 | Nonspecific | Not reported | None | 29 | Hepatotoxicity | | Lederman et al., 1983 |
| 32.5 g | Nonspecific | 159.5 mg/L | None | 29 weeks | Liver necrosis, | Premature delivery, RSD, death at 3 mos | Lederman et al., 1983 |
| 35 | None | Not reported | None | 31 | Hepatorenal failure | Death | Wang et al., 1997 |
| 36 | N-acetylcysteine | Not reported | None | 16 | Uncomplicated | Normal | Robertson et al., 1986 |
| 36 g | N-acetylcysteine | 340 mg/L | None | 16 weeks | Normal | Normal | Robertson et al., 1986 |
| 37.5 g | Nonspecific | 170 mg/L | None | 7–8 weeks | No symptoms | Spontaneous abn 2 weeks later | McElhatton et al., 1997 |
| 40–50 g | Nonspecific | 214 mg/L | None | 32–34 weeks | Not reported | Normal | McElhatton et al., 1997 |
| 47.5 g | N-acetylcysteine | 87 mg/L | None | 3 weeks | Not reported | Normal | McElhatton et al., 1997 |
| 5 g | Nonspecific | Not reported | None | 40 weeks | Not reported | Normal | McElhatton et al., 1997 |
| 5–10 g | Nonspecific | Not reported | Antidepressant | 10 weeks | Not reported | Normal | McElhatton et al., 1997 |
| 5–6 g | Nonspecific | Not reported | None | 39 weeks | Not reported | Normal | McElhatton et al., 1997 |
| 50 | N-acetylcysteine | Not reported | None | 32 | Uncomplicated | | Rosevear and Hope, 1989 |
| 50 g | Nonspecific | Not reported | None | 18 weeks | Not reported | Elective abortion | McElhatton et al., 1997 |
| 50 g | N-acetylcysteine | 448 mg/L | None | 32 weeks | Hepatic injury, recovered | Hypoglycemia, jaundice | Rosevear and Hope, 1989 |
| 6 g | Nonspecific | Not reported | Aspirin, hepatitis B at 16 weeks | 36 weeks | Not reported | Term delivery, 8 weeks of age | McElhatton et al., 1997 |

| | | | | | | | |
|---|---|---|---|---|---|---|---|
| 6 g | Nonspecific | 18 mg/L | None | 35 weeks | Not reported | Normal | McElhatton et al., 1997 |
| 6 g | Nonspecific | <5 mg/L | Chlorpheniramine | 36 weeks | Not reported | Normal | McElhatton et al., 1997 |
| 6.5 g | Nonspecific | Not reported | None | 5–6 weeks | Not reported | Normal | McElhatton et al., 1997 |
| 64 | N-acetylcysteine | Not reported | None | 15 | Hepatotoxicity | | Ludmir et al., 1986 |
| 64 g | N-acetylcysteine | 198.5 mg/L (10 h later) | Vitamin K | 15.5 weeks | Hepatic necrosis, RSD | Premature delivery (32 weeks) | Ludmir et al., 1986 |
| 7.5 g | Nonspecific | 59 mg/L | Cefadroxil, codeine, co-danthramer, a | 26 weeks | Not reported | Term delivery, spina bifida occulta, strabism | McElhatton et al., 1997 |
| 7.5 g | Nonspecific | Not reported | None | 20 weeks | Not reported | Normal | McElhatton et al., 1997 |
| 7.5 g | Nonspecific | 50 mg/L | Ipecac | 37 weeks | Not reported | Normal | McElhatton et al., 1997 |
| 70 | Nonspecific | Not reported | None | 17 | Vaginal Bleed | Sp. ab | Payen et al., 2011 |
| 75 | Nonspecific | Not reported | None | 9 | Uncomplicated | El. ab | Payen et al., 2011 |
| 8.4 X 10 days | N-acetylcysteine | Not reported | Codeine | 19.5 | Liver transplant | Fetal Demise | Thornton and Minns, 2012 |
| 9 g | Nonspecific | 51 mg/L | None | 17 weeks | Not reported | Normal | McElhatton et al., 1997 |
| 9.5 g | Nonspecific | 35 mg/L | None | 8 weeks | Not reported | Normal | McElhatton et al., 1997 |
| Not reported | N-acetylcysteine | 176 mg/L | None | 37 weeks | Recovered | Discharged w/o evidence of liver injury | Horowitz et al., 1997 |
| Not reported | N-acetylcysteine | Term | None | Unknown | Recovered | Discharged w/o evidence of liver injury | Horowitz et al., 1997 |
| Not reported | Nonspecific | Not reported | None | 8 weeks | Not reported | Large perineal mass, death at day 7 | Williams et al., 1983 |
| Not reported | Nonspecific | Not reported | None | Preconception to 10–12 weeks | Not reported | Anophthalmia (n) | Golden et al., 1982 |
| Not reported | Nonspecific | Not reported | None | 29 weeks | Normal | Congenital cataracts | Harley et al., 1964 |
| Unknown | N-acetylcysteine | 69 mg/L | None | 12 weeks | Not reported | Premature delivery at 33 weeks, RSD | McElhatton et al., 1997 |
| Unknown | N-acetylcysteine | 363 mg/L | None | 10 weeks | Nausea and vomiti | Spontaneous | McElhatton et al., 1997 |
| Unknown | Nonspecific | Not reported | None | 3 weeks | Not reported | Elective abortion | McElhatton et al., 1997 |
| Unknown | N-acetylcysteine | 225 mg/L | Methionine | 37 weeks | Not reported | Normal | McElhatton et al., 1997 |
| Up to 1.2 g/day, chronic | Nonspecific | Not reported | Aspirin, caffeine | 0–6 weeks | Not reported | Single umbilical artery/vein, dextrocardia, li | McNeil, 1973 |

# 15 Miscellaneous Drugs during Pregnancy

## *Tocolytics, Immunosuppressants, and Biologic Therapeutics*

## TOCOLYTICS

In 2014, 3.99 million women delivered infants in the USA, of whom 9.61 percent were preterm (Hamilton *et al.*, 2021). In 2020 during the COVID-19 pandemic, 3.61 million babies were delivered in the US. Approximately 10.1 percent of women delivered prematurely (Hamilton *et al.*, 2021). No tocolytic agent is universally effective, although more than 100,000 pregnancies receive tocolysis therapy annually. Physicians do not universally accept efficacy of tocolytic agents. Gravidas treated with tocolytics are at increased risk for serious cardiopulmonary complications directly attributable to the tocolytic drug. Tocolytic therapy invariably occurs outside embryogenesis, therefore, risk of congenital anomalies is not an issue. With tocolysis, the primary concern is adverse maternal, fetal, and neonatal effects (Sanchez-Ramos *et al.*, 2000). Three main indications for tocolysis in the treatment of preterm labor are (1) prophylaxis, (2) acute therapy, and (3) maintenance.

Instances exist when exposure to tocolytic agents occurs during organogenesis. Some tocolytic agents are used for other indications: terbutaline for asthma, indomethacin for pain, and nifedipine for hypertension. Use of these drugs for other indications is discussed in the chapters on antiasthma (Chapter 5), analgesics (Chapter 8), and cardiovascular drugs (Chapter 3).

### PHARMACOKINETICS OF TOCOLYTIC DRUGS

Pharmacokinetic data on tocolytic drugs in pregnancy are limited to five studies of four drugs (Table 15.1). Half-life and steady state concentrations are generally not different between pregnant and non-pregnant states.

**TABLE 15.1**

**Pharmacokinetics of Tocolytic Agents during Pregnancy**

| Agent | n | EGA (weeks) | Route | AUC | $C_{max}$ | $C_{SS}$ | $t_{1/2}$ | Cl | PPB | Control group[a] | Source |
|---|---|---|---|---|---|---|---|---|---|---|---|
| Fenoteral | 4 | 30–32 | IV | ↑ | = | = | = | | | No | Mandach *et al.* (1995) |
| Ritodrine | 91 | 28–36 | IV, IM, PO | ↓ | = | = | = | | | Yes (1) | Van Lierde *et al.* (1984) |
| Ritodrine | 10 | 20–34 | IV | ↓ | ↓ | = | = | | | Yes (1) | Caritis *et al.* (1989) |
| Salbutamol | 7 | 16–33 | IV, PO | ↓ | = | = | = | = | | Yes (3,4) | Hutchings *et al.* (1987) |
| Terbutaline | 8 | 27–35 | IV | | = | ↓ | | ↑ | | Yes (4) | Berg *et al.* (1984) |

*Abbreviations:* EGA, estimated gestational age; AUC, area under the curve; $V_d$, volume of distribution; $C_{ss}$, peak plasma concentration; $C_{ss}$, steady-state concentration; $t_{1/2}$- half life; PPB, plasma protein binding; PO, by mouth; ↓ denotes a decrease during pregnancy compared to nonpregnant values; ↑ denotes an increase during pregnancy compared to nonpregnant values; = denotes no difference between pregnant and nonpregnant values; IV, intravenous; IM, intramuscular.
*Sources:* Little BB. *Obstet Gynecol*, 1999; **93**: 858.

DOI: 10.1201/9780429160929-15

## BETA-ADRENERGIC RECEPTOR AGONISTS

Ritodrine and terbutaline, beta-adrenergic agonist drugs used as tocolytics, are structurally related to epinephrine. Fenoterol is another drug in this class that is used in Europe.

Several other beta-agonists used for tocolysis are currently not approved for tocolysis, or not available in the US (Box 15.1).

---

### BOX 15.1   TOCOLYTIC AGENTS

**Beta-adrenergic receptor agonists**

- Fenoterol
- Hexoprenaline
- Ritodrine[a]
- Solbutanol[a]
- Terbutaline

**Magnesium sulfate**

- Magnesium sulfate

**NSAIDs/Prostaglandin synthetase inhibitors**

- Indomethacin
- Sulindac

**Calcium channel blockers**

- Nifedipine
- Verapamil

**Nitric oxide donor drugs**

- Nitroglycerin

**Oxytocin analog**

- Atosiban

[a] Not available in the United States.
*Source:* Adapted from ACOG, 2016.

---

Beta-adrenergic tocolytic drugs bind to beta-adrenergic receptors on the outer myometrial cell membrane and activate adenylate cyclase, which catalyzes conversion of ATP to cAMP. Increased intracellular cAMP levels activate cAMPase-dependent protein kinase and decreases intracellular calcium concentration, reducing myometrial contractility (Caritis *et al.*, 1989; Roberts, 1984). Phosphorylation of myosin light chain kinase, another pathway, inactivates the enzyme, thus inhibiting subsequent phosphorylation of the myosin light chain. Maternal metabolic abnormalities (gluconeogenesis, hypokalemia, and hyperglycemia), and cardiopulmonary complications (tachycardia, hypotension, arrhythmias, myocardial ischemia, pulmonary edema) are associated with beta-agonist tocolysis (Box 15.2). Apprehension, electrocardiogram (EKG/ECG) changes (S-T segment depression) and maternal death are associated with beta-adrenergic agonist tocolytic agents. Every beta-agonist is associated with an increased frequency of pulmonary edema, occurring among <5 percent of pregnant women who use these drugs (Boyle, 1995; McCombs, 1995).

---

### BOX 15.2   MATERNAL ADVERSE EFFECTS OF BETA-ADRENERGIC RECEPTOR AGONIST THERAPY

| | |
|---|---|
| Cardiac arrhythmia | Hypotension |
| Chest discomfort/pain | Pulmonary edema |
| Hyperglycemia | Shortness of breath |
| Hypokalemia | Tremors |
| | Tachycardia |

Ritodrine is not available in the US; contraindications include tachycardia-sensitive maternal disease, hypertension, uncontrolled hyperthyroidism, and poorly controlled maternal diabetes mellitus.

---

Maternal beta-adrenergic agonist tocolytic therapy was associated with neonatal hypoglycemia and tachycardia, and with several fetal and neonatal cardiovascular adverse effects (Katz and Seeds, 1989; ACOG, 2016) (Box 15.3). Decreases in umbilical artery systolic/diastolic ratios were reported in fetuses whose mothers used terbutaline or ritodrine (Brar *et al.*, 1988; Wright *et al.*, 1990).

---

### BOX 15.3   POSSIBLE ADVERSE FETAL EFFECTS OF MATERNAL BETA-ADRENERGIC RECEPTOR AGONISTS THERAPY

**Adverse effects**

- Hypoglycemia
- Hypotension and tachycardia
- Other cardiovascular effects[a]
- Cardiac dysrhythmia
- Decrease in umbilical artery systolic/diastolic ratios
- Heart failure
- Myocardial ischemia
- Neonatal death
- Ventricular hypertrophy

**Contraindications**

- Tachycardia-sensitive maternal disease
- Poorly controlled maternal diabetes mellitus

**Possible long-term postnatal effects**

- Autism in exposed offspring was reported for ritodrine and terbutaline

[a] From Brar *et al.*, 1988; Hill, 1995; Katz and Seeds, 1989.

## Ritodrine

The US FDA no longer approves Ritodrine for obstetric use for tocolysis. Ritodrine was approved for tocolytic use in 1980, and was available as a tocolytic agent in 23 foreign countries (Barden *et al.*, 1980). Ritodrine FDA approval was withdrawn in 1996.

Ritodrine hydrochloride is a beta-adrenergic agonist with beta-receptor effects that relax smooth muscle in the arterioles, bronchi, and uterus.

In the longer term, preterm labor is not effectively prevented by tocolysis. We analyzed national ritodrine sales over a seven-year period and found no evidence that treatment of preterm labor with ritodrine hydrochloride was associated with a decreased incidence of low birth weight (LBW) infants in the United States (Leveno *et al.*, 1990). This drug is no longer marketed in the United States because of serious side effects associated with its use (Iams *et al.*, 2009).

### MATERNAL EFFECTS

Acute maternal pulmonary edema, hypokalemia, and hyperglycemia, were reported among gravidas given ritodrine to prevent preterm delivery. Concomitantly, steroids administered to accelerate fetal lung maturation seem to increase the risk for maternal pulmonary edema (see Box 15.2). Nearly 5 percent of women treated with terbutaline for preterm labor had severe maternal cardiovascular complications (Katz *et al.*, 1981). The risk of pulmonary edema among women receiving ritodrine or other beta-mimetics is increased among gravidas with maternal infection, excessive intravenous hydration, multifetal gestation, or underlying cardiac disease increase (ACOG, 2016).

Beta-mimetics alter glucose tolerance and are associated with ketoacidosis in diabetic women with poorly controlled insulin-dependent glycemia. Maternal deaths are reported in association with beta-mimetic therapy.

### FETAL EFFECTS

Fetal tachycardia and arrhythmias are associated with beta-mimetic therapy, including ritodrine (Barden *et al.*, 1980; Hermansen and Johnson, 1984). Protracted ritodrine therapy was associated with increased septal thickness in exposed neonates (Nuchpuckdee *et al.*, 1986), but seem to be frequent complications of ritodrine, or other beta-mimetic, therapy.

Beta-adrenergic agonist tocolytic therapy, including ritodrine, was associated with a 2.5-fold increased risk of periventricular-intraventricular hemorrhage (Groome *et al.*, 1992), but grade 3 and 4 were not increased. In another investigation, no association of ritodrine with intraventricular-periventricular hemorrhage was found (Box 15.3) (Ozcan *et al.*, 1995).

Beta-mimetics are generally not used during the period of organogenesis, with the exception of terbutaline for asthma. No reports of birth defects associated with ritodrine in humans are published.

Autism was increased in frequency among children exposed to ritodrine during gestation (Chae *et al.*, 2021), increasing the incidence from 0.70 percent to 1.37 percent, nearly doubling its frequency (1.98 percent).

## Terbutaline

The FDA approved terbutaline for tocolytic therapy in 2012, but in 2017 issued a warning against use of terbutaline to treat preterm labor (FDA, 2017). It is the most commonly used beta-mimetic for tocolysis, approved for use or off label. Terbutaline was used to manage symptomatic placenta previa in pregnancies remote from term (Besinger *et al.*, 1995), and to manage uterine hypotonus, particularly with presence of a non-reassuring fetal heart rate pattern. Terbutaline was also used to induce uterine relaxation prior to external cephalic version (Fernandez *et al.*, 1996).

Neonatal myocardial dysfunction and necrosis were associated with terbutaline tocolytic therapy (Fletcher *et al.*, 1991; Thorkelsson and Loughead, 1991), but the association may not be causal (Bey *et al.*, 1992; Kast and Hermer, 1993). Terbutaline tocolytic therapy late in pregnancy was associated with transient neonatal hypoglycemia and fetal tachycardia (Peterson *et al.*, 1993; Roth *et al.*, 1990; Sharif *et al.*, 1990). Among infants born to women given terbutaline tocolysis, neonatal organizational behavior was transiently altered (Thayer and Hupp, 1997).

## MATERNAL EFFECTS

Terbutaline was associated with maternal cardiovascular effects (including pulmonary edema) similar to those associated with ritodrine (Katz *et al.*, 1981). One review of cardiopulmonary effects of low-dose continuous terbutaline infusion in 8709 women found 47 women (0.5 percent) developed one or more adverse cardiopulmonary effects. Twenty-eight women (0.3 percent) developed pulmonary edema (Perry *et al.*, 1995). Among 1,000 women who were given intravenous terbutaline and magnesium sulfate tocolysis, side effects were negligible (Kosasa *et al.*, 1994). Terbutaline hepatitis in pregnancy was reported in two cases (Quinn *et al.*, 1994), but cited in multiple sources. ACOG recommends use of terbutaline inpatient and for no more than 48 hours. (ACOG, 2016). The FDA placed a Boxed Warning on use of terbutaline during pregnancy for treatment of preterm labor, citing significant maternal complications (cardiac arrhythmias, myocardial infarction, pulmonary edema, hypertension, and tachycardia) and risk for death.

## Ethanol

Ethyl alcohol should not be used during pregnancy because it is associated with both teratogenic and fetal effects. Ethanol agent is reviewed in detail in Chapter 16.

## Magnesium Sulfate

Magnesium sulfate (MgSO) inhibits uterine contractions by antagonizing calcium flow into myometrial cells. Magnesium sulfate has no proven efficacy in delaying delivery beyond 24–48 hours (Cotton *et al.*, 1984; Cox *et al.*, 1990; Kimberlin *et al.*, 1996). A review of 23 studies including 2,000 patients showed no efficacy of magnesium sulfate (Grimes and Nanda, 2006).

## MATERNAL EFFECTS

The most frequent adverse effects of hypermagnesemia include cutaneous flushing, nausea, vomiting, respiratory depression, intracardiac conduction delays. MgSO levels 12 mEq/L or greater are associated with respiratory arrest. Protracted therapy with MgSO for preterm labor increases calcium loss and may decrease bone mineralization (Smith *et al.*, 1992). Prolonged but not clinically significant bleeding time during pregnancy may be associated with magnesium sulfate therapy (Fuentes *et al.*, 1995). Magnesium sulfate is not associated with a "peripheral vascular steal" syndrome, and apparently does not decrease placental perfusion (Dowell and Forsberg, 1995). Use of this drug with indomethacin before 32 weeks for short periods are suggested in some cases (ACOG, 2016).

## FETAL EFFECTS

Magnesium sulfate crosses the placenta and, in extremely large doses, may cause neonatal cardio-respiratory depression and transient loss of beat-to-beat variability (Hallak *et al.*, 1999; Hiett *et al.*, 1995; Idama and Lindow, 1998; Wright *et al.*, 1996). If these symptoms become severe, calcium gluconate can reverse cardiorespiratory symptoms.

Magnesium sulfate treatment for more than a week prior to delivery was associated with transient fetal-neonatal osseous lesions (metaphyses, costochondral junctions, skull) (Malaeb *et al.*, 2004; Tsukahara *et al.*, 2004). Lesions are resorbed within months of life (Santi *et al.*, 1994; Tsukahara *et al.*, 2004).

## NONSTEROIDAL ANTI-INFLAMMATORY AGENTS

### Indomethacin

Indomethacin is a prostaglandin synthetase inhibitor used to delay labor (Carlan *et al.*, 1992; Niebyl *et al.*, 1980; Zuckerman *et al.*, 1974). Indomethacin is efficacious as a tocolytic for short periods of time (Niebyl *et al.*, 1980), but it may be associated with significant adverse fetal effects: oligohydramnios, ductus arteriosus constriction, persistent fetal circulation, neonatal hypertension, intracranial hemorrhage, necrotizing enterocolitis, anemia, cystic renal changes, and neonatal death (Csapo *et al.*, 1978; Goldenberg *et al.*, 1989; Manchester *et al.*, 1976; Moise *et al.*, 1988; Norton *et al.*, 1993; Rubattelli *et al.*, 1979; Rudolph, 1981; van der Heijden *et al.*, 1994).

Indomethacin plus MgSO is an option before 32 weeks (ACOG, 2016).

### MATERNAL EFFECTS

Indomethacin resulted in few maternal side effects when used as a tocolytic. Potential relatively rare adverse maternal effects include interstitial nephritis, acute renal failure, peptic ulcer disease, decrease in platelets, and prolonged bleeding time (Clive and Stoff, 1984; Lunt *et al.*, 1994; Norton *et al.*, 1993). Indomethacin may exacerbate hypertension (Gordon and Samuels, 1995).

Among 83 women who received indomethacin during pregnancy, no adverse maternal or fetal effects were noted, except for oligohydramnios, which resolved spontaneously (Sibony *et al.*, 1994). Review of 28 studies included 1621 infants born to women treated with indomethacin tocolysis indicated no significantly increased risks (Loe *et al.*, 2005).

### FETAL EFFECTS

The review of 28 studies of indomethacin for tocolysis (n = 1621 exposed infants), the risk for adverse neonatal outcomes was not increased (Loe *et al.*, 2005). Necrotizing enterocolitis and patent ductus arteriosus were reported with late pregnancy exposure to indomethacin (Abbasi *et al.*, 2003; Norton *et al.*, 1993; Parilla *et al.*, 2000; Soraisham *et al.*, 2010; Sood *et al.*, 2011). Only three randomized clinical trials were included in the review, and statistical power was low, limiting the literature survey analysis of indomethacin effects on infant outcome. A recent review concluded that, if indomethacin is given for >48 hours, regular ultrasound assessments to evaluate the fetus for oligohydramnios and potential narrowing of the fetal ductus arteriosus (Patel and Ludmir, 2019).

### Sulindac

Sulindac, another prostaglandin synthetase inhibitor was similar to controls when used to treat preterm labor in 34 women (Carlan *et al.*, 1992). In another study of sulindac tocolysis, there was no difference in gestational age in 46 women who took sulindac (Humphrey *et al.*, 2001). Sulindac was as effective as indomethacin in tocolysis, but had fewer adverse fetal effects in a randomized prospective study of 36 women in preterm labor (Carlan *et al.*, 1992). No epidemiological studies of sulindac during pregnancy have been published, but it is probably associated with potential adverse effects similar to indomethacin (Patel and Ludmir, 2019).

## CALCIUM CHANNEL BLOCKERS

### Nifedipine

Nifedipine, a calcium channel blocker, promotes smooth muscle relaxation by reducing intracellular calcium. It also has vasodilation actions. Smooth muscle relaxation may lead to maternal hypotension and subsequent decreased uteroplacental perfusion. However, human studies have not provided evidence that nifedipine compromises the fetus through reduced uteroplacental perfusion (Ray and Dyson, 1995).

An early study comparing nifedipine and ritodrine suggested that nifedipine was associated with fewer maternal and fetal side effects than ritodrine (van Dijk *et al.*, 1995). A case report of severe maternal hypotension and fetal death associated with nifedipine tocolysis was published (van Veen *et al.*, 2005). As with case reports, other investigators have noted that the association is probably not causal (Johnson and Mason, 2005; Kandysamy and Thomson, 2005; Papatsonis *et al.*, 2005).

In a study comparing nifedipine to no treatment for possible preterm delivery, the drug group (n = 37) delivered 10.4 days later than the no treatment group (n = 38), which was a significant delay of birth (Sayin *et al.*, 2004). A placebo controlled clinical trial of nifedipine tocolysis did not significantly delay delivery or improve outcomes (Lyell *et al.*, 2008). In a review, women treated with nifedipine pregnancy significantly prolonged by an average 5.4 days in four trials (n = 275 women). No differences were found frequency of births <36 weeks' gestation, <28 weeks' gestation, birth within seven days of treatment, or gestational age at birth (Gaunekar *et al.*, 2013). Neonatal morbidities were not significantly different in frequency between the nifedipine and control groups for any secondary neonatal morbidities reported (Gaunekar *et al.*, 2013). The ACOG bulletin on preterm birth states nifedipine does not prevent preterm birth (ACOG, 2016).

## Verapamil

As discussed in Chapter 3, verapamil is a calcium channel blocker used as an antiarrhythmic, antihypertensive, and tocolytic agent. No epidemiologic studies on the safety of this agent during pregnancy are published. Maternal hypotension and resultant decreased uterine blood flow are the major risks from the use of this agent.

## Oxytocin Antagonists

Atosiban, unavailable in the United States, inhibits oxytocin-induced uterine contractions by competing with oxytocin for myometrial binding (Shubert, 1995). Atosiban is a nonapeptide oxytocin analog with competitive oxytocin antagonist action. Consistent reduction in uterine activity during the infusion of atosiban has been observed (Goodwin *et al.*, 1995). No systematic studies regarding the safety of this agent are published.

## Nitric Oxide Donor Drugs

Among 13 women given nitroglycerin patches, the drug was effective in preventing preterm birth, but maternal side effects involved hypotension and sedation (Lees *et al.*, 1994).

No difference in tocolytic efficacy was noted in a randomized investigation comparing intravenous nitroglycerin with magnesium sulfate (Clavin *et al.*, 1996). Parenteral nitroglycerin is associated with severe maternal hypotension, which suggests that placental hypoperfusion may be a serious risk. Insufficient evidence is published upon which to base routine administration of nitric oxide donors to treat threatened preterm labor. Nitric oxide donors were compared with only a limited number of other types of tocolytics (beta-mimetic, MgSO, calcium channel blockers) (Duckitt *et al.*, 2014).

## Special Considerations

Whether tocolytic therapy is efficacious and which agents to use remains controversial. Concerns over efficacy of specific agents and whether these agents can effectively delay labor for greater than 48 hours (i.e., for 1 week or longer) remain unresolved. Tocolytics appear to be effective to delay labor for short intervals (24–48 hours), and possibly for relieving hypertonic contractions. No tocolytic agent has consistently delayed birth for a week or more. The short period of efficacy may benefit fetal lung maturation corticosteroid therapy.

## Premature Labor

The most commonly used agents for treating premature labor are ritodrine, terbutaline, and magnesium sulfate. The usual doses of ritodrine and terbutaline are shown in Boxes 15.4 and 15.5, respectively.

Magnesium sulfate treatment is an initial loading intravenous dose of 4 g of a 20 percent solution, followed by an infusion of 2–3 g/hour until uterine contractions cease (Cox *et al.*, 1990). Duration of infusions are usually 12–24 hours.

---

### BOX 15.4   PROTOCOL FOR INTRAVENOUS RITODRINE

- Initial: 50–100 µg/min
- Incremental increases: 50 µg/min every 20 min
- Maximum dose: 350 µg/min

*Source:* From manufacturer's recommendations, 1995.

---

### BOX 15.5   PROTOCOL FOR TERBUTALINE

| Intravenous | Subcutaneous |
|---|---|
| Initial: 2.5 mg/min | Dose, 250 µg every hour until contractions stop |
| Increases: 2.5 mg/min every 20 min | Oral |
| Maximum: 20 mg | Dose, 2.5–5 mg q 4–6 h |

---

Indomethacin is given in an initial oral dose of 100 mg followed by 25 mg orally every four hours for 48 hours (Carlan *et al.*, 1992). Sulindac is given in an oral dose of 200 mg every 12 hours for 48 hours (Carlan *et al.*, 1992).

The ACOG (2016) MgSO and indomethacin tocolysis as "a potential option."

### Uterine Hypertonus or "Fetal Distress"

Before FDA approval was withdrawn, the usual ritodrine dose in a clinical setting was previously an intravenous bolus of 1–3 mg over two minutes, and for terbutaline, 0.25 mg subcutaneously or intravenously. Magnesium sulfate can also be given in a 4 g intravenous bolus with indomethacin.

### External Versions of Breech Presentation

Terbutaline, and ritodrine previously, may be used to relax the uterus prior to attempting external version of breech presentations. Preference has been to use terbutaline in a dose of 0.25 mg intravenously. If ritodrine is chosen, a dose of 1–3 mg intravenously over two minutes should be used (Fernandez *et al.*, 1996).

## IMMUNOSUPPRESSANTS DURING PREGNANCY

The only indication for immunosuppressants use during pregnancy is therapy for specific life-threatening conditions for which no other options exist. Three primary indications for immunosuppressant use during pregnancy are (1) organ transplant maintenance, (2) treatment of autoimmune disease, and (3) systemic lupus. One of the most common post-transplantation immunosuppressive regimens include prednisone with either azathioprine or cyclosporine. This raises the issue of the possible small risk of cleft palate associated with prednisone during pregnancy (see Chapters 4 and 13). Virtually all the known immunosuppressants (Box 15.6), even proximate metabolites of the very large molecule cyclosporine, cross the placenta (Little, 1997). An exposure to immunosuppressant drug(s) as a fetus makes the neonate at high risk for transiently compromised immune system. Risk of opportunistic infection is a danger until the infant's immune system recovers following intrauterine exposure to immunosuppressant therapy. Long-term effects on the infant's immune system are unknown.

### BOX 15.6   IMMUNOSUPPRESSANT AGENTS

| | |
|---|---|
| Adrenocorticoids | Gold salts (Myochrysine, Ridaura, Solganol) |
| Azathioprine (Imuran) | Monoclonal antibodies |
| Chloroquine (Aralen) | Muromonab-CD3 (Orthoclone OKT3) |
| Corticosteroids | Tacrolimus |
| Cyclosporine (Samdimmune) | |

## IMMUNOSUPPRESSANT AGENTS

Immunosuppressants reduce the immune response by toxic effects on, downregulation of, and/or decreased production of immune system components, especially T cells. A higher incidence of neoplastic disease is associated with chronic long-term use of immunosuppressants with risk increasing above the general population within five years of transplant (Nasser-Ghodsi *et al.*, 2021). The relevance of this association with exposure *in utero* is unknown.

### Azathioprine

Azathioprine is a 6-mercaptopurine derivative and a purine antimetabolite that acts by suppression of T-lymphocytes and cell-mediated immunity. *In vivo*, the drug is metabolized to mercaptopurine. It is used to treat autoimmune diseases and to prevent transplant rejection. Dose-dependent maternal side effects include bone marrow suppression, increased susceptibility to infection, alopecia, rash, gastrointestinal disturbances, arthralgias, hypersensitivity, pancreatitis, and toxic hepatitis (Berkowitz *et al.*, 1986).

Among 154 infants born to renal transplant recipients treated with azathioprine and prednisone throughout gestation, congenital anomalies occurred among 9 percent (four of 44) and 6.4 percent (seven of 110), respectively (Penn *et al.*, 1980; Registration Committee, 1980). No pattern of anomalies was present. It is not possible to determine whether this rate of congenital anomalies is higher than expected because these mothers took other drugs in addition to azathioprine, and were ill.

The frequency of birth defects was not increased among 481 infants with 30 congenital anomalies (6.2 percent) in the Swedish Medical Register whose mothers used azathioprine during organogenesis. the frequency was significantly increased for cardiac septal defects (Cleary and Kallen, 2009). The majority of mothers in this study had inflammatory bowel disease. In the UK, the frequency of birth defects (n = 5, 6.8 percent) was not increased in 74 infants born to women who took azathioprine during the first trimester (Ban *et al.*, 2014). No birth defects were reported in 87 infants born to women who took azathioprine during embryogenesis (Saavedra *et al.*, 2015), but one may expect three congenital anomalies due to background risk. The Swedish Birth Defects Registry reported 1,110 infants exposed to azathioprine during the first trimester, and 70 birth defects (Kallen, 2019). Notably, the risk for cardiac septal defects was significantly increased, nearly doubled, as in the prior study from Swedish medical registries. Fetal growth retardation and prematurity were increased in frequency among infants born to renal transplant recipients treated with azathioprine compared to infants born to healthy untreated women (Penn *et al.*, 1980; Pirson *et al.*, 1985; Registration Committee, 1980). The need for renal transplantation may be responsible in part for prematurity and growth retardation. Conditions resulting in chronic renal failure, such as maternal hypertension, diabetes, and other vascular diseases, were associated with an increased frequency of prematurity and/or growth retardation in offspring.

An increased frequency of congenital anomalies (limb defects, ocular anomalies, and cleft palate) occurred among the offspring of experimental animals born to mothers treated with azathioprine in doses similar to those used medically in humans (Davison, 1994; Rosenkrantz *et al.*, 1967; Tuchmann-Duplessis and Mercier-Parot, 1964; Williamson and Karp, 1981), but not in other studies (Fein *et al.*, 1983; Rosenkrantz *et al.*, 1967; Tuchmann-Duplessis and Mercier-Parot, 1964).

Fatal neonatal pancytopenia of an infant born to a renal transplant recipient treated with azathioprine and prednisone during pregnancy was a published case report (DeWitte *et al.*, 1984). Neonatal lymphopenia and thrombocytopenia in several children born to women who received similar therapy was reported (Davidson *et al.*, 1985; Lower *et al.*, 1971; Penn *et al.*, 1980; Price *et al.*, 1976; Rudolph *et al.*, 1979). Perinatal infant disorders are similar to those observed in adults on immunosuppressive medications.

Frequencies of acquired chromosomal breaks and rearrangements were increased in somatic cells of renal transplant recipients receiving azathioprine therapy and, transiently, in the infants of women who were given such treatment during pregnancy (Price *et al.*, 1976; Sharon *et al.*, 1974). One child with two separate *de novo* constitutional chromosomal anomalies was born to a woman treated before and during pregnancy with azathioprine and prednisone (Ostrer *et al.*, 1984). Relevance of either observation to clinical situations is unclear. Importantly, chromosome abnormalities in somatic cells cannot be extrapolated to interpret possible gonadal effects.

## Cyclosporine

Cyclosporine is a large molecule (cyclic polypeptide) of fungal origin. It is an immunosuppressant in the prevention and treatment of allograft rejection, and acts on cell-mediated immunity and T-cell-dependent humoral immunity (Hou, 1989). Cyclosporine, a large molecule (>1,000 in molecular weight), metabolizes to several amino acids ranging from 300 to 500 molecular weight, a range that easily crosses the placenta and produces detectable fetal levels of the drug (Claris *et al.*, 1993; Lewis *et al.*, 1983). Maternal cyclosporine use risks include hypertension, nephrotoxicity, hepatotoxicity, tremor, hirsutism, paresthesias, seizures, gout, and gingival hypertrophy (Berkowitz *et al.*, 1986). Cyclosporine need not be increased during pregnancy to maintain therapeutic levels, although body weight and blood volume increase substantially during pregnancy. One study found that cyclosporine doses needed to be lowered during the later stages of pregnancy (Flechner *et al.*, 1985). Cyclosporine has been detected in breast milk, with breastfeeding contraindicated in patients who remain on cyclosporine (Flechner *et al.*, 1985). Blood levels of cyclosporine decline to 50 percent at 48 hours postpartum and should be undetectable at one week (Berkowitz *et al.*, 1986). Thus, suppression of the infant's immune system should be short-lived (Rose *et al.*, 1989). One report found persistent (one to three months) hematologic abnormalities in newborns from renal transplant mothers receiving cyclosporine A, azathioprine, and methylprednisolone (Takahashi *et al.*, 1994).

The frequency of birth defects (n = 5, 3.1 percent) was not increased in 161 infants exposed to cyclosporine during organogenesis (Kallen, 2019). The frequency of preterm deliveries and of abortions (spontaneous and induced) was higher among cyclosporine-exposed pregnancies (Haugen *et al.*, 1994).

The frequency of congenital anomalies was not increased among offspring of rats and rabbits whose mothers were treated with doses within several multiples of the usual human therapeutic doses of cyclosporine. Fetal growth retardation, intrauterine deaths, and maternal toxicity, were increased in frequency in both species at doses at or slightly greater than the maximum human therapeutic dose (Brown *et al.*, 1985; Mason *et al.*, 1985; Ryffel *et al.*, 1983).

## Mycophenolate

Mycophenolate mofetil (MMF, CellCept) is a prodrug form of mycophenolic acid, a reversible inhibitor of inosine monophosphate dehydrogenase (IMPDH). MMF is used as an immunosuppressant, and sometimes combined with drugs such cyclosporine or corticosteroids to prevent organ rejection after solid organ transplantation (liver, kidney, heart). It is also used to treat systemic lupus. A case report of MMF use in pregnancy stated the infant had hypoplastic nails and short fifth digit (Pergola *et al.*, 2001). A report of two severely malformed MMF exposed infants included one neonate with esophageal atresia and major cardiovascular defect and eye malformation. The second infant had gastroschisis (Kallen *et al.*, 2005). Four of 15 infants (26.7 percent) born after MMF exposure had birth defects (Sifontis *et al.*, 2006), which is high but the sample is very small. A possible pattern of microtia and cleft lip/palate was described in an infant whose mother took mycophenolate, and other medications, during the first trimester (Sebaaly *et al.*, 2007). Seven infants without external ear canals were described (Perez-Aytes *et al.*, 2008) In 10 cases, other congenital anomalies (congenital heart disease, eye defects, minor digit and facial anomalies) were described (Vento *et al.*, 2008). Four of 26 live-born infants exposed to MMF had birth defects, and two had severe malformations (Hoeltzenbein *et al.*, 2012). Review of evidence for mycophenolate teratogenicity included: external ear anomalies, absent ear canal, cleft lip or cleft lip/palate, ocular anomalies including anophthalmia/microphthalmia and iris defects. Congenital heart defects, distal limb anomalies including hypoplastic nails, esophageal atresia, vertebral malformations, diaphragmatic hernia, kidney, and CNS malformations were less frequent (Perez-Aytes *et al.*, 2017). The authors proposed these anomalies constitute a mycophenolate embryopathy.

## Tacrolimus

Tacrolimus is a macrolide immunosuppressant, used to prevent solid organ rejection after transplantation (Scott *et al.*, 2003). Tacrolimus decreases T-cell production through binding to an immunophilin, FK506 binding protein (FKBP), inhibiting calcineurin phosphatase. This inhibits downstream calcium-dependent events, such as interleukin-2 gene transcription, nitric oxide synthase activation, cell degranulation, and apoptosis, inhibiting T-cell production. Several small case series or case reports of the use of tacrolimus during pregnancies of transplant patients are published (Jain *et al.*, 1993; Laifer *et al.*, 1994; Yoshimura *et al.*, 1996). No birth defects or adverse pregnancy outcomes were reported, except for slightly reduced birth weight and transient immunocompromise.

Among 71 infants born following tacrolimus exposure during embryogenesis, four (5.6 percent) had congenital anomalies (Kainz *et al.*, 2000), a rate not different from the rate in the general population. A clinical series of tacrolimus exposure during early pregnancy in 19 pregnancies in 16 patients reported 10 infants with no birth defects and normal birth weights, four spontaneous abortions, and 5 elective terminations for maternal disease exacerbation (Garcia-Donaire *et al.*, 2005). In the Swedish Birth Defects Registry, 60 infants exposed to tacrolimus during the first trimester had seven birth defects, an increased frequency (OR = 4.7, $p<0.001$). Three infants were exposed to multiple immunosuppressant agents. Excluding three exposed to polypharmacy, the frequency of birth defects remained significant with 4 malformed infants (Kallen, 2019). The increased risk was for cardiovascular defects (OR = 3.36). The frequency of congenital anomalies was not increased among mice exposed to the drug during embryogenesis, although litter weights were slightly reduced (Farley *et al.*, 1991).

## Prednisone and Prednisolone

Corticosteroids are among the most commonly used immunosuppressants. Use of both prednisone, which is metabolized to prednisolone, and prednisolone during pregnancy has been studied intensively (see Chapters 4 and 13). The short summary is that some studies suggest an association between cleft palate and corticosteroid use in the first trimester. If the risk exists, it is quite small, <1 percent.

## Gold Compounds

Gold salts are immunosuppressants in humoral and cell-mediated mechanisms, act as antirheumatic agents, and cross the placenta (Gimovsky and Montoro, 1991). Conception should be delayed one to two months after cessation of therapy in patients taking gold compounds. Fetal exposure to gold compounds has adverse neonatal renal and hemolytic effects.

The frequency of congenital anomalies was not increased among more than 100 infants born to women treated with gold salts during the first trimester (Miyamoto *et al.*, 1974). According to the manufacturers, gold compounds were teratogenic in some but not all animal studies.

## Chloroquine

This antimalarial agent also has some immunosuppressant properties and was for the treatment of rheumatoid arthritis. It should be avoided in pregnancy if possible (see Chapter 2).

## Biologics

## Monoclonal Antibody

T-lymphocyte monoclonal antibodies can eradicate circulating T cells within hours of administration. Acute rejection reactions to organ transplantation can be treated acutely and prophylactically with monoclonal antibodies. Untoward maternal effects include increased vulnerability to infection and neoplasm. Other side effects include tremor, headache, anaphylactic shock, chest pain, hypotension, neurospasm, pulmonary edema, gastrointestinal upset, rash, and allograft vascular thrombosis.

## Vedolizumab

Vedolizumab is a monoclonal antibody used to treat ulcerative colitis and Crohn's disease. A meta-analysis of vedolizumab use during the first trimester found that the frequency of birth defects (1 percent, 95 percent CI: 0–4 percent) was not increased among 120 infants (from 5 studies) was not increased (Nielsen *et al.*, 2020).

## Ustekinumab

Ustekinumab is a monoclonal antibody that blocks the production of inflammatory factors associated with plaque psoriasis, psoriatic arthritis, ulcerative colitis, and Crohn's disease. Meta-analysis showed no increased frequency of birth defects (5 percent, 95 percent CI: 2–8 percent) associated with first trimester exposure to ustekinumab in 216 infants whose mothers used the drug (Nielsen *et al.*, 2020).

## TNF-Inhibitors

**Anti-TNF biologics** are antibodies that inhibit an inflammatory hormone, **tumor necrosis factor** (**TNF**). White blood cells produce **TNF**, which causes inflammation. These biologics, or **medicines**, induce and help with clinical remission in patients with refractory inflammatory bowel disease (IBD). The PIANO Registry reported outcomes of 767 first trimester exposures to azathioprine (or 6-mercaptopurine), TNF-inhibitors (infliximab, adalimumab, certolizumab), or both. The overall outcome was not increased frequency of birth defects (3.5 percent) with anti-TNF exposure during embryogenesis (Mahadevan *et al.*, 2012). However, the findings were not given by only anti-TNF group, and was an abstract. Meta-analysis found no increased frequency of congenital anomalies (1 percent, 95 percent CI: 1–2 percent) in 4838 infants whose mothers took TNF-inhibitors during embryogenesis (Nielsen *et al.*, 2020). The Swedish Birth Defects Registry found no increased frequency of birth defects (n = 5, 2.3 percent) among 216 infants whose mothers used TNF-inhibitors (etanercept, infliximab, adalimumab, certolizumab, golimumab) during embryogenesis (Kallen, 2019).

## TNF-α INHIBITORS

Anti-TNF-α is used to treat IBD. Meta-analysis of 9 investigations of TNF-α inhibitors in pregnancy included 8,013 women with IBD (n = 5,212 Crohn's disease, n = 2,801 ulcerative colitis) who gave birth to 8,490 infants found no increased frequency of birth defects (Gubatan *et al.*, 2021). Biologic use during the first and subsequent trimesters of pregnancy was not associated with an increased risk of any infantile infections. Biologic use was associated with an increased frequency of infantile upper respiratory infections (1.6-fold increase). Exposure to biologics during embryogenesis and fetal growth and development was not associated with need for antibiotics neonatally or infection-related hospitalization after birth.

## SPECIAL CONSIDERATIONS

### AUTOIMMUNE DISORDERS

'All autoimmune disorders occur more frequently in women' (Gimovsky and Montoro, 1991; Angum *et al.*, 2020). Many women of reproductive age have disorders that require immunosuppressant therapy. Clinicians providing care for pregnant women can expect and can prepare to encounter gravid patients who are receiving ongoing immunosuppressant therapy.

### SYSTEMIC LUPUS ERYTHEMATOSUS

Systemic lupus erythematosus (SLE) is rare during pregnancy, ranging from approximately one in 2,952 deliveries (Gimovsky and Montoro, 1991; Gimovsky *et al.*, 1984) to one in 5,000 pregnancies (Tozman *et al.*, 1982). SLE is sometimes first manifested during pregnancy. SLE can adversely affect pregnancy with increases in abortion, prematurity, intrauterine death, and congenital heart block (Gimovsky and Montoro, 1991; Gimovsky *et al.*, 1984). Approximately 20–60 percent of gravid SLE gravidas experience disease exacerbation during pregnancy (Gimovsky *et al.*, 1984; Mintz *et al.*, 1986; Mor-Yosef *et al.*, 1984). Infants born to women who had SLE during pregnancy may develop a transient lupus-like picture and congenital heart block (Scott *et al.*, 1983; Watson *et al.*, 1984).

Treatment of SLE during pregnancy usually includes glucocorticoids (Dombroski, 1989; Gimovsky and Montoro, 1991). It would seem reasonable to continue steroid treatment of SLE as warranted if the patient was on the therapy when the pregnancy was recognized, or if steroids are required during pregnancy (Box 15.7).

---

**BOX 15.7    INDICATIONS FOR STEROID THERAPY IN PREGNANT WOMEN WITH SYSTEMIC LUPUS ERYTHEMATOSUS (SLE)**

| | |
|---|---|
| Central nervous system involvement | Nephritis |
| Hemolytic anemia | Pericarditis |
| Leukopenia | Pleuritis |
| Myocarditis | Thrombocytopenia |

*Source:* From Gimovsky and Montoro, 1991

---

Prednisone (or prednisolone) is the adrenocorticoid most frequently used to treat SLE patients. Initial dose is usually 60 mg/day, with dose adjustment increasing or decreasing as needed to control disease symptoms (Gimovsky and Montoro, 1991).

Large-dose steroid therapy at the time of delivery and early postpartum period is not a consensus treatment (Dombroski, 1989). Increased prednisone or other steroid during delivery and during the postpartum period can avoid disease exacerbations (Polic and Obican, 2020). Gravid patients asymptomatic and not on steroid therapy before the pregnancy may not necessarily require such therapy during pregnancy and postpartum. To maintain symptom management, steroid dose should be increased during pregnancy for women who are maintained on steroid therapy and/or have active disease during gestation. Intravenous hydrocortisone (100 mg) may be given every six to eight hours during labor and the first 24 hours postpartum. Beyond 24 hours postpartum, the patient may be returned to her usual maintenance steroid dose regimen. In patients with lupus anticoagulant, low-dose aspirin may be used as necessary throughout pregnancy.

Other immunosuppressants (e.g., azathioprine, cyclophosphamide—an alkylating agent) are used in pregnant women with SLE exacerbations refractory to high-dose steroids. According to the manufacturer, the dose of azathioprine is lower for patients with SLE than for patients with organ transplants. Authorities recommend avoiding alkylating agents in early pregnancy (embryogenesis, first trimester). These agents may be used during the second and third trimesters, if needed (Glantz, 1994). Hydroxychloroquine has been used to treat SLE and in usual doses (for malaria) carry little risk to the embryo or fetus (Polic and Obican, 2020; Sperber *et al.*, 2009).

Etiology, pathogenesis, and diagnosis of SLE have been expertly reviewed elsewhere (Gimovsky and Montoro, 1991).

## RHEUMATOID ARTHRITIS

Women are diagnosed with rheumatoid arthritis frequently than men. Rheumatoid arthritis is common among women of childbearing age, the more prevalence of this disease during pregnancy is unknown. Up to two-thirds of the patients with rheumatoid arthritis experience marked improvement during pregnancy (Neely and Persellin, 1977; Ostensen and Husby, 1983; Unger *et al.*, 1983), suggesting that pregnancy may improve the symptoms of rheumatoid arthritis.

The mainstay of therapy for both pregnant and non-pregnant women with rheumatoid arthritis is aspirin (Box 15.8). To achieve therapeutic blood levels of 15–25 mg/dL, patients may require up to 4 g of salicylates daily (Thurnau, 1983). However, during pregnancy lower doses of salicylates (up to 3 g per day) are recommended. Large-dose salicylate therapy during pregnancy may increase the risk for hemorrhagic complications in the fetus because salicylates cross the placenta. Hemorrhagic complications may also occur in newborns and/or mothers. Non-steroidal anti-inflammatory agents (NSAIDs) may be used in pregnant women with rheumatoid arthritis. NSAIDs may be associated with mild to moderate oligohydramnios, premature closure of the ductus arteriosus and persistent fetal circulation, as well as intracranial hemorrhage in the neonate (Chapter 8). The risk is dose-related, with higher doses conferring a higher risk. Hydroxychloroquine, as a mild immunosuppressant, was used to treat rheumatoid arthritis and SLE, but because of low efficacy, it is generally not recommended to treat pregnant women who have rheumatoid arthritis.

---

### BOX 15.8   AGENTS USED FOR THE TREATMENT OF RHEUMATOID ARTHRITIS

- Salicylates
- Nonsteroidal anti-inflammatory agents (NSAIDs)
- Steroids
- Penicillamine[a]

- Chloroquine[a]
- Gold salts

[a] Not recommended for use during pregnancy.
*Source:* Adapted from Gimovsky and Montoro, 1991.

---

Penicillamine (Cuprimine) is used to treat rheumatoid arthritis, but should not be used during pregnancy because it is a known teratogen. It is a chelating agent used to treat lead poisoning. However, its mechanism of action as an antirheumatoid agent is not understood. Penicillamine crosses the placenta and is contraindicated for use during pregnancy because it interrupts fetal collagen formation (Gimovsky and Montoro, 1991) and is considered a human teratogen (Shepard, 1989). Immunosuppressant drugs such as cyclosporine and azathioprine are used to treat rheumatoid arthritis that is refractory to high dose aspirin in non-pregnant patients (Kerstens *et al.*, 1995; Kruger and Schattenkirchner, 1994). These agents should be reserved to treat pregnant women with severe disease refractory to more commonly used agents with which there is greater clinical experience and published data.

## ORGAN TRANSPLANTATION

Organ transplantation and pharmacological therapy has advanced over the past four decades significantly. Renal transplantation and subsequent pregnancy is increasing in frequency each year, and literature on the transplants and pregnancy is growing.

## RENAL TRANSPLANTATION

Among more than 800 pregnancies (from seven reports) after renal transplantation, there were 0.5 percent maternal deaths, 6–8 percent miscarriages, 12–20 percent therapeutic abortions, 1 percent stillbirths, and 2 percent neonatal deaths (Hou, 1989; Radomski *et al.*, 1995). Three first-line medications are used to prevent rejection following renal transplantation: corticosteroids, azathioprine, and cyclosporine. Corticosteroid, cyclosporine, azathioprine, and tacrolimus therapy have been discussed earlier.

The frequency of renal transplant rejection, especially of cadaver kidneys, is decreased with cyclosporine therapy (Hou, 1989). This immunosuppressant and its metabolites cross the placenta. If the situation is life threatening, the benefits of its use clearly outweigh any potential risks. Intrauterine growth retardation and subsequent lower birth weight was observed in infants whose mothers used cyclosporine for renal transplant (Hou, 1989; Pickrell *et al.*, 1988; Radomski *et al.*, 1995), but it is not possible to differentiate drug effects from the renal disease being treated (e.g., chronic hypertension is a concomitant complication).

Pregnant women should be counseled for the increased risks of both maternal and fetal infection, and the possible increased risk of genital carcinoma associated with immunosuppressant therapy (Kossay *et al.*, 1988). Notably, women who have symptoms of rejection within three months of delivery usually progress to loss of the renal transplant within the next 24 months. The medical significance of an efficacious immunosuppressant therapy during pregnancy is emphasized by these sequelae.

A systematic review and meta-analysis of 6,712 pregnancies in 4,174 kidney transplants indicated the rate of preterm birth was high at 43.1 percent. The cesarean section rate was 62.6 percent and pregnancy-induced hypertension 24.1 percent. The average birth weight was 2,470 g and mean gestational age was 34.9 weeks (Shah *et al.*, 2019). Stillbirths were 5.1 percent. Graft rejection was not increased by pregnancy, with an average of 9.1 percent (95 percent CI: 6.4–13.7) across all studies in the meta-analysis. Unfortunately, lack of individual patient data prevented assessment of pregnancy outcomes by immunosuppression regimens. Another meta-analysis of graft rejection and pregnancy found that renal transplantation had no effect on long-term graft survival. A possible negative effect on graft function within two years postpartum was noted but may be publication bias against normal outcomes (van Buren *et al.*, 2020).

## OTHER ORGAN TRANSPLANTATION

Several reports of pregnancies following liver, heart and heart-lung, and bone marrow transplants have been published (Deeg *et al.*, 1983; Kallen *et al.*, 2005; Key *et al.*, 1989; Kossay *et al.*, 1988; Lowenstein *et al.*, 1988; Miniero *et al.*, 2004; Newton *et al.*, 1988; Rose *et al.*, 1989; Walcott *et al.*, 1978). Immunosuppressant therapy, especially with regard to cyclosporine, is utilized similarly with other organ transplants as with renal transplantation. Among 152 infants born after transplantation, a high frequency of preeclampsia (22 percent), preterm birth (46 percent), low birth weight (41 percent), infants small for gestational age (16 percent), and infant death were found for deliveries after transplantation. Congenital anomalies were not increased in frequency (Kallen *et al.*, 2005).

## Heart Transplantation

More than 40 infants have been born to women with heart transplants (Miniero *et al.*, 2004; Radomski *et al.*, 1995; Scott *et al.*, 1993). Mothers were treated with cyclosporine or azathioprine throughout gestation. Signs of organ rejection occurred in about one-quarter of mothers, and about one-third of infants were of low birth weight and premature. The pregnancies, mothers' postpartum and neonatal course were complicated by infection.

## Liver Transplantation

Among 38 pregnancies to 29 women with liver transplants, 13 percent of mothers had signs of organ rejection (Radomski *et al.*, 1995). There were 31 live births (eight abortions) and 32 percent had low birth weight, with 39 percent premature. Infection complicated >25 percent of the liver transplant pregnancies. Immunosuppression is a mainstay of treatment to prevent transplant rejection. Two of 15 infants born to liver transplant patients had birth defects (Kallen *et al.*, 2005). A review of 450 pregnancies in 306 liver transplant recipients (systematic review, 8 studies) indicated that miscarriage was 17.1 percent, pregnancy induced hypertension 21.9 percent and C-section 44.6 percent (Deshpande *et al.*, 2012). Compared to renal transplant obstetric patients, liver transplant pregnancies lasted longer (36.5 vs. 35.6 weeks) had greater birth weight (2866 g vs. 2420 g).

## Inflammatory Bowel Disease

Inflammatory bowel disease includes ulcerative colitis and Crohn's disease (regional enteritis) of unknown etiology. Corticosteroids (i.e., prednisone) have been used for the active stages of both diseases (Box 15.9). Sulfasalazine and 5-aminosalicylic acid were successfully used to treat ulcerative colitis during pregnancy (Habal *et al.*, 1993). Refractory cases of Ulcerative colitis and Crohn's disease during pregnancy refractory to corticosteroid therapy are an indication for immunosuppressive drugs, (e.g., azathioprine, 6-mercaptopurine). Meta-analysis of azathioprine/6-mercaptopurine to treat Crohn's disease found that both drugs were efficacious for treatment of active disease and remission maintenance (Pearson *et al.*, 1995). However, efficacy during pregnancy was not studied. Inflammatory bowel disease treatments (Box 15.9) include cyclosporine for Crohn's disease (Brynskov *et al.*, 1989). More potent immunosuppressants (e.g., azathioprine, 6-mercaptopurine, cyclosporine) should be reserved for pregnant women refractory to steroid therapy. The best possible maternal health is the most important milestone in optimizing child health and continuing medical therapy in IBD during pregnancy. The benefit of efficacious maternal treatment with non-teratogenic medication outweighs possible risks under most circumstances (Restellini *et al.*, 2020).

**BOX 15.9   AGENTS USED FOR THE TREATMENT
OF INFLAMMATORY BOWEL DISEASE**

**Ulcerative colitis**

- 5-aminosalicylic acid
- 6-mercaptopurine

- Azathioprine
- Prednisone
- Sulfasalazine

**Crohn's disease**

- 6-mercaptopurine
- Azathioprine
- Cyclosporine
- Prednisone

## MULTIPLE SCLEROSIS

Secondary, progressive, and relapsing multiple sclerosis is treated with immunosuppressants. Agents in current use to treat multiple sclerosis include azathioprine, cyclophosphamide, cyclosporine, glatiramer acetate, interferons, methotrexate, and natalizumab. In a meta-analysis of multiple sclerosis in pregnancy, 3629 pregnancies treated (azathioprine, cyclosporine, dimethyl fumarate, glatiramer acetate, interferons, methotrexate, natalizumab), medication specific analysis found 188 in three studies were treated with glatiramer acetate, and the frequency of birth defects was not increased. Among 143 infants born to women who used natalizumab during organogenesis the frequency of birth defects was not increased. Interferon therapy during the first trimester was not associated with an increased frequency of birth defects (Lopez-Leon *et al.*, 2020). The comparison group was 3,029 pregnancies with multiple sclerosis that were untreated during gestation. No consensus treatment for multiple sclerosis relapse is published. Treatment of multiple sclerosis relapse with immunosuppressants is controversial. Treatment of multiple sclerosis with some of these drugs (azathioprine, cyclophosphamide, methotrexate) during pregnancy is associated with an increased risk of birth defects. Importantly, a dose-related effect is noted with multiple sclerosis medications associated with birth defects and other potential adverse effects. Adverse outcomes decrease in frequency as the dose is lowered (e.g., cyclophosphamide "booster" doses).

## SUMMARY

A variety of diseases in gravidas (e.g., collagen-vascular disease, organ transplantation, multiple sclerosis, IBD) are treated with immunosuppressant agents. Steroids, azathioprine, cyclophosphamide, cyclosporine, glatiramer acetate, interferons, methotrexate, and natalizumab are agents most frequently used to treat these diseases during pregnancy.

Several of these agents (cyclosporine, glatiramer acetate, interferons, natalizumab, steroids) have been used in pregnant women with minimal risk to the fetus, and birth defects rates that are no greater than expected. Steroids seem to pose little or no risk to intrauterine development after the first trimester or to the mothers, except for the very small possible risk for cleft palate. Azathioprine in the first trimester is apparently associated with an increased frequency of birth defects. However, organ transplant rejection is life threatening and any risk is outweighed by the benefit.

# 16 Substance Abuse during Pregnancy

*How relevant is this chapter to contemporary obstetric practice? Approximately 1 in 4 or 25 percent of gravidas in your practice is using one or more of the substances discussed in Chapter 16.*

Substance abuse is a life style, and pregnancy is nine months of the preexisting practices during gestation. Substances used in their life style will determine the exposures during organogenesis because it is unusual for pregnancy to be recognized before two months. Profiling the pregnant substance abuser is difficult for several reasons, the most frequent of which is the private pay patient frequently has greater anonymity. In addition to anonymity, private pay patients also have greater access to treatment. Surveys of substance use or abuse during pregnancy very frequently use data from public hospitals and claim records from public health programs. Pregnant substance abusers are frequently reported to be dependent on public assistance for medical care (Slutsker *et al.*, 1993). Private pay patients' medical information is not included in these surveys, biases the surveys, and probably better describes the public pay patient population, rather than the private pay patient group.

A Canadian survey, The Canadian Alcohol and Drug Use Monitoring Survey, reported that of primigravidas in 2007, 10.5 percent smoked cigarettes, 10.5 percent used alcohol, and 1 percent used street drugs (O'Campo *et al.*, 2009). The 2008 Canadian Perinatal Health Report found similar prevalence of alcohol use (11 percent), and only a slightly higher smoking (13 percent) rate. Illicit drug use (5 percent) was fivefold higher among pregnant women (Cook *et al.*, 2017; Public Health Agency of Canada, 2013).

According to surveys, largely from public hospital systems, pregnant substance abusers are frequently (>50 percent) unmarried, began using prenatal care late in pregnancy or had no prenatal care, and are dependent upon public health care resources. The substances most frequently used during pregnancy include alcohol, cocaine, heroin (opiates), methamphetamine, and tobacco. Alcohol and tobacco use is a common polydrug use pattern, but some fraction of a percentage point of women use only alcohol. Use of mood-altering chemicals in non-medically supervised use of mood altering chemicals is prevalent in the USA today. According to some sources (Rouse, 1996). Prevalence was estimated at 70–90 percent of the general population and women of reproductive age (Finnegan, 1994). In 2017, it was reported that 37 percent of adults in the US were using one or more substances in a regular basis (Welty *et al.*, 2017). The take home message is that the prevalence of substance use/abuse remains at a level between 20–30 percent, but the variation can be substantial. In the 1980–1990s, the prevalence of cocaine was 10 percent or higher, but presently may be 3 percent (Kerridge *et al.*, 2019; see Figure 16.1).

Clinically important health risks exist for gravidas and their unborn children who use social and illicit substances during gestation. The most critical period for the induction of congenital anomalies (embryogenesis) is the first trimester (specifically the first 58 days post-conception) (see Chapter 1). Importantly, most women do not know that they are pregnant this early in gestation. Amenorrhea occurred among 28.8 percent of participants in a study of accuracy of menstrual history reporting (Jukic *et al.*, 2008), and cycle length >30 days in 42.2 percent of individuals (Chiazze *et al.*, 1968). Variation in cycle length (having a long period) contributes to the proportion of women who may believe they are not pregnant, probably >50 percent.

Therefore, usual life style practices (e.g., substance/alcohol use, diet, etc.) are superimposed on the critical period of pregnancy, organogenesis, without the intent to expose the developing embryo.

DOI: 10.1201/9780429160929-16

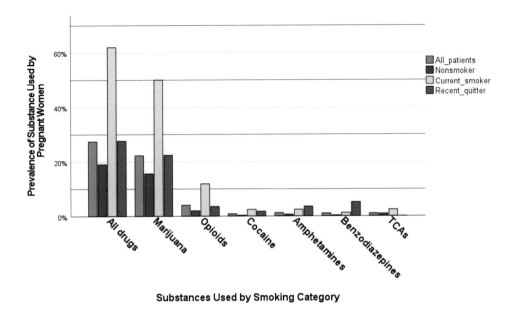

**FIGURE 16.1**    Prevalence of substance use by smoking category (All, Smoker, Non-Smoker, Recently Quit).

The results presented were verified by urine toxicology; notably, alcohol (ethanol) is not included in the survey data.

Fetal development in the second and third trimesters of pregnancy is also a time of great vulnerability, and continued substance use during this period carries the risk of atypical development (i.e., some congenital anomalies, but mainly growth retardation). The prudent practice of pre-conception birth control is the most effective way to protect possible pregnancies from being exposed to known and suspected teratogens in substances of abuse.

All substances of abuse reviewed in this chapter, for which information exists, cross the placenta (Box 16.1) (Little and Vanbeveren, 1996). Where information is not available, it is likely, given the chemical properties of alkaloid substances of abuse (low polarity, low molecular weight), these substances will likely readily cross the placenta.

---

**BOX 16.1    SUBSTANCES OF ABUSE KNOWN TO CROSS THE PLACENTA**

- Alcohol (ethanol)
- Amphetamine
- Barbiturate
- Benzodiazepines
- Cocaine
- Codeine
- Fentanyl
- Heroin
- Inhalants (organic solvents, e.g., toluene, gasoline)

- LSD (lysergic acid diethylamide)
- Marijuana
- Mescaline
- Methadone
- Methamphetamine
- Morphine
- PCP (phencyclidine)
- Tobacco (nicotine)
- Ts and Blues (pentazocine)

*Source:* Modified from Little and VanBeveren, 1996.

# CLINICAL EVALUATION

## MEDICOLEGAL CONSIDERATIONS

Certain legal obligations on the care providers' knowledge of patient use of social and illicit substances during pregnancy vary by state in the United States. It would be prudent to know these regulations as certain states place a reporting burden on the physician. The intake interview and medical history-taking process should be sufficiently thorough to discover information regarding the use of potentially dangerous substances. Upon discovery of an exposure, the important second step is to determine timing of exposures during pregnancy, and the nature and extent of the social or illicit substance use. In exposures that occurred during gestation, the obstetrician needs to know as much as possible about the teratogenic and toxic potentials of the substance or combinations of substances. Physicians may have their own resources to document the topic or may refer the patient to a specialist. The physician should disclose fully medically known risks posed by maternal substance abuse to the patient. Disclosure should be documented in the medical record in a clear and concise manner. The physician should emphasize to patients that social or illicit substance(s) use during the pregnancy is totally contraindicated.

*Not Theoretical Concerns:* These cautions are not theoretical concerns because we have assisted in the defense of physicians sued for adverse pregnancy outcomes caused by substance abuse, despite the physician's appropriate counseling that the patient chose to ignore. The risk-benefit ratio for substance abuse during pregnancy is easily explained to be *increased risk with no benefit.* Patient consultation, particularly this aspect, must be documented in the medical record to show that the risk was recognized and patient appropriately advised that substance use must be ceased during pregnancy. What happens after pregnancy is a later concern. In some institutions, patients are asked to initial or sign counseling notes regarding substance abuse during pregnancy to acknowledge that they received and understood counseling. The sections that follow published material on maternal and fetal medical risks for specific substance use in pregnancy including: alcohol, amphetamine, cocaine, heroin, inhalants, lysergic acid diethylamide (LSD), marijuana, methadone, mushrooms, methamphetamine, morphine, phencyclidine (PCP), tobacco, and Ts and blues.

## PATIENT CONSULTATION

Speaking to their physician, most pregnant women usually admit to some use of a substance, few will acknowledge they have a "problem" with social or illicit substance. Once some substance use is admitted, two tandem approaches to the history-taking process are suggested. Differences in substance use between weekdays and weekends are important to ascertain, because it is common for the user's pattern of use to differ greatly between these two periods. The patient should describe her daily activities, including any substances used, from awakening to going to sleep at night on a normal weekday. Weekend activities and substance use should be assessed similarly. The second approach is to ask about substance use in particular. The patient should be asked when she begins drinking or using drugs during the course of a day and the duration of such use. For example, does the patient use the substance as an "eye-opener" in the morning (Sokol *et al.*, 1989) and/or is it what she uses to go to sleep. Quantity is important, and the patient should be asked how much of the substance(s) is used in an average day/week and approximately how much would be consumed in an hour/day. Combined with information about the weekly pattern (weekend versus weekday), a semi-quantitative estimate of the amount and frequency of substance use can be made.

Alcohol use during pregnancy is well studied. Crude risks of fetal alcohol syndrome can be estimated using the average daily dose. With other less well-researched substances used during pregnancy, daily dose information can be used only to assess the severity of maternal addiction. Serious dependencies are associated with more severe adverse effects. The physician should explain that the purpose of obtaining this personal and private information is to better manage the pregnancy, i.e., to give medical care more suited to the patient's specific needs. Reassured that this information is confidential is protected by Federal Law (CFR 37). Attorneys emphatically state that no release should ever be signed and that each person must protect their individual rights to privacy assertively.

Another important aspect of patient consultation is to provide information regarding specific risks from substance use (Tables 16.1 and 16.2). It is important that this information be as accurate as possible. "Scare" tactics or exaggeration-type deterrents should be avoided because substance users are aware of this commonly employed approach. This tactic erodes trust in the physician and his/her credibility will be lost. Ethical and legally sound approach is to provide information that may be verified directly with the medical literature. A standardized summary from a computerized database, Teratogen Information System (TERIS), may be purchased, or a Teratogen Information Service may be contacted (see Chapter 1). TERIS summaries are detailed and documented. Ultimately, the clinical conclusion/treatment is that **social and illicit substance use during pregnancy is contraindicated** because of associated maternal and embryo-fetal risks.

The need for services to assist pregnant substance users is being recognized, and programs exist in most areas. For assistance in locating such a treatment program, the physician can contact their local substance abuse service, or their state's commission on substance abuse that accredits treatment facilities. In some states, Medicaid pays for treatment. Ideally, an obstetrician or maternal-fetal medicine specialist in conjunction with an addiction specialist manages the pregnant substance user with a treatment program designed to promote abstinence at least during pregnancy. The medical positions of abstinence and treatment are the only appropriate ones clinically and legally.

**TABLE 16.1**

**Summary of Embryo-Fetal Effects of Social and Illicit Substance Use during Pregnancy**

| Substance | FGR | Congenital Anomalies | Withdrawal Syndrome | Perinatal Morbidity | Documented Syndrome |
|---|---|---|---|---|---|
| Alcohol | + | + | + | + | + |
| Amphetamines | + | + | + | + | — |
| Barbiturates | + | ?(—) | + | + | + |
| Benzodiazepines | ?(+) | ?(—) | + | + | — |
| Cocaine | + | + | + | + | — |
| Codeine | + | + | + | + | — |
| Heroin | + | + | + | + | — |
| Inhalants | + | + | + | + | + |
| LSD | ? | (—) | ?(—) | ? | ? |
| Marijuana | + | — | — | + | — |
| Methadone | + | — | + | + | — |
| Methamphetamine | + | — | + | + | — |
| Morphine | + | (—) | + | + | — |
| PCP | + | ? | + | + | ? |
| Tobacco | + | — | — | + | — |
| Ts and Blues | + | (—) | + | + | — |

+, Documented, positive; —, documented, negative; (—) data inconclusive but suggestive of a negative finding; (+) data inconclusive but suggestive of a positive finding; ?, unknown.

*Abbreviations:* FGR, fetal growth restriction; LSD, lysergic acid diethylamide; PCP, phencyclidine.

*Source:* Modified from Little *et al.*, 1990b.

## PATIENT EVALUATION

*Note*: Use of "legal, legally, etc." is not intended as a substitution for legal advice and the reader is cautioned to contact a licensed attorney when confronted with questions concerning issues of the law and its application in the situation confronted, as noted in Chapter 1. Laws vary from state to state and from nation to nation. One's medical malpractice insurance provider is often the most economical and efficient source of legal information as this service has been a provision of a medical malpractice policy.

The **pregnant substance user is a high-risk obstetric patient**. Pregnant substance users are at increased risk for a number of complications, including sexually transmitted diseases (STDs), hepatitis, poor nutrition, and bacterial endocarditis. Chronic use of the substances reviewed in this chapter is an indication for syphilis, gonorrhea, herpes, chlamydia, HIV, and hepatitis testing. Parenteral drug use is the greatest risk for HIV and other STDs, including hepatitis C and other hepatides. Drug injection sites on the upper forearm ('track marks') are strong evidence of a serious substance use problem, but not frequently observed. Among 122 gravid parenteral substance users (intravenous drug abusers, IVDAs), only one woman presented with track marks on the forearm; the 121 remaining IVDA women used hidden sites of injection (veins in breasts, thighs, calves, and ankles) (Little *et al.*, 1990b). Poor weight gain during pregnancy may sometimes be associated with the anorectic effect of substance abuse. Signs of substance use during pregnancy may include new-onset "spontaneously arising" heart murmur and hypertension not associated with preeclampsia. Heart murmurs occur with increased frequency among women who are chronic substance users. Bacterial endocarditis is associated with IVDA. Bacterial endocarditis or a history of this disease is also associated with heart murmurs. Chronic substance use can induce hypertension in the non-pregnant adult, although not all substances are studied for hypertensive effects during pregnancy. Cocaine, heroin, amphetamines, and tobacco use is associated with hypertension during pregnancy (Abel, 1980a, 1980b; Little *et al.*, 1989b, 1990a; Stillman *et al.*, 1986; Cox *et al.*, 2008). In addition, abruptio placentae or a history of this serious complication is also an indication that substance use may be a factor. Risk of abruptio placentae may be as high as 1–2 percent among substance abusers compared to 0.1 percent (one in 830) in the general population (Cunningham *et al.*, 1997). The risk was 1 in 185 in a study of amphetamine use in pregnancy (Cox *et al.*, 2008). Stillbirths are increased in frequency with substance use during pregnancy. Combined with other risk factors, a history of stillbirths is a clue substance abuse is a complicating factor.

## HIDDEN RISKS OF SUBSTANCE ABUSE: IMPURITIES

Even our prescriptions from the pharmacy are diluted with other substances, frequently micro-crystalline cellulose, and it is called vehicle. Our digestive systems could not tolerate pure doses of drugs. In most instances, we consume 3 percent or less of a pure substance when taking a tablet, caplet, or capsule. All substances of abuse, even alcohol, may be contaminated by certain impurities that may not be pharmacologically inert. 'Moonshine' (illegally distilled alcohol) can contain significant amounts of lead and cause heavy metal poisoning in the mother and fetus. Amphetamine and methamphetamines may contain impurities, such as lead oxides (Allcott *et al.*, 1987). Leaded gasoline is sometimes used as an organic solvent. The result is lead contamination of the cocaine paste extracted of from cocoa leaves. Production of illicit drugs, such as PCP, involve cyanohydrin intermediate reactions. Cyanide or other impurities may be contained in the final product because illicit laboratories are usually crudely equipped for purification, with no quality control. Lead and cyanide poisoning resulted from using illicitly manufactured substances. These adulterants are associated with significant maternal—fetal morbidity and mortality. Incomplete amination of lysergic acid or failure to purify the product in manufacture of LSD results in lysergic acid toxicity (peripheral neuropathy and progressive necrosis). Lysergic acid toxicity in humans and animals includes rapid onset (days) peripheral gangrene from impeded circulation, and eventual death (Rall and Schleifer, 1985). Drugs available as tablets, caplets, or capsules (for example, codeine, metha-done, morphine, benzodiazepines, pentazocine) contain a significant amount of the tablet/capsule vehicle agent (> 97 percent), typically microcrystalline cellulose. Preparation for parenteral use frequently consists only of heating powder and dissolving in water. Usually no attempt is made to separate the drug from the vehicle, or sometimes a cotton ball is used as a crude filter. The resultant solution of mostly dissolved microcrystalline cellulose is injected. It has a high potential for pulmo-nary emboli, placental infarcts, and other maternal vascular blockages.

Aromatic (benzene ring-containing) substances, such as toluene or gasoline, are abused as inhal-ants. In addition to the resonant ring, substances such as lead or nitriles may also be present and can cause toxicity. Marijuana may contain dangerous vegetable contaminants such as nightshade, poison sumac, poison ivy, and poison oak, known to cause serious pulmonary-cardiac morbidity or even death when smoked. Herbicides (e.g., paraquat) and/or pesticides (i.e., chlordane) may be in marijuana itself, the result of treatment during production in plant's growth as production practices have no quality control (Klaassen, 1985). Death has been associated with smoking marijuana con-taminated with herbicides.

### OTHER DRUGS AND CHEMICALS AS DILUTANTS

Chemicals are used by dealers to "cut" or dilute illicit drugs to increase their profits. Sometimes the dilutant is more dangerous than the illicit drug. Cocaine is cut with lidocaine, amphetamines, and sometimes fine glass beads. In Dallas in the early 1900s, lidocaine with no trace of cocaine was being sold as the drug of abuse. Amphetamines are diluted, sometimes heavily, with antihistamines or ephedrine. Heroin has been cut with diverse compounds: talcum, confectioner's sugar, and even finely ground sawdust. Perhaps the most notorious case of the dilutant being more dangerous than the substance of abuse is cutting heroin with warfarin, leading to a cluster of warfarin embryopathy cases that were never published. Some dilutants may be teratogenic and others may cause serious maternal and/or placental vascular complications, especially when used parenterally. Strychnine and arsenic have been intentionally added to amphetamine, methamphetamine, cocaine, heroin, and LSD to enhance their effects, although the 'intensification' is actually due to subclinical/clinical strychnine/arsenic toxicity.

## TREATMENT OF SUBSTANCE USE DURING PREGNANCY

Non-pregnant adults with substance use problems normally includes withdrawal. Opiates are the exception because methadone, buprenorphine, and naltrexone therapy are available for such drugs as heroin. Adjunct regimens have been used an adjunct to assist in actual withdrawal include a ben-zodiazepine plus an antidepressant (e.g., diazepam and amitriptyline). Others have used diazepam and fluoxetine. A different pharmacological strategy is suppression of alpha-adrenergic action with drugs, such as clonidine, and to alleviate withdrawal symptoms, sometimes with a benzodiazepine or barbiturate (Nembutal) adjunct. Such regimens are given in doses adjusted to the individual case to facilitate asymptomatic withdrawal, and the dose is gradually decreased over periods ranging from 10 days to 1–6 months.

Substance addiction is a psychological phenomenon as well as physical. Both aspects must be addressed for successful treatment. Early in treatment planning, specialists in addiction psychology/ psychiatry should be involved. Recommendations they may offer include private and/or group coun-seling, such as Narcotics Anonymous (NA) or Alcoholics Anonymous (AA). Physicians support use of these programs because they increase patient abstinence success rate.

We reported gravid patients in substance abuse treatment during pregnancy was associated with increased birth weight and head circumference, and fewer perinatal complications compared to untreated matched substance-abusing pregnant controls (Little *et al.*, 2003). Prenatal care, psycho-logical therapy and routine substance abuse screening was part of the inpatient program.

## OBSTETRICAL GOALS OF SUBSTANCE ABUSE TREATMENT

Reducing maternal and fetal/infant morbidity and mortality is the obstetrical goal of substance abuse treatment during pregnancy. Prenatal care is very important. It was the major determinant of pregnancy outcome in substance abusers, more important than attaining abstinence (MacGregor *et al.*, 1989). Regular prenatal care was associated with better pregnancy outcomes than those who did not have prenatal care regardless of continued substance use. The primary medical goal in treatment of gravid substance user (risks to both the mother and the fetus) is thus to increase prenatal care use, early and regularly.

Treatment for the pregnant substance abuser involves assessment of risks from continued substance use (for example, maintenance) versus risk of withdrawal, and the benefits of withdrawal (i.e., improved fetal growth) must be evaluated. Recommendations that withdrawal from heroin or methadone not be attempted after 32 weeks of gestation because of the possible risk of abruptio placentae, preterm labor, premature rupture of membranes (PROM), or fetal death in more advanced pregnancies is based on anecdotal data from the 1970s (Rementeria and Nuang, 1973). Recent clinical experience does not support increased risks with withdrawal (Luty *et al.*, 2003). Currently, withdrawal of the gravid patient from substances of abuse is generally advocated but remains controversial. No generally accepted regimen exists for use during pregnancy. As with non-pregnant adults, a benzodiazepine and antidepressant or a benzodiazepine and a low-dose alpha-blocker (e.g., clonidine) regimen was to assist pregnant women withdrawing from a variety of substances (e.g., alcohol, cocaine, methamphetamine, amphetamine). The primary danger of the alpha-blockers is maternal hypotension, possibly impeding placental perfusion. In France, buprenorphine was used, with no increase in the incidence of adverse pregnancy outcomes compared to controls (Auriacombe *et al.*, 2004). Neonatal withdrawal was reported with buprenorphine (Marquet *et al.*, 1997). Therefore, only minimal effective dose levels are used. Blood pressure and fetal heart rate should be monitored closely with this regimen. Doppler flow studies may prove useful for monitoring umbilical blood flow in these patients.

Naltrexone has been used to treat several substance dependencies during pregnancy without apparent untoward effects, but no long-term follow-up studies have been published (Hulse *et al.*, 2001). An alternative therapy with little or no potential for abuse is buprenorphine/naloxone (Suboxone), but there are no studies of its use during pregnancy. Disulfiram (Antabuse), a deterrent for alcohol abuse, should not be used at any time during pregnancy because of its strong copper-chelating properties. Copper is essential to normal fetal neuronal formation and migration, and any impediment in these processes may result in fetal brain malformations. Notably, this is a theoretical risk.

## ALTERNATIVES TO TRADITIONAL TREATMENT FOR SUBSTANCE DEPENDENCE DURING PREGNANCY

Substance abuse during pregnancy can be treated without the use of substances that are potentially addicting. New approaches for detoxification have included drug combinations, such as clonidine and naltrexone, and other drug regimens (Hulse *et al.*, 2001; Rayburn and Bogenschutz, 2004). A combined regimen of these two drugs has been successfully employed for rapid opioid withdrawal for outpatient treatment. The combination of naloxone with midazolam or methohexitone (methohexital) can be used for inpatient settings. Investigators also found that this treatment can be used by using the partial opioid-receptor agonist buprenorphine for either heroin or methadone addiction. Limited experience with clonidine transdermal patches has shown that these can be successfully applied in suppressing symptoms of withdrawal (MacGregor *et al.*, 1985). Low-dose Nembutal as an adjunct may assist in sleep. Importantly, the use of low-dose clonidine does not seem to be associated with adverse effects on the course of pregnancy (Boutroy, 1989). Moreover, limited experience with this regimen seems to indicate that it is effective and does not pose serious risks to advanced pregnancies (beyond 32 weeks). However, these results come from uncontrolled, anecdotal studies and the ability to extrapolate is very limited. In 1993, the US FDA approved a drug for the treatment of opioid dependence: levo-alpha-acetyl-methadol (LAAM). This drug has a slower onset and a longer half-life than methadone, and because it is a prodrug, its onset is slower when administered intravenously than when given orally. This reduces its potential for abuse (Rowe, 1993).

### Risks of Withdrawal

Data from the 1970s suggested an increased frequency of fetal deaths and maternal morbidity associated with opiate withdrawal, especially later in pregnancy (Finnegan *et al.*, 1977; Rementeria and Nunag, 1973). Pregnancies reported in these case reports and series were complicated by several other factors in addition to heroin addiction (i.e., hypertension, syphilis, and chorioamnionitis).

### Risks of Maintenance

The most common maintenance protocol for heroin-addicted gravidas involves the use of methadone. The efficacy of this regimen in such pregnancies is somewhat controversial (Edelin *et al.*, 1988). Babies born to mothers on methadone, as with heroin, may experience withdrawal symptoms. Methadone withdrawal symptoms occur much later (i.e., at or after 1 week after the birth) because of methadone's much longer half-life (30–40 hours) compared to heroin (8–10 hours). Furthermore, withdrawal symptoms of methadone-exposed infants are more severe than those of heroin-exposed infants. Methadone neonatal withdrawal is associated with a higher frequency seizures and a greater number of days with symptomatic withdrawal (Blinick *et al.*, 1973). In addition, it was found that fetal growth retardation is more severe among methadone-exposed infants than among heroin-exposed infants (Blinick *et al.*, 1973), a finding that was not supported by other studies (Lifschitz *et al.*, 1983; Soepatimi, 1986). Methadone withdrawal using dose tapering employing adjuvants such as Nembutal were not associated with adverse pregnancy outcomes in a more recent study in a large public hospital where a number of studies of substance abuse were undertaken (Dashe *et al.*, 1998, 2002).

## SPECIFIC SOCIAL AND ILLICIT SUBSTANCES USED DURING PREGNANCY

Substance use during pregnancy has not been studied as extensively as it should be to assess fully the risks to the embryo/fetus and to the mother. The available information is often confounded by many factors, including poor maternal health, lack of prenatal care, malnutrition, presence of infectious diseases, and the use of a myriad of substances. It is rare that a gravid substance user takes only one substance. The sections that follow are a summary of the known maternal-fetal effects of the 16 social and illicit substances most commonly used during pregnancy. This chapter concludes with a section that summarizes the complex issues that attend polydrug use during pregnancy. Each substance is described, highlights of human embryo-fetal risks are reviewed, and perinatal effects are defined. A summary of the embryo-fetal effects is given in Table 16.1 and a summary of the maternal effects in Table 16.2. Details underlying Tables 16.1 and 16.2 are discussed in the sections that follow.

### Alcohol Use during Pregnancy and Maternal Alcoholism

Alcohol is a central nervous system depressant and its abuse during pregnancy has adverse effects on both the mother and the fetus. It is now a well-known human and animal teratogen, a fact that was discovered in the US in 1973 (Jones *et al.*, 1973) **and in France in 1968** (Lemoine *et al.*, 1968).

**TABLE 16.2**

**Summary of Maternal Effects of Social and Illicit Substance Use during Pregnancy**

| Substance | Abruption | CNS Damage | ICH | Metabolic Acidosis | Anorexia | Hepatorenal Damage | Endocarditis (Parenteral Use) |
|---|---|---|---|---|---|---|---|
| Alcohol | + | + | — | + | + | + | NA |
| Amphetamines | + | + | + | ? | + | + | + |
| Barbiturates | — | + | + | ? | + | + | ? |
| Benzodiazepines | — | + | — | ? | + | + | ? |
| Cocaine[a] | + | + | + | ? | + | + | + |
| Codeine | — | + | — | ? | + | ? | + |
| Heroin | + | + | + | ? | + | + | + |
| Inhalants | ? | + | — | + | + | + | NA |
| LSD | ? | + | — | ? | + | ? | NA |
| Marijuana | — | (—) | — | ? | — | — | — |
| Methadone | + | + | — | ? | + | + | + |
| Methamphetamine | + | + | ? | ? | + | + | + |
| Morphine | + | + | — | ? | + | + | + |
| PCP | ? | (+) | (+) | ? | + | + | ? |
| Tobacco | + | (—) | — | ? | + | + | NA |
| Ts and Blues[a] | (+) | (+) | (+) | ? | + | + | + |

+, Documented, positive; —, documented, negative; (—) data inconclusive but suggestive of a negative finding; (+) data inconclusive but suggestive of a positive finding; ? unknown; NA, not applicable/not available.

[a] Infarction/embolism.

*Abbreviations:* CNS, central nervous system; ICH, intracranial hemorrhage; LSD, lysergic acid diethylamide; PCP, phencyclidine.

*Source:* Modified from Little *et al.*, 1990b.

## Prevalence and Epidemiology

Up to 70 percent of the adult population in the USA use alcohol socially, but the rate of alcohol abuse during pregnancy is unknown. Early reports found alcohol use during pregnancy ranged from <2 percent to >70 percent (Abel and Sokol, 1987; NIAAA, 1983). The prevalence of drinking four or more drinks [2 ounces (59 ml) of absolute alcohol] per day was estimated to be 1.4 percent in a large urban public hospital in Texas (Little *et al.*, 1989a).

Considering only women who are alcoholic during pregnancy (>8 drinks per day), an estimated 30–50 percent of infants whose mothers are alcoholic have fetal alcohol syndrome (FAS) (Jones, 1989). An 80-percent FAS rate was observed in offspring of frankly alcoholic women (i.e., eight or more drinks per day) at Parkland Memorial Hospital (Little *et al.*, 1990a). Prevalence of FAS varies between countries. It is estimated that one per 100 live births in northern France has FAS (Daehaene *et al.*, 1977), one per 600 in Sweden (Olegard *et al.*, 1979), and one per 750 in Seattle (Hanson *et al.*, 1978). An estimated average of 1.9 per 1,000 live births worldwide are FAS (Abel and Sokol, 1987). FAS prevalence in the US is an estimated 1.95 per 1,000 live births (Abel, 1995). Estimated FAS prevalence was approximately one per 1,000 live births was seen in Dallas, Texas (Little *et al.*, 1990b).

Meta-analysis of the prevalence of alcohol use (n=23,470 studies) reviewed 328 studies to estimate the prevalence of alcohol use during pregnancy, 9.8 percent (95 percent CI: 8.9–11.1) (Popova *et al.*, 2017). A meta-analysis and systematic review of 62 infants outcome studies (selected from n=11,110 reports) estimated the global prevalence of FAS was 14.6 per 10,000 births (Popova *et al.*, 2017), or 0.15 percent. It was estimated that one in 67 women who use alcohol during pregnancy will have a child with FAS, or approximately 1.5 percent. Importantly, this estimate spans the spectrum from any use to abusive consumption, and is clear that high levels of ethanol consumption increased FAS risk.

An estimated 2–3 percent of pregnant women drink heavily enough to cause FAS (Abel and Sokol, 1987; NIAAA, 1983). In 1993, the rate of infants born with FAS was estimated to be 6.7 per 1,000 births (MMWR, 1995). As many as 5 percent of all congenital anomalies may be caused by maternal alcohol intake during pregnancy (Sokol, 1981), although precise estimates of alcohol-induced birth defects are difficult to ascertain. A recent review estimated FAS prevalence of 0.5 to two cases per 1,000 live births (Vorgias and Bernstein, 2020). Some authorities estimated **alcohol abuse during pregnancy is the most frequent known teratogenic cause of mental retardation** (Abel and Sokol, 1987; Clarren and Smith, 1978).

## MATERNAL EFFECTS

Use or abuse of alcohol abuse during pregnancy negatively affects the course of pregnancy with higher frequencies of adverse pregnancy outcomes including stillbirths, premature deliveries, decreased placental weight, and spontaneous abortion (Parazzini *et al.*, 1994). Low levels of alcohol consumption (< four drinks per day) are associated with adverse pregnancy outcomes (Little, 1977; Plant, 1984; Sokol *et al.*, 1980; Streissguth *et al.*, 1981). "Binge" drinking during pregnancy is associated with an increased frequency of congenital anomalies and physical and intellectual development abnormalities. Studies of alcohol use of varying durations in pregnancy found that occasional binge drinking by moderate drinkers did not negatively affect birth outcome (Autti-Ramo *et al.*, 1992; Tolo and Little, 1993). However, exposure to alcohol throughout gestation was associated with an increased rate of alcohol-related birth defects and developmental abnormalities (Autti-Ramo and Granstrom, 1991; Coles *et al.*, 1991). Continued alcohol drinking throughout pregnancy showed a dose-response of ethanol on the embryofetus (Halmesmaki, 1988). Sexually transmitted diseases and other infections occur at a higher frequency among women who abuse alcohol during pregnancy, compared to women who did not drink during pregnancy.

## EFFECTS ON INTRAUTERINE DEVELOPMENT

The fetal alcohol syndrome (FAS) was described in the English literature in 1973 (Jones *et al.*) and reported eight children born to mothers with chronic alcoholism. FAS was first described in 127 infants from France (Lemoine *et al.*, 1968). Anomalies (growth deficiency, mental deficiency, and syndromic facial features) were consistently observed among infants born to women who were chronic alcoholics during pregnancy (i.e., eight or more ethanol beverages per day) (Clarren and Smith, 1978; Larroque, 1992; Sokol *et al.*, 1986; Streissguth *et al.*, 1980, 1981, 1985).

FAS diagnostic features include (1) pre- and postnatal growth deficiency (Faden and Graubard, 1994; Greene *et al.*, 1991; Larroque *et al.*, 1993); (2) mental retardation (Autti-Ramo *et al.*, 1992a; Jacobson *et al.*, 1993); (3) behavioral disturbances (Coles *et al.*, 1987); and (4) typical recognizable facial appearance (Box 16.2) (Autti-Ramo *et al.*, 1992b; Lewis and Woods, 1994). Congenital heart defects (Loser *et al.*, 1992) and brain anomalies (Mattson *et al.*, 1992) are the most frequent structural congenital anomalies. Structural heart anomalies were found in 43 (57 percent) of 76 children evaluated diagnosed with FAS in one series (Sandor *et al.*, 1981). Other major congenital anomalies (e.g., spina bifida, limb defects, genitourinary defects, eye anomalies, airway obstructions, renal hypoplasia) are associated with FAS (Carones *et al.*, 1992; Froster and Baird, 1992; Hinzpeter *et al.*, 1992; Lewis and Woods, 1994; Taylor *et al.*, 1994; Usowicz *et al.*, 1986). When the full FAS syndrome is not present, but mild to moderate mental development delay and physical growth retardation are termed fetal alcohol effects (FAE) (Jones, 1989). Other published categories include fetal alcohol spectrum disorder (FASD), or fetal alcohol disorder (FAD), partial FAS (pFAS), alcohol related neurodevelopmental disorder (ARND), neurobehavioral disorder associated with prenatal alcohol exposure (ND-PAE), alcohol related birth defects (ARBD) (Vorgias and Bernstein, 2020), and Fetal alcohol spectrum disorders (FASD) (Hoyme *et al.*, 2021).

---

**BOX 16.2   FEATURES OF FETAL ALCOHOL SYNDROME**

- Craniofacial anomalies
- Absent-to-hypoplastic philtrum
- Broad upper lip
- Flattened nasal bridge
- Hypoplastic upper lip vermillion
- Micrognathia
- Microphthalmia
- Short nose
- Short palpebral fissures

---

#### EFFECTS ON POSTNATAL DEVELOPMENT

Fetal alcohol spectrum disorders (FASD) describes the continuum of disabilities ranging from mild symptoms to very severe presentation with major structural birth defects and intellectual deficits. The most severe cases of FAS have growth restriction, distinct facial dysmorphology with attendant cognitive and/or neurobehavioral effects, full-blown FAS. At the other end of the continuum are individuals exposed to alcohol prenatally who have neurobehavioral and cognitive deficits, but minimal or no growth or physical signs (alcohol-related neurodevelopmental disorder). FASD probably occurs more frequently than prior studies estimated. Prospective studies in United States schools estimate FASD affects 11.3–50.0 /1000 children (1–5 percent). In the foster care system it is estimated that ~169 / 1000 (~17 percent) suffer from FASD (Hoyme and Shah, 2021). However, foster care is a biased sample biased toward affected individuals who have disrupted living and social environments. Children born to women who abused alcohol during pregnancy had postnatal physical growth delays of 2 years. The long-term consequences of intrauterine alcohol exposure on the child's physical and cognitive development at 5 years of age had an increased frequency of alcohol-related deficits compared to offspring of non-alcohol exposed children, or compared to children whose mothers stopped drinking in the second trimester of pregnancy. Transient withdrawal symptoms (tremors, hypertonia, and irritability), have been observed among infants whose mothers drank ethanol chronically in late pregnancy (Coles *et al.*, 1984), In another study at Parkland Memorial Hospital, we found similar sequelae for prenatal alcohol exposure (Little *et al.*, 1990a).

Chronic prenatal exposure to alcohol during gestation resulted in postnatally smaller head circumferences, lower IQs, other deficits in intellectual functioning (short-term memory and encoding), problems in abstraction, arithmetic, and speech (Autti-Ramo and Granstrom, 1991; Becker *et al.*, 1990; Caruso and ten Bensel, 1993; Coles *et al.*, 1991; Spohr *et al.*, 1993; Streissguth *et al.*, 1985, 1991a, 1991b).

Poor protein-calorie nutrition, vitamin deficiencies, and alcohol contaminants (e.g., lead) are frequent complications associated with maternal alcohol abuse, and likely play an etiological role. Genetic polymorphisms for alcohol dehydrogenase suggest a pharmacogenetic etiologic role in the severity of FAS effects, and imply that acetaldehyde may in fact be the proximate teratogen, not ethanol per se.

### Counseling

Women who abuse alcohol during pregnancy should be counseled to stop drinking completely. Medical and psychological support for drinking cessation should be offered. Many of women who abuse alcohol may also use/abuse other substances; in ranked order by frequency substances used during pregnancy are tobacco, marijuana, benzodiazepines, methamphetamines, cocaine and opiates. Counseling should include advice to stop using these agents as well because every one of the substances used non-medicinally/abused counts toward the risk of a poor outcome.

## ALCOHOL SUMMARY

Fetal alcohol syndrome is one of the three leading causes of mental retardation. **FAS** is the only cause of mental retardation that is **potentially preventable**. FAS is a leading cause of poor pregnancy outcome and childhood morbidity (congenital anomalies, including mental retardation). **Advice against any use of alcohol during pregnancy must be strongly emphasized**. Low level alcohol maternal consumption (<3 drinks per day) was associated with mild to moderate decrease in IQ scores among infants (Streissguth *et al.*, 1981) and with prenatal growth retardation (Larroque, 1992; Larroque *et al.*, 1993).

# AMPHETAMINE ABUSE DURING PREGNANCY

Dextroamphetamines (D-amphetamine, amphetamine) and methamphetamines are sympathomimetic agents used medically during pregnancy to treat narcolepsy. Amphetamines are stimulants used illicitly known by a number of street names. Approximately 6 percent of pregnant women had positive urine toxicology for methamphetamines, often in combination with other drugs such as cocaine at delivery in two studies (Little *et al.*, 1988a; Ramin *et al.*, 1994). The majority of drug positive women were White (Little *et al.*, 1988a, 1988b). Prevalence of illicit methamphetamine use during pregnancy in Hawaii was 0.7 percent (Derauf *et al.*, 2003). In four major US cities, participating in a multicenter study (Los Angeles, CA, DeMoines, IA, Tulsa, OK, Honolulu, HI) the prevalence of methamphetamine use was 5.2 percent. Methamphetamine use in pregnancy increased over time, and reaching a high prevalence of 24 percent (Terplan *et al.*, 2009). Factors that complicate extrapolation results across studies of illicit use or abuse include (1) dose regimens in illicit use are not controlled and purity is unknown, (2) doses likely involve amounts much greater than those used therapeutically, and (3) harmful impurities (e.g., dilutants or poor chemical purification) may be present in illicit amphetamines or methamphetamines. Methylphenidate (Ritalin), dextroamphetamine (Dexedrine), a medicinal cocktail of amphetamine salts (Adderall) are stimulants with potential for abuse that are often represented as amphetamine or methamphetamine by those who distribute illegal drugs. Another drug that has similar effects is modafinil, but its potential for abuse was judged low (Malcolm *et al.*, 2002). Modafinil is, however, associated with an increased frequency of birth defects in one large study (Kaplan *et al.*, 2021) but not in another study (Cesta *et al.*, 2020).

## AMPHETAMINES

### Human Congenital Anomalies

Birth defects were not increased in frequency among 69 infants whose mothers abused amphetamines during the first trimester, but the rates of, preterm delivery and perinatal mortality were increased (Eriksson *et al.*, 1981). Fifteen percent were delayed in academic achievement in school at follow-up (Eriksson *et al.*, 2000).

Medically supervised use of amphetamines during pregnancy is not convincingly associated with an increased frequency of congenital anomalies among several thousand infants exposed during the first trimester (Heinonen *et al.*, 1977; Milkovich and van den Berg, 1977; Nelson and Forfar, 1971; Nora *et al.*, 1967, 1970).

## Animal Studies of Amphetamines

At maternally lethal amphetamine doses, cardiac, eye, and other congenital anomalies were increased in frequency in mice (Nora *et al.*, 1965). The relevance of these findings to human amphetamine use is unknown.

### METHAMPHETAMINES

## Human Congenital Anomalies

Like amphetamines, methamphetamines are sympathomimetic agents with potent central nervous system stimulant properties. They are prescribed medically to treat ADHD, obesity, and narcolepsy. Illegal methamphetamines are known as 'designer drugs' because they are synthesized by novel site methylation along the carbon chain and ring in a one-step reduction process. This "design" creates molecules different from pharmaceutical forms of the drug. Methamphetamines are a popular class of recreational drug, but are occasionally used to 'cut' or dilute other illicit drugs (e.g., cocaine). The stimulant effects of methamphetamines keep the partygoers awake, although some varieties of this drug may cause hallucinations or other altered states of consciousness. In 2021, parties sometimes called "raves" go on for 36+ hours with the pharmacological assistance of methamphetamines.

Methamphetamine use during pregnancy was 5.2 percent in one large cohort in a public hospital, and the typical user was a single White woman with no or few prenatal visits and who was dependent on public health care (Arria *et al.*, 2006), consistent with other studies (Catanzarite and Stein, 1995; Ho *et al.*, 2001; Little *et al.*, 1988b). Prevalence of methamphetamine use has not decreased over 10–15 years (Buchi *et al.*, 2003).

Among 52 pregnancies complicated by methamphetamines, we found symmetric fetal growth retardation was increased compared to controls. Congenital anomalies were not significantly increased in frequency among infants born to methamphetamine users (Little *et al.*, 1988b). No increase in perinatal infant and maternal complications was found. The small sample (n=52) of methamphetamine-exposed infants seriously limits the ability to extrapolate these 1988 findings. Methamphetamine and cocaine use in pregnancy were associated with lower birth weight but not with anomalies in several studies (Oro and Dixon, 1987; Chomchai *et al.*, 2004; Ramin *et al.*, 1994). Methamphetamine use throughout pregnancy was associated with fetal growth retardation but no difference in birth weight was found when drug use was discontinued after the second trimester (Smith *et al.*, 2003). In a study from Thailand, lower birth weight was associated with maternal methamphetamine use during pregnancy among 47 infants (Chomchai *et al.*, 2004).

Medically supervised use of methamphetamines in 89 infants born to women who took the drug during embryogenesis had a frequency of congenital anomalies no different from controls. No birth defects were reported among 320 infants born to women who used the drug outside organogenesis (Heinonen *et al.*, 1977). Medically supervised use of methamphetamines cannot be compared to effects of the drug's abuse that employ much higher doses.

Meta-analysis of 8 studies that included 626 infants born to women who used methamphetamines socially/illicitly during pregnancy EGA was reduced by 0.9 weeks, birth weight was 244 grams lower, head circumference was 0.9 cm lower, and birth length was 0.9 cm shorter (Kalaitzopoulos *et al.*, 2018).

## Intracerebral Hemorrhage

Intracerebral hemorrhage and other cardiovascular accidents are markedly increased in frequency among methamphetamine abusers and their fetuses/infants (Catanzarite and Stein, 1995; Dixon and Bejar, 1989; Keogh and Baron, 1985; Sachdeva and Woodward, 1989), often resulting in maternal and/or infant death (Perez *et al.*, 1999; Stewart and Meeker, 1997). Among young adults in 77 studies reviewed, a preponderance of strokes were associated with methamphetamine use (Lappin *et al.*, 2017). In three cases of methamphetamine use during pregnancy, mother and fetus suffered drug-associated brain injuries. Maternal and fetal/neonatal death occurred in two of three cases (Chin and Bartholomew, 2020).

### Long-Term Effects of Prenatal Amphetamine Exposure on Child Development

Children whose mothers took amphetamines during pregnancy followed postnatally had slightly lower IQ scores, were more aggressive, and were delayed in academic achievement (Billing *et al.*, 1985; Cernerud *et al.*, 1996; Eriksson and Zetterstrom, 1994; Eriksson *et al.*, 2000). In 146 children prenatally exposed to methamphetamine who were followed at 7.5 years of age, frequency of behavior problems (aggressiveness, rule breaking) was increased, but early childhood adversity was a major mediator. It was suggested that poor postnatal environment might be a major contributor to adverse outcomes, in addition to prenatal methamphetamine exposure (Eze *et al.*, 2016). In a small study of 23 children prenatally exposed to methamphetamine, a variety of cognitive measures (IQ, memory, fine motor coordination, visual-motor integration were significantly reduced compared to non-exposed children, after controlling for postnatal environmental effects (Kwiatkowski *et al.*, 2018). In 171 children exposed to methamphetamine prenatally, caregiver psychological symptoms accounted for all the cognitive and behavioral deficits observed (Chu *et al.*, 2020), suggesting no measurable effect of maternal drug use.

### Animal Studies

Doses of methamphetamine similar to those used for narcolepsy were not associated with an increased frequency of congenital anomalies in non-human primates (macaque monkeys) (Courtney and Valerio, 1968). Congenital anomalies (brain, anencephaly, eye, cleft palate) were increased in frequency among mice and rabbits whose mothers were given methamphetamines during organogenesis at doses up to 20 times the usual human therapeutic dose (Kasirsky and Tansy, 1971; Martin *et al.*, 1976; Yamamoto *et al.*, 1992).

### SUMMARY OF AMPHETAMINE/METHAMPHETAMINE USE

Medically supervised use of amphetamines and methamphetamines during pregnancy apparently does not pose significant risks for increased frequencies of congenital anomalies or maternal—fetal complications. Risks for congenital anomalies and pregnancy complications for those who abuse this class of drugs exist and probably involve serious complications secondary to vascular disruption and other cardiovascular accidents.

## CANNABINOID USE DURING PREGNANCY

More than 22 million people in the USA use marijuana or its derivatives [hash, hash oil, Thai sticks, tetrahydrocannabinol (THC)] regularly. Fifty percent or more of users are women of reproductive age. An estimated 3 percent of the population uses marijuana daily and as many as 10–15 percent of Americans use the drug on a monthly basis (CDC, 2017). Estimated prevalence rates of cannabinoid use during pregnancy from 41 studies indicates a wide range, from 0.24 to 22.6 percent of gravidas (Singh *et al.*, 2020).

### MATERNAL EFFECTS

Preterm labor was increased in frequency among women who smoked marijuana during pregnancy in several investigations (Fried *et al.*, 1984; Gibson *et al.*, 1983; Hatch and Bracken, 1986), but other investigators have failed to confirm this observation (Fried, 1980; Hingson *et al.*, 1982; Shiono *et al.*, 1995; Tennes *et al.*, 1985; Zuckerman *et al.*, 1989). In one small uncontrolled study (n = 35), prolonged labor and meconium-stained amniotic fluid was seemingly increased in frequency in women who smoked marijuana late in pregnancy (Greenland *et al.*, 1982). Labor was not prolonged and meconium stained amniotic fluid was not increased with cannabis use during pregnancy in several other controlled studies with larger sample sizes (Fried *et al.*, 1983; Greenland *et al.*, 1983; Witter and Niebyl, 1990). Preeclampsia and gestational diabetes were compared between cannabis using gravidas and nondrug users in three studies, but no clear association was identified (Singh *et al.*, 2020). Three (Corsi *et al.*, 2019; Burns *et al.*, 2006; Hayatbaksh *et al.*, 2012) of nine studies reviewed reported an increased frequency of preterm birth (Singh *et al.*, 2020).

## PERINATAL INFANT EFFECTS

Significantly lowered birth weights have been reported among infants whose mothers used marijuana during pregnancy in three studies (Cornelius *et al.*, 1995; Hingson *et al.*, 1982; Zuckerman *et al.*, 1989; Campbell *et al.*, 2018; Hayatbakhsh *et al.*, 2012; Crume *et al.*, 2018). In several other studies birth weight was not decreased with marijuana use during pregnancy (Fried, 1980; Greenland *et al.*, 1983; Linn *et al.*, 1983; Shiono *et al.*, 1995; Witter and Niebyl, 1990; Reichman and Teitler, 2003; Bada *et al.*, 2005; Conner *et al.*, 2016; Van Gelder *et al.*, 2010). Most investigations report no increased frequency of congenital anomalies with prenatal marijuana use (Day *et al.*, 1991; Fried, 1980; Gunn *et al.*, 2016; Kharbanda *et al.*, 2020) Among more than 1200 infants whose mothers smoked marijuana during pregnancy, 137 during the first trimester, the frequency of major congenital anomalies was not increased (Linn *et al.*, 1983). An increased frequency of anencephaly (OR=1.9) was reported among infants born to women who used marijuana during pregnancy in the National Birth Defects Prevention Study (van Gelder *et al.*, 2010). In another large study (California Birth Defects Monitoring Program), the frequency of gastroschisis was increased among infants whose mothers used cannabis during pregnancy (Lam and Torfs, 2006). The data on cannabis use during pregnancy and birth defects is confounded by poly drug use and other social/environmental factors (e.g., poor to no prenatal care, poor nutrition). The risk of birth defects with marijuana use during pregnancy cannot be ruled out until better controlled investigations are published. In the interim, marijuana use is apparently not a potent teratogen, but a very small risk of congenital anomalies can be excluded (Grant *et al.*, 2020).

A not generally accepted "syndrome" (fetal growth retardation, craniofacial and other minor dysmorphologic features) was proposed in a clinical case series that included five infants born to women who used two to 14 joints (cigarettes) of marijuana daily throughout pregnancy (Qazi *et al.*, 1985). The infants probably had fetal alcohol syndrome as alcohol and cocaine exposures confounded these findings, which have not been replicated.

A number of investigations analyzing marijuana and THC use during gestation were conducted in pregnant rats, mice, hamsters, and rabbits (Abel, 1980a; Schardein, 2000). Most animal teratology studies of marijuana are negative, particularly if dosing (amount, route of intake) was comparable to the human situation.

## META-ANALYSIS

Meta-analysis of 24 studies of women who used cannabis during pregnancy and their infants shows a decrease in birth weight of 109 grams and an increased odds (OR=1.77) of low birth weight (Gunn *et al.*, 2016).

## WITHDRAWAL SYMPTOMS

Among infants born to women who used marijuana near the time of delivery, certain neonatal neurobehavioral abnormalities (tremulousness, abnormal response stimuli) were found (Fried, 1980;

Fried and Makin, 1987), but other studies found no differences (Tennes *et al.*, 1985). Nonetheless, these withdrawal-like effects are transient and resolve spontaneously without complications or need for medical management.

## SUMMARY OF CANNABINOID USE

Mild fetal growth retardation and maternal lung damage are the adverse outcomes that can reasonably be attributed to marijuana use during pregnancy. Importantly, women who use marijuana during pregnancy frequently use other substances known to be harmful (i.e., alcohol and/or cocaine) (Cornelius *et al.*, 1995; Shiono *et al.*, 1995) because illicit substance abuse is often polydrug use, not a single substance exposure (Little *et al.*, 1990c). Polypharmacy in substance use further compounds the confounding associated with social and illicit substance use. Dose of cannabis is unknown, purity is unknown, cocaine timing in pregnancy is usually not known, and use of harmful substances in a poly drug regimen poses even further unknown risks

## Cocaine Abuse during Pregnancy

Cocaine use is widespread among those of reproductive age. Cocaine use is not limited to Western society. It was detected in the urine of people from around the world, and among residents in areas as remote as the Arctic. The epidemic began in the mid to late 1970s, and the population of users expanded to include members every age, sex, ethnic, and socioeconomic sub-group. Approximately half of these users are women of reproductive age (GAO, 1990). Cocaine use is widely known to be dangerous during pregnancy, delaying intrauterine development and causing vascular disruption related birth defects (**not a syndrome**), fetal growth retardation/low birth weight, and transient withdrawal symptoms. Postnatal intellectual development may be adversely affected by prenatal cocaine exposure.

## COCAINE USE AMONG PREGNANT WOMEN

Prevalence of cocaine use during pregnancy was estimated at 9.8 percent in one of the nation's largest hospitals (Little *et al.*, 1988a). In other public hospitals, cocaine use during pregnancy ranged from 11 to 31 percent (Brody, 1989; Nair *et al.*, 1994; Ostrea *et al.*, 1992), and a high rate of 48 percent in a San Francisco public hospital was reported (Osterloh and Lee, 1989). Widely varying estimates of the prevalence of cocaine use in pregnancy (0.1–20 percent) center on about 9 percent. The professional community was not prepared for the large number of cocaine-exposed fetuses over the last decade (Landry and Whitney, 1996; Kuczkowski, 2005). Approximately 77 percent of pregnant cocaine abusers at a large public hospital used other drugs of abuse and/or alcohol (Little *et al.*, 1990d). Another group reported 90 percent of female cocaine users were of reproductive age (Kuczkowski, 2005).

We reported that cocaine crosses the placenta and is metabolized by placental plasma cholinesterase to ecgonine methyl ester, a major active metabolite (Roe *et al.*, 1990). Cocaine actions on the vasculature precipitates a number of untoward effects. Even very low doses of cocaine cause coronary artery vasospasm and arrhythmias (Lange *et al.*, 1989). Cocaine can cause myocardial infarction, congestive heart failure, dilated cardiomyopathy, or severe ischemic events in the heart or brain (Box 16.3). Cocaine can exacerbate vascular weakness and cause serious cerebrovascular accidents (intracerebral infarctions, intracerebral hemorrhages, acute ischemic brain events). Cocaine toxicity (death) is usually preceded by hyperpyrexia, shock, unconsciousness, respiratory/cardiac depression. Chronic cocaine use is associated with epileptogenic seizures and cerebral atrophy (Pascual-Leone *et al.*, 1990; Karch, 2005).

---

### BOX 16.3   COMPLICATIONS AMONG PREGNANT WOMEN WHO USE COCAINE

- Abruptio placentae
- Hepatitis B and C
- Intracerebral hemorrhage
- Placental vasculitis
- Pregnancy-induced hypertension
- Premature delivery (shortened gestation length)
- Premature rupture of membranes
- Preterm labor
- Ruptured ectopic pregnancy
- Sexually transmitted diseases
- Spontaneous abortion

---

### ABRUPTIO PLACENTA

Numerous reports of the increased frequency of abruptio placentae after intravenous or intranasal cocaine use are published (Acker *et al.*, 1983; Bingol *et al.*, 1987a, 1987b; Chasnoff and MacGregor, 1987; Chasnoff *et al.*, 1985, 1987, 1989a; Cherukuri *et al.*, 1988; Collins *et al.*, 1989; Cregler and Mark, 1986; Dixon and Oro, 1987; Dusick *et al.*, 1993; Hladky *et al.*, 2002; Keith *et al.*, 1989; Little *et al.*, 1988a; Miller *et al.*, 1995; Neerhof *et al.*, 1989; Oro and Dixon, 1987; Shiono *et al.*, 1995; Townsend *et al.*, 1988; Witlin and Sibai, 2001). However, some investigators did not observe placental abruption cases among gravid cocaine users (Chouteau *et al.*, 1988; Doberczak *et al.*, 1988).

## META-ANALYSIS: ABRUPTION

Meta-analysis of abruptio placentae and premature rupture of membranes (PROM) risks show that they are strongly associated with cocaine use during pregnancy (Addis *et al.*, 2001).

## COCAINE AND EMBRYO-FETAL DEVELOPMENT

Fetal growth retardation, cerebrovascular accidents, and congenital anomalies are frequently observed in pregnancies complicated by maternal cocaine use (Box 16.4).

---

### BOX 16.4   FETAL COMPLICATIONS REPORTED TO BE ASSOCIATED WITH ANTEPARTUM COCAINE EXPOSURE

- Bradycardia
- Brain cavitations
- Brain growth retardation
- Cardiac arrhythmias
- Cerebral ischemia
- Congenital anomalies
- Fetal heart rate abnormalities
- Growth retardation
- Intracerebral hemorrhage/infarction
- Meconium staining
- Prematurity
- Tachycardia

## Estimated Gestational Age

Significantly shortened mean gestational periods and increased frequencies of preterm labor are associated with maternal cocaine use during pregnancy (Chasnoff *et al.*, 1985, 1989a; Chasnoff and MacGregor, 1987; Cherukuri *et al.*, 1988; Chouteau *et al.*, 1988; Cohen *et al.*, 1991; Dixon and Oro, 1987; Keith *et al.*, 1989; Kliegman *et al.*, 1994; Little *et al.*, 1989b, 1999; MacGregor *et al.*, 1987; Neerhof *et al.*, 1989; Oro and Dixon, 1987; Ryan *et al.*, 1986, 1987a, 1987b; Zuckerman *et al.*, 1989). An increased frequency of precipitous labor was observed in pregnant cocaine users (Bateman *et al.*, 1993; Chasnoff *et al.*, 1987). However, among 1,220 gravid women, no decrease in duration of labor was associated with cocaine use (Wehbeh *et al.*, 1995). Gestation length and frequency of preterm delivery among women who used only cocaine during the first trimester were not significantly different those of women who did not use cocaine during pregnancy (Chasnoff *et al.*, 1989a). Other investigators found no association between preterm labor or low birth weight with cocaine use when other obstetric complications were statistically controlled (Miller *et al.*, 1995; Shiono *et al.*, 1995).

## Birth Weight, Length, and Head Circumference

A number of studies have found that *in utero* cocaine exposure adversely affects fetal growth parameters such as birth weight, length, and head circumference (Bateman *et al.*, 1993; Bauchner *et al.*, 1987, 1988; Bingol *et al.*, 1987a, 1987b; Chasnoff and MacGregor, 1987; Chasnoff *et al.*, 1985, 1987, 1989b; Cherukuri *et al.*, 1988; Chouteau *et al.*, 1988; Dixon and Oro, 1987; Donvito, 1988; Eyler *et al.*, 1994; Fulroth *et al.*, 1989; Hadeed and Siegel, 1989; Keith *et al.*, 1989; Little *et al.*, 1988a; MacGregor *et al.*, 1987; Madden *et al.*, 1986; Neerhof *et al.*, 1989; Oro and Dixon, 1987; Petitti and Coleman, 1990; Ryan *et al.*, 1986, 1987a, 1987b; Zuckerman *et al.*, 1989).

Importantly, head circumference is significantly reduced among infants exposed to cocaine prenatally (Chasnoff *et al.*, 1992; Bateman *et al.*, 1993; Bateman and Chrirboga, 2000). Head circumference was reduced proportionately more than birth weight among 80 infants whose mothers used only cocaine during pregnancy, exhibiting a pattern of brain growth similar to that observed in 67 infants whose mothers had used only alcohol during pregnancy (Little and Snell, 1991a).

Serial ultrasound examinations (two to four) found retarded fetal growth, and reduced head circumference/biparietal diameter among cocaine exposed fetuses, but estimated fetal weight was not significantly reduced (Mitchell *et al.*, 1988).

## Cerebrovascular Accidents and Related Cocaine Toxicity

Adult cocaine use and death is widely published but have frequently been reported. However, only four cases are documented of pregnant women with cocaine associated stroke (Burkett *et al.*, 1990; Greenland *et al.*, 1989; Henderson and Torbey, 1988), although many have occurred among pregnant women and are not published. Of the published cases, two were due to subarachnoid hemorrhage resulting from ruptured aneurysms and a third case involved a pregnant woman admitted to the hospital in a comatose condition after about 1.5 g of cocaine had been placed in her vagina. She was maintained on life-support systems and eventually died approximately four months later, never having regained consciousness. The fourth maternal death was attributed to cardiac ischemia and arrhythmia (Burkett *et al.*, 1990). Among more than four million women studied in California, the risk of maternal mortality was more than doubled among women who used cocaine during pregnancy (Wolfe *et al.*, 2005). This is a large, reliable study whose findings are important.

## Pregnancy-Induced Hypertension and Cocaine

Two studies have reported an increased frequency of pregnancy-induced hypertension associated with cocaine use (Chouteau et al., 1988; Little et al., 1989b). Other factors, such as maternal age, race, and use of multiple substances of abuse, may have accounted for this difference, but a causal association seems likely. Finally, one study reported hepatic rupture during pregnancy associated with severe pregnancy-induced hypertension associated with cocaine use (Moen et al., 1993).

## Congenital Anomalies

Cocaine use during pregnancy was associated with a number of congenital anomalies. The parsimonious list of birth defects probably associated with cocaine use in pregnancy have a common causative mechanism, vascular disruption (Box 16.5). Pharmacologic vasoactive effects are the plausible operatative mechanism with cocaine precipitating vascular accidents. Sites of the vascular accidents may be central or peripheral. Limb reduction defects may be the result of peripheral vascular disruption. The most consistent association between cocaine use and fetal malformations involves the genitourinary tract (Buehler et al., 1996). In publications from 1985 to 2020, numerous isolated congenital anomalies have been described (Appendix I). These birth defects include ileal atresia in two infants (with bowel infarction in one) and genitourinary tract malformations in nine infants (Chasnoff et al., 1985, 1987, 1988, 1989a; MacGregor et al., 1987; Sarpong and Headings, 1992; Sheinbaum and Badell, 1992; Spinazzola et al., 1992; Viscarello et al., 1992), prune belly syndrome with urethral obstruction, bilateral cryptorchidism, absent digits 3 and 4 on the left hand in two infants, and hypospadias, female pseudohermaphroditism, hydronephrosis with ambiguous genitalia and absent uterus and ovaries, anal atresia, clubfoot, limb-body wall complex, limb deficiencies, secondary hypospadias, and bilateral hydronephrosis and unilateral hydronephrosis with renal infarction of the contralateral kidney.

---

### BOX 16.5   CONGENITAL ANOMALIES ASSOCIATED WITH COCAINE USE: VASCULAR DISRUPTION DURING PREGNANCY

- Cardiomegaly
- Horse shoe kidney
- Hypoplastic right heart
- Limb reduction/amputation
- Multiple ventricular septal defects
- Prune belly syndrome with urethral obstruction
- Renal agenesis
- Transverse limb reduction, unilateral
- Unilateral hemimelia (absent right hand and right leg below the knee)
- Ventricular septal defect

**See Appendix I for more complete list.**

---

No congenital abnormalities were observed in four studies of infants born to women who used cocaine during pregnancy (Cherukuri et al., 1988; Doberczak et al., 1988; LeBlanc et al., 1987; Townsend et al., 1988). Among 114 infants born to women who used cocaine during pregnancy, the frequency of congenital anomalies (major or minor) was not increased after controlling for other substances of abuse used and maternal characteristics known to adversely affect pregnancy outcome (Zuckerman *et al.*, 1989).

The bulk of evidence supports the association between prenatal cocaine exposure and isolated major congenital anomalies of vascular origin. Mechanisms of for these malformations is apparently vascular disruption, hypoperfusion, hemorrhage, and vascular occlusion, paralleling the known effects of cocaine on adults. During embryogenesis, effects of vascular resistance and hemodynamics may also affect structural formation.

## COCAINE SYNDROME: PROBABLY NOT ONE

**Does a fetal cocaine syndrome exist? Probably not.** Facial defects among 10 of 11 infants included blepharophimosis, ptosis and facial diplegia, unilateral oro-orbital cleft, Pierre-Robin anomaly, cleft palate, cleft lip and palate, skin tags, and cutis aplasia in a case series of infants exposed to cocaine during gestation (Kobori *et al.*, 1989). All infants had major brain abnormalities (cavitations, holoprosencephaly, porencephaly). Another study reported unusual facies similar to fetal alcohol syndrome in cocaine-exposed infants, and posed the question of whether or not a cocaine syndrome exists (Fries *et al.*, 1993). We found **no evidence of a fetal cocaine syndrome in a matched case-control study** of 50 infants chronically exposed to cocaine prenatally (Little *et al.*, 1996). Fetal growth retardation was the only significant finding in this study.

An increased risk of isolated congenital anomalies exists during the first trimester, and outside the first trimester, but not a classic dysmorphologic syndrome. Investigators reassessed a possible cocaine syndrome and concluded that physical growth deficits were associated with prenatal cocaine exposure. Our earlier study finding was replicated, showing no systematic pattern of congenital anomalies (i.e., a syndrome) characterized children exposed to cocaine prenatally (Minnes *et al.*, 2005). The existence of a fetal cocaine syndrome is not generally accepted.

## PERINATAL DISTRESS AND CEREBROVASCULAR ACCIDENTS WITH PRENATAL COCAINE EXPOSURE

Perinatal complications (tachycardia, bradycardia, respiratory problems, jaundice, elevated bilirubin, etc.) were significantly increased in frequency among infants born to cocaine abusers (Box 16.6). Maternal cocaine use is associated with major neuropathology of the fetus and newborn. The mechanisms of brain injury include vascular accidents or ischemia. The association of cocaine abuse and cerebral palsy has not been published. It is a plausible association given cocaine associated ischemia is known to occur.

---

### BOX 16.6   PERINATAL COMPLICATIONS ASSOCIATED WITH PRENATAL COCAINE EXPOSURE

- Asphyxia
- Bradycardia
- Brain lesions
- Cardiac arrhythmias
- Cerebral ischemia
- Cerebrovascular infarction/hemorrhage
- Congenital heart block
- Congenital infections [syphilis, cytomegalovirus (CMV), human immunodeficiency virus (HIV), hepatitis]

- Decreased cardiac output
- Hyperbilirubinemia
- Increased vascular resistance
- Meconium aspiration syndrome
- Myocardial infarction
- Myocardial ischemia
- Neurobehavioral abnormalities
- Neurovascular ischemia
- Respiratory depression
- Seizures
- Stillbirth
- Tachycardia
- Tachypnea
- Withdrawal symptoms (inconsolable, shrill cry, opisthotonic posturing, hyperirritability, hyperresponsiveness, poor feeding behavior)

*Sources:* Bauer *et al.*, 2005; Chasnoff *et al.*, 1985, 1986, 1987, 1989a; Cherukuri *et al.*, 1988; Dixon and Bejar, 1988, 1989; Dixon and Oro, 1987; Dixon *et al.*, 1987; Doberczak *et al.*, 1988; Geggel *et al.*, 1989; Hadeed and Siegel, 1989; Kapur *et al.*, 1991; Keith *et al.*, 1989; Kobori *et al.*, 1989; Little *et al.*, 1989; MacGregor *et al.*, 1987; Madden *et al.*, 1986; Miller *et al.*, 1995; Neerhof *et al.*, 1989; Oro and Dixon, 1987; Ryan *et al.*, 1986, 1987a, 1987b; Spence *et al.*, 1991; Sztulman *et al.*, 1990; Telsey *et al.*, 1988; Tenorio *et al.*, 1988; van de Bor *et al.*, 1990a, 1990b; Wang and Schnoll, 1987a, 1987b.

## NEUROBEHAVIORAL ABNORMALITIES IN THE PERINATAL PERIOD

Neonates exposed to cocaine *in utero* have significant neurobehavioral impairment in the neonatal period including increased irritability, tremulousness and muscular rigidity, vomiting, diarrhea, seizures, EEG abnormalities, and behavioral abnormalities on the Brazelton Assessment (Chasnoff *et al.*, 1985, 1987, 1989a, 1989b, 1992; Cherukuri *et al.*, 1988; Dixon *et al.*, 1987; Doberczak *et al.*, 1988; Feng, 1993; Kandall, 1988; LeBlanc *et al.*, 1987; Little and Snell, 1991b; Little *et al.*, 1989b; Nair and Watson, 1991; Neerhof *et al.*, 1989; Oro and Dixon, 1987; Ryan *et al.*, 1986, 1987a, 1987b).

## PERINATAL MORTALITY AMONG COCAINE-EXPOSED BABIES

Increased perinatal mortality among cocaine-exposed infants compared to controls was reported (Bauchner *et al.*, 1988; Chasnoff *et al.*, 1987, 1989a; Critchley *et al.*, 1988; Davidson *et al.*, 1986; Kandall *et al.*, 1993; Neerhof *et al.*, 1989; Ryan *et al.*, 1987a, 1987b).

The number of neonatal hospital days was significantly increased among infants born to women who used cocaine during pregnancy (Neerhof *et al.*, 1989). The number of days may be biased because treating physicians had knowledge of prenatal drug exposure status, which could influence discharge decisions.

## POSTNATAL FOLLOW-UP OF INFANTS WHOSE MOTHERS USED COCAINE DURING PREGNANCY

A common finding among prenatally cocaine-exposed infants is growth and development delays and intellectual deficits (Box 16.7).

## BOX 16.7   SUMMARY OF FOLLOW-UP STUDIES OF COCAINE-EXPOSED INFANTS

- Decreased cognitive function (correlated with reduced head circumference)
- Delayed mental and motor development
- Delays in all domains (Fagan test)
- Language development impairments
- Lower IQ
- Lower verbal reasoning
- Mental and psychomotor development delay
- Motor performance deficits
- Poor perseverance
- Reduced height and weight
- School performance poor
- Small head circumference

*Sources:* Angelilli *et al.*, 1994; Azuma and Chasnoff, 1993; Chasnoff *et al.*, 1992; Ernhart *et al.*, 1987; Frank *et al.*, 2005; Griffith *et al.*, 1994; Gross *et al.*, 1991; Hack *et al.*, 1991; Hurt *et al.*, 2005; Lewis *et al.*, 2004a, 2004b; Miller-Loucar *et al.*, 2005; Nulman *et al.*, 1994; Singer *et al.*, 2004; VanBeveren *et al.*, 2000.

### META-ANALYSES: POSTNATAL FOLLOW-UP OF COCAINE-EXPOSED INFANTS

However, other risks (birth defects, low birth weight, prematurity, decreased length, and lower head circumference) can be attributed to polydrug use and to cocaine use in pregnancy (Addis *et al.*, 2001). Meta-analysis of low birth weight and preterm birth in 31 studies showed weight was reduced 492 grams and gestation age was reduced by 1.5 weeks (Gouin *et al.*, 2011). Among 91 infants exposed to cocaine who were followed at 4 to 9 years of age, male IQ was lower by four to six points (abstract reasoning, short term memory, verbal reasoning) on the Stanford-Binet at all ages (Bennett *et al.*, 2008). Meta-analysis of nine cocaine (crack form, smoked) studies included 201 to 1,480 mother-infant dyads found risk of low birth weight, preterm delivery and placental displacement were more than doubled, and odds of small for gestational age was quadrupled (dos Santos *et al.*, 2018). Among 192 cocaine exposed children assessed at 9 years old, perceptual IQ was significantly lowered, but school performance was not affected (Singer *et al.*, 2018).

### ANIMAL MODELS OF COCAINE

Animal models of the possible teratogenicity of cocaine have yielded inconsistent results.

### SUMMARY OF COCAINE DURING PREGNANCY

In summary, the use of cocaine during pregnancy is a risk factor for serious adverse outcomes in mothers, fetuses, and newborns. Cocaine use in pregnancy is compounded by frequent concomitant heavy use of alcohol and illicit drugs. Cocaine during pregnancy is associated with no/very little prenatal care, shorter gestations, premature rupture of membranes, premature labor and delivery, spontaneous abortions, abruptio placentae, decreased uterine blood flow, and maternal/fetal death. Cocaine-exposed fetuses are frequently growth-retarded, suffer perinatal complications, and have an increased mortality risk. Fetal and maternal cerebrovascular accidents are associated with maternal cocaine use in pregnancy. Major congenital anomalies are increased in frequency among cocaine-exposed infants, particularly anomalies of the brain, genitourinary tract, bowel, heart, limbs, and face.

Cocaine use during pregnancy is teratogenic and fetotoxic. The mechanisms of cocaine's adverse effects are vascular disruption and hypoperfusion for gross abnormalities, but molecular level mechanisms are yet to be determined.

## USE OF HALLUCINOGENS DURING PREGNANCY

Psychedelic drugs produce visual hallucinations through a disruption of higher central nervous system function. Most hallucinogens are actually functional analogs of neurotransmitters (e.g., LSD resembles serotonin). Some hallucinogens are assumed to exert their effect by displacing this or other neurotransmitters, but the molecular basis for the action of hallucinogens is not established. Tolerance of hallucinogens is rapidly developed and chronic users must increase doses rapidly over the course of the drug's use to maintain desired effects (Carroll, 1990).

Hallucinogens or psychedelic drugs are not nearly as popular in 2006 as they were 30 or so years ago. Less than 2 percent of the general population uses psychedelic drugs, based upon data that are not partitioned by sex, ethnicity, or pregnancy status. Among pregnant women at a large urban hospital in Dallas, Texas, it is estimated that approximately 1 percent used psychedelic drugs (LSD, mescaline, psilocybin) during gestation.

### Specific Hallucinogens

### Lysergic Acid Diethylamide

Lysergic acid amides or lysergides, including LSD (lysergic acid diethylamide) are amine alkaloids obtained only through chemical syntheses and have a variety of street names. Under medical supervision, lysergide and ergotamine are used to treat psychiatric illness. A closely related drug. LSD stimulates the sympathetic nervous system, often producing increased heart rate and blood pressure, and a rise in body temperature. Recreational LSD also has powerful hallucinogenic effects. Hallucinations usually last 8–36 hours, depending upon LSD dose and formulation. Published studies of LSD use during pregnancy are uncontrolled and involve medically unsupervised administration of this drug class. Clinical experiments in non-pregnant adults are published.

Birth defects in infants born to women who used LSD before or during pregnancy show no consistent pattern of anomalies, and are highly heterogeneous (Cohen and Shiloh, 1977/78; Long, 1972). Congenital anomalies reportedly associated with maternal LSD exposure are unlikely caused by LSD use drug during pregnancy. Limb reduction defects were the most frequently reported congenital anomaly type among LSD exposed infants. Limb reduction defect types lacked a pattern. Eight infants had a heterogeneous group of congenital anomalies among 86 infants born to women who used LSD at undetermined times during gestation, (Jacobson and Berlin, 1972). Five exposed infants had central nervous system defects, but only two were exposed to LSD during embryogenesis (2/86 or 2.3 percent). No convincing evidence is published that LSD is causes birth defects. LSD use is associated with polydrug use and lifestyle practices probably harmful to intrauterine development (e.g., tobacco and alcohol use).

Three groups of investigators reported increased frequencies of chromosomal breakage in somatic cells of individuals who used LSD (Cohen and Shiloh, 1977/78; Hulten *et al.*, 1968; Long, 1972), but other researchers reported no increased frequency of chromosome breakage. Importantly, chromosomal aberrations in somatic cells are not clinically relevant to risks of congenital anomalies in the children of parents who used LSD. Somatic cell chromosomal abnormalities are not heritable.

Illegally produced LSD may contain lysergic acid with no amination, and can cause peripheral neuropathy, gangrene, and necrosis, resembling toxic shock syndrome. Toxic human exposures to lysergic acid are rare. Peripheral neuropathy, gangrene, and necrosis were observed among cattle and sheep that consumed wheat grain infected with the fungus *Claviceps pupurea*, which produces lysergic acid. LSD produced illegally has no quality control or routine assurance measures are taken to assure LSD purity, as is the case with most illegal drugs,

## MESCALINE

Mescaline is a naturally occurring hallucinogenic alkaloid that is concentrated in the 'buttons' of the peyote cactus, *Lophophora williamsii*. Mescaline also occurs in the San Pedro cactus (*Trichocereus pachanoi*) and the Peruvian torch (*Trichocereus peruvianus*). Flattened, dried seedpods from these cacti are called "peyote buttons" or simply "peyote." Buttons are ingested for recreational use. Members of the Native American Church may use mescaline legally in their religious rituals and ceremonies. Naturally occurring mescaline is often contaminated with strychnine, which may heighten the excitement sensation. Mescaline from natural sources is associated with severe nausea and vomiting. Mescaline is available from chemical synthesis. Mescaline effects are similar to LSD effects, but some mescaline users report much more vivid and intense hallucinations. Auditory hallucinations are reported with mescaline but not with LSD. The hallucinogenic effects usually last about 12 hours, but some users report much longer (20–40 hours) periods of hallucination, probably depending mainly upon dose and drug concentration.

No studies of mescaline use during organogenesis and congenital anomalies in infants born to mothers who used mescaline during pregnancy are published. A case report of an infant with a birth defect with ritual peyote use was reported, but causality cannot be inferred from a report (Gilmore, 2001). Neural tube defects were increased in frequency among the offspring of hamsters whose mothers were given mescaline during pregnancy at 10 percent to 20 percent the usual human dose, but the frequency of birth defects was not dose related (Geber, 1967). Neonatal weight was decreased among hamsters born to mothers injected with mescaline during pregnancy (Geber and Schramm, 1974). Importantly, no neural tube defects were found in animal studies by other investigators who employed doses three to six times the usual human recreational dose (Hirsch and Fritz, 1981). An increased frequency of intrauterine death was found in animal studies of mescaline exposure in early pregnancy.

## PSILOCYBIN

Psilocybin is a naturally occurring hallucinogenic alkaloid present in several species of psychedelic mushrooms belonging to the genus *Psilocybe*. *P. mexicana* is the classic source of the drug and is known as the magic mushroom. It is most commonly found in Mexico, particularly in the Valley of Oaxaca, and southern Texas. However, other species occur north of Mexico in the southern United States and elsewhere, particularly in dairy pastures in the spring. Psilocybin typically grows in highly organic media, such as cow feces (cow patties) and usually in the springtime. Psilocybin mushrooms are eaten, used as a food additive, a tea, or a drink additive for hallucinogenic effects. The hallucinogenic effects usually last six to eight hours, although some sources quote times as short as an hour. Ingestion of these hallucinogenic mushrooms has become a popular form of substance abuse among some adolescents and young adults (Schwartz and Smith, 1988). The effects of psilocybin ingestion include hallucinogenic visions, altered states of consciousness, and a pronounced pyrogenic effect. Several surveys have indicated that mushroom use is more prevalent among high school and college students than is the LSD use.

The frequency of congenital anomalies in the offspring of mothers who ingested psilocybin during pregnancy has not been published for human studies or animal experiments. Psilocybin crosses the rat placenta and reaches concentrations close to maternal levels in the fetal compartment (Law *et al.*, 2014).

## SUMMARY OF HALLUCINOGENS

Hallucinogen use during pregnancy is studied and unknown risks may exist. Purported association of LSD with limb defects in children born to women who used LSD during pregnancy is probably not causal. The pyrogenic effects of hallucinogens and nonmedical use of other substances are cause for concern in use of these agents during pregnancy. Note: the basis for concerns about birth defects and hallucinogen use during pregnancy are theoretical because published information does not exist on which to make evidence-based conclusions.

## OPIATE ABUSE DURING PREGNANCY

Opiates are a class of drugs with sedative and analgesic effects derived from white, milky secretions of the flower bud of the opium poppy plant (*Papaver somniferum*). Medically, opiates are used to treat moderate to severe pain. Synthetic opioids are also available (e.g., meperidine). Opiates (natural and synthetic) are pharmacological narcotics, not to be confused with the legally defined narcotic class that includes such nonnarcotic drugs as marijuana, amphetamines, and methamphetamines. Narcotics include opium, morphine, oxycodone, codeine, meperidine, paperavine, thebaine, and heroin. Opiates act on opioid receptors to produce analgesia and euphoria. A severe opiate withdrawal syndrome occurs after discontinuation of chronic use, medical or illicit. Importantly, withdrawal occurs in adults and neonates chronically exposed to these opiates. An increasingly more common source of opiates for abuse is prescription drugs such as oxycodone and hydrocodone, obtained either legally or illegally.

Methadone is a synthetic opioid analog and is used as an alternative to heroin in abuse, and as a treatment. Fentanyl is sometimes used to cut heroin. Fentanyl is 40 to 100 times more potent than opiates, and are associated with a high proportion of opiate overdose deaths. Fortunately, naloxone is the antidote to fentanyl. An intranasal form is available for use in emergency out of hospital resuscitation.

### HEROIN

Heroin is a narcotic analgesic available in many countries (e.g., UK), but it cannot be prescribed in the USA (i.e., is a schedule I drug). Heroin abuse occurs worldwide. Most population studies report the prevalence of heroin use during pregnancy is 2 to 5 percent. In the Netherlands where illegal drug use is tolerated, an estimated 20 percent of adults use heroin. Among pregnant women in Dallas at a large public hospital, 2.5 percent reported using heroin (unpublished data).

Studies of heroin use during pregnancy are of illicit use only. The health effects of heroin use are confounded because users often abuse other drugs (alcohol, cocaine), use tobacco, and have poor health and nutritional status. Heroin purity, dose, frequency, duration, and trimesters of use are usually unknown in studies of drug use during pregnancy. Notably, prescription use of opioids during pregnancy was significantly associated with birth defects (Chapter 8).

Several investigators reported the frequency of congenital anomalies was not increased among infants born to heroin-addicted mothers compared to the rate expected among infants born in the general population (Kandall *et al.*, 1977; Little *et al.*, 1990e; Naeye *et al.*, 1973; Stimmel and Adamsons, 1976; Stone *et al.*, 1971). No pattern of congenital anomalies was found among infants born to heroin users (Rothstein and Gould, 1974). A large cohort study (830 heroin-exposed infants) found heroin abuse in pregnancy was associated with an increased frequency of congenital anomalies (3.5 percent) compared to controls (Ostrea and Chavez, 1979). However, the significant finding was because of a non-representative control sample with an unrealistically low frequency of congenital anomalies among control group infants (0.5 percent). Recall from Chapter 1 that the background rate is 3.5–5 percent in human populations. Among 890 infants with neonatal abstinence syndrome (NAS-withdrawal) and 4250 infants with major congenital anomalies, neonates with a birth defect were 1.9 times more likely to have a malformation than those without NAS (Fornoff and Sandidge, 2021). This aligns with the finding that opiate analgesia is associated with an increased frequency of birth defects (See Chapter 8). Frequencies of acquired chromosomal aberrations in peripheral blood lymphocytes were elevated above background frequency in narcotic addicts (Amarose and Norusis, 1976; Kushnick *et al.*, 1972). These findings were replicated in infants of narcotic-addicted women in one study (Amarose and Norusis, 1976), but not in another (Kushnick *et al.*, 1972). Aberrations in somatic cells and risks to reproduction are not related. Hepatides (B and C) and sexually transmitted infections (syphilis, HIV, gonorrhea) are correlated with intravenous drug abuse IVDA and occur with increased frequency among pregnant heroin addicts and infants (Perez-Bescos *et al.*, 1993). Birth weight and other growth measures (head circumference, birth length) are consistently decreased among infants born to heroin addicts compared to drug-free controls (Fricker and Segal, 1978; Kandall *et al.*, 1977; Lam *et al.*, 1992; Lifschitz *et al.*, 1983; Little *et al.*, 1990a, e; Oleske, 1977; Zelson *et al.*, 1971). Miscarriages, perinatal death, and a variety of perinatal complications were increased in frequency among heroin-exposed children (Fricker and Segal, 1978; Kandall *et al.*, 1977; Lifschitz *et al.*, 1983; Little *et al.*, 1990e; Oleske, 1977, Zelson *et al.*, 1971). Fetal exposure to heroin is confounded by the generally poor health and nutritional status of heroin-using mothers.

Child postnatal growth in height and weight of those exposed to heroin prenatally seems normal compared to controls and reference data (Little *et al.*, 1991a), except for head circumference. It was smaller among heroin exposed children compared to children not exposed to heroin prenatally in several studies (Chasnoff *et al.*, 1986; Lifschitz *et al.*, 1985). As noted for all substances of abuse discussed in this chapter, heroin crosses the placenta freely, with fetal drug concentrations quickly reaching maternal levels. Importantly, if the mother is heroin addicted, her fetus is also addicted. Heroin (opiates) rapidly crosses the placenta and enters fetal circulation. Neonatal withdrawal symptoms (tremors, irritability, jitteriness, diarrhea, seizures, poor feeding, high-pitched, shrill cry, irregular sleep patterns, sneezing, respiratory distress, fever, vomiting) occur among 40–80 percent of infants born to heroin-using gravidas (Alroomi *et al.*, 1988; Fricker and Segal, 1978; Kandall *et al.*, 1977; Rothstein and Gould, 1974). Withdrawal symptoms may present shortly after birth, or take from 6 to 10 days to develop. This depends on the time needed for the infant to metabolize heroin present at birth to a no effect level. Opiate withdrawal symptoms can have prolonged duration, persisting for less than 3 weeks. Treatment is sometimes with tincture of opium (paregoric) in downward tapering doses to avoid introducing additional addictive drug exposures to the neonate.

Ultimately, postnatal environment is the apparent major determinant of postnatal cognitive and behavioral development in heroin exposed infants (Ornoy *et al.*, 1996; van Baar and de Graff, 1994; van Baar *et al.*, 1994). Postnatal environment seems to be the major influence on postnatal infant/child development for most substances of abuse, except alcohol and perhaps cocaine.

## METHADONE

Methadone is a synthetic opiate narcotic structurally similar to propoxyphene. Methadone is principally used medically is as opiate maintenance therapy for heroin addiction. It is also used illegally as a substitute for heroin. No studies of methadone abuse are published. Published studies include only pregnant women on regimented-dose maintenance therapy in treatment who took methadone of known pharmacological purity.

Congenital anomalies were not increased in frequency compared to the background rate among infants born to heroin-addicted women treated with methadone during pregnancy (Fundaro *et al.*, 1994; Kempley, 1995; Soepatmi, 1994; Stimmel and Adamsons, 1976; van Baar *et al.*, 1994; Vering *et al.*, 1992). Methadone infant withdrawal symptoms occurred frequently (up to 80 percent) and birth weights were significantly lower (2,600 g) than drug unexposed infants among methadone-exposed infants (n=278) (Connaughton *et al.*, 1977). Neonatal complications occurred at a high frequency, and included: asphyxia neonatorum, transient tachypnea, aspiration pneumonia, congenital syphilis, jaundice, meconium staining, and neonatal death. Adverse maternal effects associated with heroin addiction include prolonged rupture of membranes, breech presentation, abruptio placentae, preeclampsia, and postpartum hemorrhage (Naeye *et al.*, 1973). An unusually high frequency of sudden infant death syndrome (SIDS) (17) occurred among infants in a group of 688 drug-using mothers followed (Chavez *et al.*, 1979). 14 of 17 SIDS infants were born to mothers who were enrolled in a methadone treatment program, but continued other drug use. Effects of methadone maintenance during pregnancy on neonatal outcome indicate two consistent findings across studies: withdrawal symptoms (70–90 percent) and lowered gestational age (two to four weeks) and birth weight (600 g to 900 g) of infants in the drug-exposed group compared to a control group (Behnke and Eyler, 1993).

## TREATMENT OF OPIATE DEPENDENCE DURING PREGNANCY

Medically assisted treatment of opiate addiction includes four preparations: (1) Buprenorphine, (2) methadone, (3) naltrexone, and (4) buprenorphine and naloxone. Opiate withdrawal during pregnancy remains controversial. Dose tapering to avoid withdrawal perinatally optimizes neonatal and maternal outcomes if there is sufficient gestation time and patient cooperation.

## DEVELOPMENTAL OUTCOMES OF HEROIN- AND/OR METHADONE-EXPOSED CHILDREN

Children prenatally exposed to heroin- and methadone achieved lower scores than unexposed comparison groups in motor coordination, attention and focus, and activity level domains. Abnormal behavior, emotional disturbances, and behavioral problems (aggression, anxiety, and rejection) were increased in in frequency in the prenatal opiate-exposed group (Behnke and Eyler, 1993; Davis and Templer, 1988; De Cubas and Field, 1993; Deren, 1986; Kaltenbach and Finnegan, 1984; Wilson *et al.*, 1979). Meta-analysis of 26 studies including 1455 children exposed to opiates of abuse prenatally indicated cognitive scores were significantly lower for younger (6 months–6 years.) and not older children. Motor development was delayed in all ages in the opiate exposed group (Yeoh *et al.*, 2019), but delays were mild-moderate.

## SUMMARY OF OPIATES DURING PREGNANCY

Opiate abuse during pregnancy seemingly does not significantly increase the risk of congenital anomalies, but prescription opiate use during early pregnancy is associated with an increased frequency of congenital anomalies (see Chapter 8). Adverse pregnancy outcomes among opiate abusers increased in frequency include abruptio placentae, neonatal withdrawal, preterm birth, and fetal growth retardation. Differences were found in cognitive abilities, motor development and behavior between opiate-exposed children and nondrug-exposed children. Postnatal environment for a child with a drug-abusing mother must be considered in such studies because the environment is a very important factor. Maternal personality traits, degrees of life stress, the quality of the mother-child relationship, and assessment of the health and nutritional environment must be considered.

# INHALANT (ORGANIC SOLVENT) ABUSE DURING PREGNANCY

## EPIDEMIOLOGY

Use of inhalants during pregnancy is 1 percent, somewhat lower than other substances of abuse (for example, cocaine, marijuana, and tobacco). Inhalants included toluene, spray paint, gasoline, freon, and other organic solvent substances during pregnancy (Madry *et al.*, 1991). Women who use inhalants during pregnancy are primarily Hispanic or American Indian, with an age range of 15–29 years (Goodwin, 1988; Wilkins-Haug and Gabow, 1991).

## FETAL SOLVENT SYNDROME

The "fetal solvent syndrome" was observed among infants born to women who "huffed" or "sniffed" toluene, gasoline, benzene, and other aromatic liquids during pregnancy. The solvent syndrome is associated with prenatal growth retardation (low birth weight, microcephaly), dysmorphic facial features (facies) that similar to FAS, and digital malformations (short phalanges, nail hypoplasia). Gravidas who use a substance of abuse during pregnancy, including inhalants, frequently use other substances, including alcohol (ethanol). This makes it difficult to attribute effects to a single causative agent. Case reports support an independent inhalant syndrome such as toluene or gasoline, independently of concurrent use of other substances of abuse. Anecdotal evidence suggests that the fetal solvent syndrome is associated with significant mental retardation, IQs less than 70. Occupational exposure to organic solvents cannot be compared to inhalant abuse because doses in occupational exposure are much lower. A total of 14 cases of CNS abnormalities in infants whose mothers abused organic solvents during pregnancy were reported in Finnish health registry (Holmberg, 1979).

## ANIMAL STUDIES

The frequency of congenital anomalies was not increased among rats whose mothers were exposed to high levels of toluene, but growth retardation was observed (Gospe *et al.*, 1994; Ono *et al.*, 1995). Forebrain cell counts were reduced by 15 percent in offspring whose mothers were exposed to toluene during pregnancy, including organogenesis (Gospe *et al.*, 1994). Among rat pups whose mother were exposed to binge toluene exposure during pregnancy, birth weight and developmental milestones were significantly delayed compared to controls (Bowen *et al.*, 2005).

## SPECIFIC INHALANTS

### Gasoline

Gasoline is a fuel mixture of volatile hydrocarbon and aromatic compounds, sometimes containing tetraethyl lead, methanol, and other agents. Gasoline is sometimes "sniffed" or "huffed" by inhalant abusers to produce a euphoric effect. Acute poisoning by gasoline is associated with pneumonitis, shock, cardiac arrhythmias, convulsions, coma, and death.

Two infants in a published case report had profound mental retardation, neurological dysfunction, and minor dysmorphic features ("fetal gasoline syndrome") born to women who had abused gasoline by inhalation throughout pregnancy (Hunter *et al.*, 1979). It has not been possible to assess a causal relationship based upon two children in a case report, but features are similar to the fetal solvent syndrome.

### Toluene

Toluene is an aromatic organic solvent found in paint thinner, printing liquids, and adhesives. Toluene is a substance of abuse used by "huffing" or "sniffing." It produces a euphoric effect. In non-pregnant adults, toluene use is associated with organic brain syndrome and cerebral atrophy (Allison and Jerrom, 1984; Cooper *et al.*, 1985; Filley *et al.*, 1990; King, 1982; Larsen and Leira, 1988; Lowenstein, 1985; Pearson *et al.*, 1994). Adult brain damage parallels the damage associated with toluene exposure *in utero*.

Unusual dysmorphic features described in three children who were born to women who frequently inhaled large amounts of toluene throughout pregnancy suggest a ***toluene embryopathy*** (Hersch, 1989; Hersch *et al.*, 1985). Toluene associated dysmorphic features are strikingly similar to FAS (Pearson *et al.*, 1994). Among 35 infants with the toluene embryopathy phenotype, 42 percent were premature, 52 percent had low birth weight, and 32 percent were microcephalic. Postnatally, they were below the fifth percentile for all measures postnatally for physical and neurodevelopment milestones. Most had dysmorphic facies (Arnold *et al.*, 1994). Preterm delivery, perinatal death, and prenatal growth retardation are associated with toluene huffing during pregnancy (Wilkins-Haug and Gabow, 1991). Two cases of renal tubular dysfunction and metabolic acidosis (including hyperchloremic acidosis and aminoaciduria) were recently reported in infants whose mothers chronically abused inhalants containing toluene (Lindemann, 1991). Childhood growth and development were also significantly delayed among toluene-exposed infants (Wilkins-Haug and Gabow, 1991), and has typical signs of the toluene embryopathy at follow up (Arnold *et al.*, 1994). Four of five neonates born to women who abused toluene during pregnancy had low birth weight (<2500 g), but only one had a congenital anomaly (Goodwin, 1988).

## SUMMARY OF SOLVENTS DURING PREGNANCY

Solvent huffing or sniffing during pregnancy poses significant, irreversible risks to the pregnancy and the developing embryofetus. A fetal solvent syndrome probably exists and consists of dysmorphic facial features, severe growth retardation, and developmental delay (below the fifth percentile). Maternal distal renal tubular acidosis and hyperchloremic metabolic acidosis should be expected in solvent using pregnant women, and may precipitate preterm labor. Toluene toxicity predicts premature labor. Fetal/neonatal metabolic acidosis (arterial pH less than or equal to 7.0), respiratory difficulties, and renal function abnormalities were observed, in addition to the usual complications of prematurity.

## Tobacco Use in Pregnancy

Native Americans grew and smoked tobacco in pre-Columbian times. However, tobacco native to North America is not the tobacco used today because it was too bitter to be smoked or chewed alone, and was mixed with a variety of other substances for use, including willow bark, mushrooms, and wild lettuce. The tobacco, *Nicotiana tabacum*, is widely used by smoking, chewing, or dipping, and is a hybrid of South and North American species. Tobacco smoke comprises several-hundred different chemicals, including nicotine and carbon monoxide in greatest abundance. There are several thousands of publications on the risks of tobacco use during pregnancy, including extensive reviews (Fredricsson and Gilljam, 1992; Landesman-Dwyer and Emanuel, 1979; McIntosh, 1984a, 1984b; Nash and Persaud, 1988; Rosenberg, 1987; Stillman *et al.*, 1986; Streissguth, 1986; Surgeon General, 1979).

Approximately 15–20 percent of pregnant women smoke tobacco (Rantakallio *et al.*, 1995; Vega *et al.*, 1993). The earliest finding among pregnant smokers was increased frequencies of prematurity (estimated by lowered birth weight) (Simpson, 1957). Later investigations confirmed the association of tobacco smoking and decreased birth weight (Herriot *et al.*, 1962; Lowe, 1959; Ravenholt and Lerinski, 1965). Lowered birth weight was later determined to be due to intrauterine growth retardation, and not due to prematurity (Rubin *et al.*, 1986).

## LOW BIRTH WEIGHT

Several hundred thousand women who smoked during pregnancy have been studied (Cnattingius *et al.*, 1993; Fox *et al.*, 1994; Hjortdal *et al.*, 1989; McIntosh, 1984a; Stillman *et al.*, 1986). Lowered birth weight was definitely associated with maternal tobacco smoking during pregnancy. Smoking more heavily during pregnancy results in infants that are more growth retarded. In addition, passive exposure to tobacco smoke was associated with reduced birth weight (Bardy *et al.*, 1993; Fortier *et al.*, 1994; Haddow *et al.*, 1989, 1993; Martinez *et al.*, 1994; Mathai *et al.*, 1992; Ogawa *et al.*, 1991; Rebagliato *et al.*, 1995; Seidman and Mashiach, 1991; Day *et al.*, 1994; Jacobson *et al.*, 1994). Importantly, birth weight was unaffected in infants whose mothers ceased smoking early in pregnancy (i.e., during the early second trimester) (Ahlsten *et al.*, 1993; Li *et al.*, 1993; Olsen, 1992). Meta-analysis of 210 studies (of 13,189 studies) of tobacco smoking during pregnancy indicate small for gestational age infants was significantly increased in frequency (Quelhas *et al.*, 2018).

## INTELLECTUAL DEVELOPMENT AND BEHAVIOR

Very mild, insignificant reductions in IQ (1–5 points) were found among children whose mothers smoked during pregnancy (Davie *et al.*, 1972; Dunn *et al.*, 1977; Fried, 1989, 1992, 1993; Fried *et al.*, 1992; Olds *et al.*, 1994; Rush and Callahan, 1989). However, socioeconomic status (SES) and maternal education were lower among women who smoked.

## BIRTH DEFECTS

The possibility that tobacco is a teratogen was been analyzed in hundreds of epidemiological studies, involving over one million children (McIntosh, 1984a; Stillman *et al.*, 1986; Hackshaw *et al.*, 2011). Major congenital anomalies are generally not increased in frequency among mothers who smoke tobacco during pregnancy (Andrews and McGarry, 1972; Christianson, 1980; Erickson, 1991; Evans *et al.*, 1979; Hemminki *et al.*, 1983; Kullander and Kallen, 1976; Malloy *et al.*, 1989; Pradat, 1992; Seidman *et al.*, 1990; Shiono *et al.*, 1986; Tikkanen and Heinonen, 1991, 1992, 1993; Van Den Eeden *et al.*, 1990; Werler *et al.*, 1990, 1992).

Some investigators found significant associations between cigarette smoking and birth defects, such as craniosynostosis (Alderman *et al.*, 1994). A non-specific collection of birth defects (gastroschisis, limb reduction defects, strabismus, and congenital heart disease) was increased in frequency among infants born to pregnant smokers (Aro, 1983; Christianson, 1980; Czeizel *et al.*, 1994; Fedrick *et al.*, 1971; Goldbaum *et al.*, 1990; Haddow *et al.*, 1993; Hakim and Tielsch, 1992; Himmelberger *et al.*, 1978). Cleft palate and orofacial clefts were increased in frequency among offspring of smokers (Andrews and McGarry, 1972; Ericson *et al.*, 1979; Hwang *et al.*, 1995; Khoury *et al.*, 1989; Shaw *et al.*, 1996), but not all large studies found an association (Frazier *et al.*, 1961; Lowe, 1959; Underwood *et al.*, 1965; Yerushalmy, 1964). One study found no association with maternal tobacco smoking among 288 067 infants, of whom 10 223 had congenital anomalies (Malloy *et al.*, 1989). Among 67 609 pregnancies, an increased frequency of anencephalic infants was found in infants whose mothers who smoked heavily during gestation (greater than 20 cigarettes per day) (Evans *et al.*, 1979). White cigarette smokers gave birth to anencephalic infants at 1.72 per 1,000, while White non-smokers had a rate of 1.0 per 1,000 (Naeye, 1978). Black women who smoke during pregnancy have a lower rate of anencephaly than do White women. No association with maternal smoking was found for anencephaly among Black women.

Meta-analysis of 173 687 birth defects cases and 11.7 million controls showed that birth defects were significantly increased in frequency (Hackshaw *et al.*, 2011). Specific birth defects included: cardiovascular/heart defects (OR = 1.09), musculoskeletal defects (OR = 1.16), limb reduction defects (OR = 1.26), missing/extra digits (OR = 1.18); clubfoot (OR 1.28); craniosynostosis (OR = 1.33); facial defects (OR = 1.19), eye defects (OR = 1.25), orofacial clefts (OR = 1.28), gastrointestinal defects (OR = 1.27) gastroschisis (OR = 1.50), anal atresia (OR = 1.20), hernia (OR = 1.40) and undescended testes (OR = 1.13). Notably, hernia and undescended testes are associated with preterm delivery.

## CHILDHOOD CANCER

Very weak evidence suggests that cancer during childhood is associated with *in utero* exposure to maternal tobacco smoke (McKinney *et al.*, 1986; Schwartzbaum, 1992; Stjernfeldt *et al.*, 1986). Associations are equivocal and other studies contradict the findings (Gold *et al.*, 1993; John *et al.*, 1991; McCredie *et al.*, 1994; Pershagen, 1989; Pershagen *et al.*, 1992). Among >785,000 children, childhood acute myeloid leukemia and fibrosarcoma were weakly associated with tobacco smoke exposure prenatally (Auger *et al.*, 2019). In 19 case-control studies, maternal smoking before, during, or after pregnancy was not significantly associated with childhood ALL or AML (Chunxia *et al.*, 2019).

## PREGNANCY COMPLICATIONS

Premature rupture of membranes was increased among women who smoked during pregnancy (Underwood *et al.*, 1965). Abruptio placentae, placenta previa, and amniotic infections were increased among gravidas who were heavy smokers (Naeye, 1979). Smoking during pregnancy was a risk factor for spontaneous abortion, pregnancy toxicosis, premature delivery, and chronic fetal hypoxia (Sheveleva *et al.*, 1986). Preterm delivery, placenta previa, perinatal mortality, and other complications of pregnancy were increased in frequency among women who smoke (English and Eskenzai, 1992; Guinn *et al.*, 1994; Handler *et al.*, 1994; Little and Weinberg, 1993; McIntosh, 1984b; Meis *et al.*, 1995; Raymond and Mills, 1993; Stillman *et al.*, 1986; Wilcox, 1993).

Meta-analysis of 991 publications that included 9,094,443 participants found an association between maternal smoking during pregnancy and placenta previa (OR=1.42) (Shobeiri *et al.*, 2017a). Another meta-analysis (1,167 publications, 4,309,610 participants) found that smoking during pregnancy is associated with an increased risk of abruptio placenta (OR=1.80) (Shobeiri *et al.*, 2017b).

## ANIMAL STUDIES

Nicotine and cigarette smoking in animals has also been studied and reduced fetal weight was found. Notably, a very early study showed that rabbits exposed to the equivalent of 20 cigarettes per day gave birth to fetuses that were 7 percent lighter than controls (Schoeneck, 1941).

## SUMMARY OF TOBACCO DURING PREGNANCY

Tobacco smoke adversely affects pregnancy, and even passive tobacco smoke exposure negatively affects fetal growth. However, catch-up growth in the neonatal period was observed, and at least partly compensates for fetal growth retardation in children born to active smokers.

# PHENCYCLIDINE USE IN PREGNANCY

PCP of phencyclidine is recreationally used orally, intravenously, intranasally, or smoked. It was formerly used as an anesthetic and analgesic in humans but mainly veterinary medicine. Ketamine is usually used instead of PCP currently.

The frequency of congenital anomalies was not increased above background risk (3.5–5 percent) among 57 infants whose mothers took PCP during pregnancy, including the first trimester, (Wachsman *et al.*, 1989). Congenital anomalies were not increased in frequency in 131 infants exposed to PCP in the first trimester in two controlled studies (Golden *et al.*, 1987; Tabor *et al.*, 1990). A case report was published of an infant with intracerebral abnormalities who was exposed to PCP during gestation (Michael *et al.*, 1982), but case reports have no causal meaning. Birth weights and head circumferences were growth delayed in another report; >40 percent of PCP-exposed infants were <10th percentile for reference data (Lubchenco *et al.*, 1966). A one-year postnatal follow-up for 36 infants exposed to PCP *in utero* showed 24 percent of children were <10th percentile for growth standards (Wachsman *et al.*, 1989). In another investigation, low birth weight and microcephaly were increased in frequency among 505 infants exposed to cocaine and PCP during gestation (Rahbar *et al.*, 1993).

Withdrawal symptoms (tremors, jitteriness, irritability) were observed in approximately 50 percent of infants exposed prenatally to PCP (Wachsman *et al.*, 1989), but none of seven infants in another case series (Chasnoff *et al.*, 1983a).

## SUMMARY OF PCP IN PREGNANCY

Phencyclidine is associated with fetal growth retardation and withdrawal symptoms, but the frequency of birth defects is apparently not increased.

## USE OF Ts AND BLUES IN PREGNANCY

Ts and blues is pentazocine (Talwin) mixed with an antihistamine, and was used as a heroin substitute in the early 1970s to 1980s. It may no longer be used to any detectable extent. "Ts and blues" is a street mixture of pentazocine (Talwin) and OTC antihistamine tripelennamine (Pyribenzamine). Pentazocine is a synthetic narcotic analgesic given medically by parenteral, oral, or rectal routes to relieve moderate to severe pain. In inner city Chicago in the early 1970s, pentazocine street combinations were in wide use because it was a "high" similar to heroin but much less expensive (Senay, 1985).

Limited data on were reported for 86 infants born to women who used Ts and blues during pregnancy (n = 13, 50, and 23) (Chasnoff *et al.*, 1983b; Little *et al.*, 1990f; von Almen and Miller, 1984, respectively). Ts and blues exposed infants have fetal growth retardation, an increased frequency of perinatal complications (withdrawal, infection, low birth weight) compared to controls (Chasnoff *et al.*, 1983b; Little *et al.*, 1990f; von Almen and Miller, 1984). Congenital anomalies were not increased among these 86 infants (Chasnoff *et al.*, 1983b; Little *et al.*, 1990f; von Almen and Miller, 1984).

Non-medicinal use of pentazocine during pregnancy in 39 infants whose mothers used the drug showed: 21 percent were premature, 31 percent growth retarded, 11 percent (four children) had major congenital anomalies, and withdrawal symptoms were seen in 28 percent (DeBooy *et al.*, 1993). Five of 19 (26 percent) had failure to thrive. Eight were removed from birth mothers and placed in foster care because of abuse and neglect. Of twenty-one children who were given intelligence tests, 17 (81 percent) scored within the normal range (IQ>85) and four children (19 percent) scored subnormal (IQ=70 to 84) range. No pentazocine-exposed children received a scored <70. These types of findings are difficult to assess because of other factors in the drug abusers' life style (poor diet, lack of prenatal care, and concomitant use of other substances of abuse, especially alcohol) contributed to low birth weight and other untoward outcomes among infants born to Ts and blues abusers observed by several investigators. Infants born to women who chronically used pentazocine in had transient neonatal withdrawal symptoms (Goetz and Bain, 1974; Kopelman, 1975; Scanlon, 1974) similar to those in neonatal withdrawal from other narcotics: irritability, hyperactivity, vomiting, high-pitched cry, fever, and diarrhea.

Another Ts and blues combination is also used, Talwin (pentazocine) and Ritalin (methylphenidate) (Carter and Watson, 1994). It was anecdotally associated with fetal growth retardation, but not birth defects (Debooy *et al.*, 1993). As with the Ts and blues mixture, alcohol abuse is highly prevalent, and FAS features are often observed in offspring exposed to this heroin substitute.

### Ts AND BLUES SUMMARY

This drug combination is rare in 2021, and unlikely to be encountered. Ts and blues use during pregnancy is associated with fetal growth retardation and withdrawal symptoms, maternal complications such as pulmonary thromboembolic disease and placental infarcts which may occur secondary to intravenous injection of tablet vehicle (microcrystalline cellulose). Infants born to Ts and blues users are at increased risk for fetal alcohol syndrome because most users of this drug combination drink alcohol heavily (> 6 drinks per day).

### Polydrug Use during Pregnancy

Pregnant women who use one substance of abuse frequently use two or more substances of abuse. Substances frequently used together include (1) cocaine, tobacco/marijuana, and alcohol, (2) heroin, tobacco/marijuana, and alcohol, (3) methamphetamine, alcohol, and tobacco/marijuana (4) hallucinogen, tobacco/marijuana, and alcohol, (5) cocaine, heroin, tobacco/marijuana, and alcohol.

Among 174 pregnant women who abused drugs during their pregnancies, 83 percent had some prenatal care. Heroin users were significantly older (28.3 years) than cocaine users (24.8 years) or methamphetamine users (23.4 years) (Little *et al.*, 1990e), and these patterns persist in 2017 (SAMHSA, 2017).

Polydrug use (more than one social/illicit drug) was reported by 130 (75 percent) of pregnant women studied. Other than tobacco, alcohol and cocaine were the most frequently used secondary and tertiary drugs. Alcohol and/or cocaine use during pregnancy differed considerably by primary drug of abuse. Heroin users drank alcohol 5.2-fold more often, respectively, than gravidas who abused methamphetamine. Heroin abusers used cocaine 8.9 times more frequently than abusers of methamphetamine or Ts and blues. Heroin abusers used alcohol plus cocaine 5.2-fold, respectively, more frequently than methamphetamine abusers.

Concomitant use of several substances of abuse that have teratogenic potential poses serious risks for mother and fetus. Growth retardation appears to be more severe, and the frequency of congenital anomalies increased in the offspring of mothers who abuse multiple substances (Oro and Dixon, 1987), especially when one of those substances is alcohol. The primarily intravenous use of these drugs increases the risk of maternal HIV infection and vertical transmission of this and other blood borne illnesses.

Heroin and cocaine users (and Ts and blues users) are also at high risk for birth defects attributable to alcohol abuse. Heroin abusers used cocaine significantly more frequently than abusers of any other drug, probably because of the popularity of a mixture called "speedball" (cocaine and heroin, and occasionally methamphetamine). Infants born to heroin abusers are 8.9-fold greater risk for cocaine-induced damage than those born to abusers of other drugs because of polydrug use. Infants born to Ts and blues abusers are at a three to 14 times greater risk of alcohol-induced damage to the embryo or fetus compared infants born to abusers of other drugs of abuse such as methamphetamine or cocaine (Little *et al.*, 1990f).

It is widely known that alcohol is a leading preventable (teratogenic) cause of birth defects (Abel and Sokol, 1987; Jones *et al.*, 1973). Cocaine is a likely teratogen (Chasnoff *et al.*, 1988; Little and Snell, 1991b; Little *et al.*, 1989b; Little and VanBeveren, 1996; VanBeveren *et al.*, 2000), and probably is ranked second to alcohol. Infants born to heroin abusers are exposed to cocaine and alcohol five times more often than those born to methamphetamine abusers. The relatively recent determination that first trimester opiate exposure is associated with an increased frequency of birth defects adds heroin to this list of teratogens among substances of abuse. Importantly, multiple substance use increases the possibility of drug-drug and drug-alcohol interactions (e.g., cocaine and alcohol become cocaethylene, a more potent form). Whether or not alcohol and cocaine interact to increase the severity of damage to the conceptus is not known, but seems likely (Hofkosh *et al.*, 1995).

Cocaine and heroin use increase the risk for abruptio placentae and premature birth for women who use cocaine (Acker *et al.*, 1983; Chasnoff *et al.*, 1985), as does tobacco use. Those who abuse cocaine, heroin, and Ts and blues, frequently abuse alcohol, and may cause such pregnancy complications as premature labor and FAS (NIAAA, 1983; SAMHSA, 2017).

## SUMMARY OF SUBSTANCE ABUSE DURING PREGNANCY

The risk for morbidity increases with the number of substances used and the frequency of their use. Not all substances of abuse cause congenital anomalies, but most substance use is associated with the use of alcohol and/or cocaine, generally acknowledged to cause birth defects. Abuse of any substance during pregnancy is associated with fetal growth retardation and possibly with neurological dysfunction. Associated risks include sexually transmitted diseases, hepatitis, and undernutrition.

**Appendix I**

**Congenital Anomalies Reported in Studies of Prenatal Cocaine Exposure**

Absent digits 3 and 4 on hand
Ambiguous genitalia, absent uterus and ovaries
Anal atresia
Atrial septal defect
Bilateral cryptorchidism
Blepharophimosis
Cardiomegaly
Cleft palate
Cleft palate[a]
Club foot
Complete heart block
Congenital hip dislocation
Cryptorchidism
Cutis aplasia
Duplex kidney
Esophageal atresia
Exencephaly[b]
Facial skin tags
Horse shoe kidney
Hydrocele
Hydrocephaly
Hydronephrosis, bilateral
Hydronephrosis, bilateral, prune belly syndrome, patent ductus arteriosus
Hydronephrosis, unilateral, contralateral renal infarct
Hydronephrosis, unilateral, incompetent ureteral orifices
Hydroureter
Hypertelorism, maxillary hypoplasia, high palate, holoprosencephaly with agenesis of corpus
    callosum
Hypoplastic right heart
Hypospadias
Hypospadias with accessory nipple
Hypospadias, one with chordee Ileal and colonic infarction
Ileal atresia
Inguinal hernia
Intracranial hemorrhage
Intraparietal encephalocele
Limb reduction/amputation
Mid-colonic atresia
Multiple ventricular septal defects
Necrotizing enterocolitis
Oro-orbital cleft, unilateral
Parietal bone malformation
Patent ductus arteriosus
Pierre–Robin anomaly[c]
Poland sequence,[d] ulnar ray deficiencies
Polydactyly
Prune belly syndrome with urethral obstruction

Ptosis and facial diplegia

Pulmonary atresia

Pulmonary stenosis

Renal agenesis

Renal and ureteral agenesis, unilateral, ambiguous genitalia, unilateral ectopic fallopian tube
and ovary, gastroschisis, eventration of abdominal contents, hypoplastic gall bladder, spina
bifida, hydrocephalus, postural scoliosis, asymmetric chest, congenital dislocation of a hip,
clubfoot, flexion deformity of knee joints, arthrogryposis of a lower limb

Renal tract dilation

Sacral exostosis and capillary hemangiomas

Sirenomelia

Transposition of great vessels

Transverse limb reduction, unilateral

Unilateral hemimelia (absent right hand and right leg below the knee)

Ventricular septal defect

[a] Associated with Trisomy 13 and causation by cocaine is not plausible.

[b] Probably really encephalocele.

[c] Pierre–Robin anomaly is cleft palate and severe micrognathia.

[d] Poland sequence is defect of pectoralis muscle with syndactyly of hand.

*Sources:* Bader and Lewis, 1990; Bingol *et al.*, 1987a, 1987b; Dominguez *et al.*, 1991; Hoyme *et al.*, 1988, 1990; Isenberg *et al.*, 1987; Kobori *et al.*, 1989; Little and Snell, 1991b; Little *et al.*, 1988; Little *et al.*, 1989; Madden *et al.*, 1986; Neerhof *et al.*, 1989; Oriol *et al.*, 1993; Porat and Brodsky, 1991; Puvabanditsin *et al.*, 2005; Ricci and Molle, 1987; Sarpong and Headings, 1992; Sehgal *et al.*, 1993; Shanske *et al.*, 1990; Telsey *et al.*, 1988; Teske and Trese, 1987.

# Index

Note: Please note that *italicized* page numbers in this index indicate tables or figures.

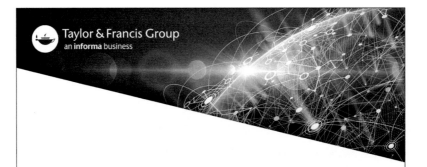